Craniofacial Pain

Brendan C. Stack Jr. • Revathi Shekar
Anthony B. Sims
Editors

Craniofacial Pain

Temporomandibular Disorders and Beyond

Springer

Editors
Brendan C. Stack Jr.
Otolaryngology-Head and Neck Surgery
Southern Illinois University School of Medicine
Springfield, IL, USA

Revathi Shekar
School of Dental Medicine
University of Pittsburgh
Pittsburgh, PA, USA

Anthony B. Sims
Ellicott City, MD, USA

ISBN 978-3-031-57562-4 ISBN 978-3-031-57563-1 (eBook)
https://doi.org/10.1007/978-3-031-57563-1

This Springer imprint is published by the registered company Springer Nature Switzerland AG
The registered company address is: Gewerbestrasse 11, 6330 Cham, Switzerland

I dedicate this work to my father Brendan C. Stack, Sr., DDS, MS (1937–2020). My father was a thought leader and private practitioner dedicated to orthodontics and temporomandibular joint (TMJ) dysfunction for over 50 years. His passion for TMJ disease was omnipresent during my upbringing. This was a significant reason I became interested in clinical care and certainly was foundational in my pursuit of a career as an otolaryngologist-head and neck surgeon. Thanks, Dad, for your love and support, your high standards for me, and your professional work for all of its benefits, direct and indirect, it had upon me and my interest in the head and neck and for TMJ/craniofacial pain practitioners and patients worldwide. Also, heartfelt thanks to Ms. Angel Biondi, who managed my father's office for many years, looked out for his best interests, and provided background material for this book.

Brendan C. Stack, Jr., MD, F.A.C.S., F.A.C.E.

Roland, AR, and Springfield, IL

With the deepest gratitude, I wish to thank every being who came into my life and illuminated me through their presence. Lassie and Ruff, thank you for making my life beautiful and meaningful. To my parents, especially my mother, Bhanumathi Shekar, for being an extraordinary woman, my inspiration, voice of reason, and the wind beneath my wings—words do little justice in conveying my gratitude and appreciation. To all my teachers and mentors, across schools and residencies, countries, and continent, thank you for giving me the courage and strength to pursue my dreams—I am forever grateful for that. To my students and residents who brighten my life and motivate me to strive to do better every day. To my patients for being my best teachers and for making life's journey worthwhile—thank you!

I am grateful to my colleagues and mentors at the SIU School of Dental Medicine and the University of Pittsburgh School of Dental Medicine for their support and guidance. I am obliged to Dr. Bruce E. Rotter, DMD, MS, Dean Emeritus, SIU School of Dental Medicine, for being the reason for my introduction to Dr. Stack 4 years ago. I cannot thank him enough for having faith in me and my abilities as we worked together on this tribute to his father. My thanks are also due to our publisher, Springer Nature, for their patience and perseverance. Lastly, to all those reading our book, thank you for valuing our words and giving us a chance.

Revathi Shekar, BDS, MDS, Dip. ABOM

Pittsburgh, PA

This book aims to do more than assemble much of the vast research on neuroanatomy related to movement disorders. The overall presentation on movement disorders in this book is felt to be unique. Many of the concepts and the information presented have resulted from our continuing goal to understand better the numerous and undeniable results witnessed from the proper knowledge of the stomatognathic system.

I want to thank, with all my heart, my wife Connie for her undaunting love and encouragement throughout our 45 years of marriage. To our children, Anthony II, Calvin, and John, you have been wonderful, and I am proud of all of you. To my grandchildren, I hope to have left a great legacy for you.

Finally, I recognize and give thanks to my teacher and mentor, Brendan C. Stack, Sr., DDS, MS, who passed on his knowledge and wisdom to his padawan.

Anthony B. Sims, DDS, ABCFP, IMD, DHS

Columbia, MD

Foreword

Brendan Stack, Sr., was one of a few dentists in TMJ and orthodontics most admired by my father Harold Gelb, DMD (1925–2022). Shortly after the founding of the American Academy of Craniomandibular Disorders, Brendan founded the rival American Academy of Craniofacial Pain (AACP, www.aacfp.org). In later years, this latter group was where my father felt at home and most welcomed. One of the greatest honors in my father's long life was receiving the **Haden-Stack** Award for his significant contributions to the advancement of knowledge and clinical practice in the diagnosis and treatment of craniofacial pain and temporomandibular joint disorders (TMDs).

Brendan was also well known globally for the Funt–Stack index, which he collaborated with Lawrence A. Funt, D.M.S.D., Bethesda, MD, and was proudly displayed on my father's operatory wall. It helped him to explain how the TMJ could affect the eyes, ears, neck, headaches, jaws, and throat and was well received around the world. It was later adapted and expanded by Bruce H. Kinnie, DDS, who renamed it the K–F–S index.

The Gelb 4/7 jaw and condyle position was the orthodontic finishing position favored by Brendan and the AACP. Harold would put in the Gelb splint, and there was no one better than Brendan to finish the case orthodontically to that position while maintaining orthopedic support. He was an excellent teacher and "professor" who passed this knowledge on to the next generation of TMJ dentists and orthodontists.

I was having lunch one day with these two giants when Brendan candidly said that there was no one that these two would least like to face as expert witnesses than each other. They were both fierce, knowledgeable, and respected experts, admired by their peers, patients, judges, and each other.

Harold and Brendan remained great friends and colleagues for over 50 years.

New York, NY, USA Michael Gelb

Foreword

I have known Brendan since we matriculated together at Georgetown Dental School in 1958. We were different people; he was single, and I was married. He was an easterner, and I hailed from Arizona. We became acquainted during dental school, and our relationship lasted for over 60 years, which expanded to include our spouses and children. I would see Brendan and his family regularly at meetings of our mutual congregation of the Church of Jesus Christ of Latter-day Saints. After graduation from dental school, I specialized in oral and maxillofacial surgery and set up practices and Brendan specialized in orthodontics and established his practices.

For 50 years, Brendan and I practiced in the same community of Northern Virginia. Brendan was well known for his focus on treating temporomandibular joint dysfunction with occlusal appliances and revision orthodontics. Brendan was well known and highly sought for his treatment success.

I am pleased to see Brendan, Jr., spearhead this book as an update on TMJ/craniofacial pain and its issues as well as a tribute to his father Brendan.

Irvine, CA, USA — N. Ken Coleman

Foreword

"We stand on the shoulders of giants." The statement is well known and frequently used by my colleagues that have dedicated their lives to treating craniofacial/orofacial pain patients. Dr. Brendan Stack was a giant in the field of craniofacial pain diagnosis and management. Dr. Stack literally educated thousands of dentists, but treating patients with complex pain was his passion. Dr. Stack pioneered treatment modalities, which helped countless number of suffering patients.

Dr. Stack was also a founder and inaugural President of the American Academy of Craniofacial Pain. The Academy's most prestigious award bears Dr. Stack's name along with Dr. Jack Haden. The **Haden-Stack** Award is dedicated to individuals who have the unselfish desire to educate others and for their exemplary and extraordinary contributions to the advancement of knowledge and clinical practice in the fields of craniofacial pain and temporomandibular disorders. It was my great honor to receive the Haden-Stack Award in the summer of 2021.

I am proud to say that Dr. Stack was my friend and personal giant in this field. He mentored, educated, and guided me to want to become a better doctor. I received this award because of the assistance and education from this great giant.

Hurricane, WV, USA — Jeanne K. Bailey

Past Presidents of the AACP

Dr. Brendan C. Stack, Sr., was a founder of the American Academy of Craniofacial Pain. This organization began in 1985. More information can be found at https://www.aacfp.org/page/About. The list of the past AACP presidential leadership is below:

Dr. Brendan Stack, DDS, MS 1985–1990	*Dr. Robert Talley, DDS* 2006–2008
Dr. Robert Talley, DDS 1990–1992	*Dr. Donald Warren, DDS* 2008–2010
Dr. Jack Haden, DDS 1992–1994	*Dr. Jamison Spencer, DMD, MS* 2010–2012
Dr. Gerald Murphy, DDS 1994–1996	*Dr. Terry Bennett, DMD* 2012–2014
Dr. Charles Holt, DDS 1996–1998	*Dr. Jeffrey McCarty, DDS* 2014–2016
Dr. Wesley Shankland, DDS, MS 1998–2000	*Dr. Steven R. Olmos, DDS* 2016–2018
Dr. Clifton Simmons, DDS 2000–2002	*Dr. Jeanne K. Bailey, DDS* 2018–2020
Dr. Larry Tilley, DMD 2002–2004	*Dr. Jeffrey McCarty, DDS* 2020–2022
Dr. Steven Kilpatrick, DDS 2004–2006	

Previous Haden-Stack Award Recipients

Dr. Wesley Shankland
Dr. Charles Holt
Dr. Ed Spiegel
Dr. Robert Talley
Dr. Jerry Murphy
Dr. Harold Gelb
Dr. Clifton Simmons
Dr. Peter Neff
Dr. Noshir Mehta
Dr. Steve Olmos
Dr. Ron Auvenshine
Dr. Barry Glassman
Dr. Riley Lunn
Dr. Allen Moses
Dr. Terry Spahl
Dr. Jamison Spencer
Dr. Larry Tilley
Dr. Ed Lipskis
Dr. Cris Simmons
Dr. Mayoor Patel
Dr. Pamela Steed
Dr. Jeanne K. Bailey
Dr. Reda Abdel-Fattah

Contributions of Brendan C. Stack, Sr., to the Dental/Medical Literature

Sims AB, Stack BC, Demerjian GG. Spasmodic torticollis: the dental connection. Cranio. 2012;30(3):188–93. https://doi.org/10.1179/crn.2012.029. PMID: 22916671.

Demerjian GG, Sims AB, Stack BC. Proteomic signature of temporomandibular joint disorders (TMD): toward diagnostically predictive biomarkers. Bioinformation. 2011;5(7):282–4. https://doi.org/10.6026/97320630005282. PMID: 21364835; PMCID: PMC3043347.

Sims AB, Stack BC. An intraoral neurocranial vertical distractor appliance provides unique treatment for Tourette's syndrome and resolves comorbid neurobehavioral problems of obsessive compulsive disorder. Med Hypotheses. 2010;75(2):179–84. https://doi.org/10.1016/j.mehy.2010.02.014. Epub 2010 Mar 19. PMID: 20303668.

Stack BC. Intraoral orthotics for treatment of TMD. Funct Orthod. 2004;21(2):16–22. PMID: 15453014.

Stack BC. Why unnamed in Concepts editorial? Cranio. 2004;22(1):5. PMID: 14964332.

Stack BC Jr, Stack BC. Under utilization of MRI. A suggested protocol. Cranio. 1998;16(3):131–2. PMID: 9852805.

Stack BC. Comment on righting the wrong paradigm. Am J Orthod Dentofacial Orthop. 1997;111(4):29A. https://doi.org/10.1016/s0889-5406(97)80003-0. PMID: 9109568.

Stack BC. Higher levels of orthodontic and dental excellence. Funct Orthod. 1997;14(1):11–3. PMID: 9610284.

Stack BC. Response to comment on TMD. Am J Orthod Dentofacial Orthop. 1995;108(4):19A. PMID: 7572840.

Stack BC. Functional forum: do we treat the "asymptomatic" click? Funct Orthod. 1994;11(4):20–1. PMID: 8613101.

Stack BC. Comments on pediatric internal derangements. Am J Orthod Dentofacial Orthop. 1994;105(3):28A; author reply 39A. PMID: 8135214.

Stack BC Jr, Stack BC Sr. Temporomandibular joint disorder. Am Fam Physician. 1992;46(1):143–50. PMID: 1621626.

Stack BC. Temporomandibular joint dysfunction. J Tenn Dent Assoc. 1992;72(3):13–5. PMID: 1528059.

Stack BC. Journal of functional orthodontics interviews Dr. Brendan Stack on TMJ. Interview by Dr. Jimi Mehta. Funct Orthod. 1990;7(5):20–1, 24–5. PMID: 2097251.

Stack BC. Temporomandibular joint diagnosis. Funct Orthod. 1989;6(5):31–40. PMID: 2639849.

Stack BC. TM therapy: avoiding legal pitfalls. J Macomb Dent Soc. 1989;26(5):38. PMID: 2600537.

Stack BC. Temporomandibular joint diagnosis. J Macomb Dent Soc. 1989;26(5):34–5, 37. PMID: 2600536.

Phillips DJ Jr, Walters PJ, Rogal OJ, Stack BC, Weiner LB, Klemons IM. Recommended guide to the evaluation of permanent impairment of the temporomandibular joint. Cranio. 1989;7(1):13–21. https://doi.org/10.1080/08869634.1989.11678263. PMID: 2611894.

Stack BC. Dr. Brendan C. Stack: an interview with the 1988 AAFO Man of the Year. Interview by Craig Stoner. Funct Orthod. 1989;6(1):6–7, 9–19. PMID: 2599434.

Given BK, Stack BC, Hickey JA. TM dysfunction in children: the development of a screening instrument and parent questionnaire. Cranio. 1987;5(1):79–86. https://doi.org/10.1080/08869634.1987.11678178. PMID: 3467871.

Given BK, Stack BC. Temporomandibular joint dysfunction syndrome in children. J Sch Health. 1986;56(3):86–9. https://doi.org/10.1111/j.1746-1561.1986.tb05702.x. PMID: 3634134.

Stack BC. TMJ from an orthodontic perspective using cephalometric laminagraphy. Basal Facts. 1985;7(2):161–71. PMID: 2931072.

Stack BC. Orthodontic treatment methods. Part II. Funct Orthod. 1984;1(4):22–3, 26–7, 29 passim. PMID: 6596279.

Stack BC. Orthodontic treatment methods. Part I. Funct Orthod. 1984;1(3):11–4, 17–8, 20 passim. PMID: 6593283.

Stack BC, Funt LA. Temporomandibular joint dysfunction in children. J Pedod. 1977;1(3):240–7. PMID: 270575.

Stack BC, Funt LA, Mann GE. The diagnosis of TMJ disorders using laminographic radiography. Va Dent J. 1977;54(2):10–6. PMID: 269571.

Stack BC, Funt LA, Mann GE. The diagnosis of TMJ disorders using laminographic radiography. J Md State Dent Assoc. 1977;20(1):18–23. PMID: 267709.

Stack BC, Funt LA. TMJ dysfunction from myofunctional prospective. Int J Oral Myol. 1977;3(1):11–26. PMID: 275222.

Mann GE, Stack BC, Funt LA. The diagnosis of TMJ disorders using laminographic radiography. Ariz Dent J. 1977;23(1):14–8. PMID: 270306.

Professional Recollections of Brendan C. Stack, Sr., DDS, MS

Brendan was a gifted teacher, mentor, and the finest TMJ clinician. I studied with him for over 25 years with annual visits to Old Courthouse Road (office) and Oberon Way (home). I owe him a huge debt of gratitude and think of him often. He had a wicked sense of humor and the heart of a lion, an extraordinary man who pursued learning in order to provide his patients with care par excellence!

Patrick Grossmann, BDS, LDS, D.Orth, RCS
London, England, UK

I had reached the oral examination stage in my quest for AACP honors. Along with other nervous AACP members who had passed rigorous written test and were facing this last hurdle to lifelong recognition, I was ushered into a large room. Tables, with three chairs at each, dotted the room. I was directed to the remaining chair at a table where my two examiners awaited, Brendan Stack and someone else who paled into insignificance alongside the great man.

A few introductory questions were easily answered. Then came the big one. "Can you give us causes associated with TMJ problems in young women?" inquired Brendan. I mentioned the usual: trauma, mandibular displacement from thumb sucking, and estrogen. Then I added, "at this first consultation it is probably not appropriate to suggest to the mother of a 14-year-old girl that ethinyl estradiol in oral contraceptives is linked to TMJ dysfunction."

"Don't worry about it," Brendan snorted. "The 14-year-old girls are all out there, mating (sic) like bunny rabbits."

One of my fellow candidates remarked to me later, "I knew you had passed when I heard your roar of laughter in that uninviting room."

John Burford, BDS, DFAACP
Auckland, New Zealand

After discussing the care of a mutual patient with Dr. Stack, he invited me to come to his office to learn more about how he treats his patients. I was not sure what this experience was going to entail, but I was certain that it was going to be life-changing after watching how he interacted with people in ways that I had never experienced before in my career. He reminded me of the M&M candy: a hard shell on the outside was required to protect the soft inside that could melt under certain conditions. His sometimes gruff exterior could be easily misunderstood as aggressive, but I quickly realized that to be the leader that he needed to be for all that followed him, this toughness was necessary. The soft, caring inside was easy to see as he gave his all in caring for his patients.

As we came near to the end of our time together during that particular office visit, he took me aside, looked me straight in the eyes, and told me that our profession needed people like me to continue pushing this field forward. He told me that you can always tell the leaders by the arrows that they have stuck in their backs. I quickly realized the challenge that I had been asked to rise to and decided to show my mentor that I was able to gain the respect of the man that had just thrown down a gauntlet that I had no choice but to pick up.

When he and I reconnected several years later at an AACP conference, when his memory had started to falter, I reminded him of our previous meeting, and it brought back every detail and conversation that we had ever discussed. I have done my best to follow in his footsteps, and I have gathered the quiver of the arrows in my back. I am constantly grateful for his leadership, wisdom, and friendship.

Angie Tenholder DMD, FAACP, DABCDSM, FAGD
President, American Board of Craniofacial Dental Sleep Medicine
Education Committee Co-chairperson, American Academy of Craniofacial Pain
Fellow, American Academy of Craniofacial Pain and Academy of General Dentistry
Board Certified, American Board of Craniofacial Dental Sleep Medicine
Columbia, IL, USA

I have been a member of the American Academy of Craniomandibular Pain (AACP) since 2004, but I first heard Dr. Stack in the early 1990s at a meeting of the American Equilibration Society in Chicago, where he lectured and participated in a round table with the other two most prominent orthodontists of that time regarding our specialty and orthodontics. It was memorable.

I again met Dr. Stack while we were both lecturing in Argentina in 2004, for what was then the Latin American chapter of the AACP, and I invited him to lecture in my country for the 2006 chapter meeting, and he immediately accepted. As always, we learned so much from him, and we even lost him during the social events, because he visited more parts of the country than planned. Later, I learned that his two dental assistants were originally from Panama, and he went and bought them many souvenirs.

During a meeting of the AACP and some years before Dr. Stack retired, I mentioned to him that I was going to spend some time in Washington, DC, and asked him if I could stay a day in his office. Of course, he accepted, and I still help my patients with what I learned that day and remember him every time.

The last time I saw Dr. Stack was in an AACP meeting in Orlando in 2017, and unfortunately, he was already in a wheelchair. He was by himself waiting to be called to be given one of the many honors he deserved, and I asked him if I could accompany and escort him. He was very happy, and I was honored but sad at the same time to see him not well.

Dr. Stack always treated me like family, student, and colleague, and he will always be in my heart and mind.

Dr. Fernando R. Jaén, Odontólogo

Panama City, Panama

I was attending an IAO meeting in VA in the 1980s where Brendan was speaking, and I asked so many questions that a doc in the front turned around and yelled, "You need to take his training!" Brendan was not teaching anything in the United States, and I could not go to the UK or Europe, so I called his office and signed in as a patient. That began our relationship, with me driving down from northeastern PA and arriving before my appointment, staying until the end of his day, and learning from him as he treated my TMD and he saw his other patients. I completed the multi-year program he gave with Jay Gerber and Dick Greenan later on. We trained together with Gerald Smith to learn about Darick Nordstrom's ALF appliance. We collaborated on some movement disorder cases.

Brendan was my savior and became my close friend and professional and personal mentor for decades. I loved him and miss him frequently. When I have a tough case, I still ask, "What would Brendan do?" and the answer always comes.

Rebecca L. Griffiths, DMD

Phoenix, AZ, USA

As the retired founder and owner of Rideau Orthodontic Mfg. Ltd., a Canadian orthopedic/orthodontic laboratory, I met Dr. Brendan Stack 40 years early on in his orthodontic career. Dr. Stack, a true pioneer for "treating the cause not the symptoms" of cranial facial pain and TMJD, provided opportunities to organize dental seminars in Canada for several thousand Canadian dentists whose patients benefited from Dr. Stack's teachings and that of other leaders as well. Brendan seldom took holidays, although following a couple of Ontario lectures, he visited my family home on the Big Rideau Lake for fishing.

Rideau Orthodontic fabricated the **A**lternative **L**ightwire **F**unctional (ALF), lower splint devices, upper four way sagittal to "explode the maxilla," in addition to Brendan's luted upper/lower Hawley-style retainers to maintain orthodontic alignment while supporting AP/TMJ correction throughout sleep. I was blessed to have Dr. Brendan Stack as a mentor and dear friend for so many years.

It is a wonderful tribute for his final textbook to be published by his loving namesake son, which also compliments Brendan's extensive video series entitled "Stack of Knowledge."

Emmett Griffiths

Smith Falls, Ontario, Canada

I knew Dr. Stack well. He was more than a friend; he was like my brother. When I could not get paid by the motor vehicle insurance companies for TMJ injuries, I began to sue them. I needed to have experts I could rely on to testify on the patient's behalf and he did that. Dr. Brendan Stack came out to Denver and testified at least four times. The opposing lawyers knew that they were in for it when he testified. I won those cases. He helped put TMJ on the map with respect to whiplash injuries.

I took each of his classes two or three times because I wanted to learn as much as I could. At one class, he called me out and said, "Is this correct, you took this same class last month and my office informs me that you're registered in the same class two months from now?" I answered yes and he asked why. I showed him my notes from the previous class and how I was now taking the notes that I missed from that last class. At a break later on in the day, he asked if there were any questions, and most of the participants had already left the room when I asked my question. I asked my question, and he answered it, but one doctor came forward and asked him to explain it. So, he explained his answer. The doctor then said, "No, I don't understand the question, can you explain the question?" The point of this is to show how deeply Dr. Stack went into the topic when he was teaching it. It was necessary to take the same class several times to get the full depth of the instruction because he was giving out so much information. Dr. Stack was a brilliant man and a great teacher and clinician.

To this day, there are times that I wish I could still ask him questions about a patient's treatment. I have three fellowships in TMJ and am a diplomate from the American Academy of Integrative Medicine. I have been treating TMJ patients for 46 years and for a total of almost 5000 patients, and I still do not know as much as Dr. Stack. He was a great man, a great teacher, and a great friend. I really miss him.

Roger Druckman DDS
Denver, CO, USA

Dr. Brendan Stack pioneered patient-centered, comprehensive collaborative therapies long before others in our profession followed his lead. He consistently challenged orthodoxies in orthodontics with upgraded and advanced craniofacial-cervical chronic pain management for orthodontic and facial orthopedic patients.

General Patton said: "When everyone is thinking alike, no-one is doing much thinking." Brendan thought outside the box without getting lost out there. He shined light on facial pain/TMD co-management and provided higher levels of whole body/system optimization, with truly comprehensive orthodontic treatments. However, he was often challenged by colleagues who did not yet know.

All truth passes through three stages: First, it is ridiculed. Second, it is vehemently opposed. Third, it is accepted as being self-evident (Arthur Schopenhauer). As Winston Churchill pointed out, you can see adversity in every opportunity, or you can see the opportunity in every adversity. Dr. Stack's chapter in the Orthodontics for the TMJ-TMD Patient textbook (Grummons) stands apart from the writings by others of us who had the privilege to advance the message and methods of interdisciplinary therapeutics.

Countless patients live better lives, and doctors treat as thinkers because of Dr. Stack's contributions and influences. Worthy thanks have been earned by him from professional and patient communities.

Respectfully shared,

Duane Grummons, DDS, MSD, ABO
American Board Certified in Facial Orthopedics and Orthodontics
Spokane, WA, USA

Some Additional History on TMD and Movement Disorders, Recollections from Dr. Stack …

"I have difficulty remembering my first Tourette's patient, but the successful treatment of that patient resulted in word spreading throughout the Tourette's (community) sic, and more Tourette's patients began to knock on my door. I have enjoyed success, as well as personal satisfaction, in treating these children without having to use medications, behavior modification, etc.", Brendan C. Stack, DDS, MS published (reference below).

"For a century and a half, Tourette's syndrome has been a mystery to the medical profession, with physicians first believing that it was a psychological disorder, then a neurological/brain disorder, and then an infectious disease caused by streptococcus. What was never considered was that this disorder was due to a structural abnormality, which would manifest itself as a neurological problem. What has since been discovered is that Tourette's syndrome is neither psychological, infectious, genetic, nor environmental in origin, but is what we have termed a structural-reflex disorder. It has been shown in a pilot study of multiple cases how and why Tourette's, and its multiple comorbid disorders, can be discontinued with an intraoral orthotic device that requires no medicine or surgery."

"Tourette's syndrome is defined as an inherited neurological disorder that is a chronic idiopathic syndrome, characterized by the presence of multiple motor tics and vocal tics that have their beginning before adulthood (usually with an onset in childhood between ages 5 and 8). Tics are repetitive, stereotypical movements or phonetic events, which are nonrhythmic and involuntary (motor tics), such as blinking, coughing, sniffing, shoulder shrugging, neck stretching, throat clearing, etc."

"Tourette's syndrome was originally thought to be a rare and severely bizarre disorder, most often associated with coprolalia, which occurs in approximately 10% of those with Tourette's. Now T.S. is understood to be less rare and is often classified as a condition having a wide range of severity. It is currently treated with medications that seem to incapacitate the patient or by frequent psychological counseling that teaches behavior modification when a promontory urge is felt immediately prior to the tic(s)."

"Tourette's patients seem to have normal intelligence and a normal life expectancy. The most common disability is within a social setting, and those with T.S. find it embarrassing when severe movements or vocalizations occur. People with Tourette's can achieve success in all walks of life, from athletics to professional careers. Prejudice or ostracizing is very common at school or at work."

"In February of (sic 2012), Dr. Anthony B. Sims and I made a presentation explaining my technique to the Board of Directors of the National Tourette's Association in New York City. We were well-received. They were interested because of the many phone calls received from parents of patients asking why they were still being treated with medications and/or psychological counseling when they had personally experienced the results of my treatment techniques. These calls originated not only from the United States, but also from Europe as a result of my having lectured there. The Tourette's Association of America is currently in the process of formulating grant proposals to test my methodology, which will probably be funded in the near future."

"As word of my treatment successes spread, other people approached me with different types of movement disorders. These were older patients, many of whom had been diagnosed with Parkinson's or pre-Parkinson's type tremors or had not yet received an official diagnosis by a neurologist, or who were trying to avoid being labeled as Parkinsonian. Their thinking was that if I could treat someone's head from shaking back and forth, then I should be able to treat their arms from flailing up and down. I then began to think about the treatment of Parkinson's movement disorder patients. Applying these same principles, I successfully treated a number of Parkinson's patients."

Stack BC. My journey from orthodontics to craniofacial pain and TMJ to movement disorders. Cranio. 2012;30(3):156–8. https://doi.org/10.1179/crn.2012.023.

Preface

The concept of this book started about 10 years ago, preceding my father's passing in 2020. The core concept of the book was to describe the arc of evolution and understanding about TMJ dysfunction over the past 50 years and my father's role in it. The book would cover the current state of basic knowledge (diagnosis, imaging, and therapeutics). It would then proceed to advanced concepts and the leading edge of TMJ therapeutics.

Unfortunately, these discussions initiated after my father's health had started to decline. We worked on outlines and a list of possible contributors, valued professional colleagues of my father, but progress was slow. Many people who my father had wanted to include as authors in the book had retired from clinical practice and/or were otherwise occupied from engaging in the book opportunity. My father's energy in the last years of his life was quite limited. Other distractions to the project presented themselves. Then came the COVID-19 pandemic and intercurrent illness of my father. My father passed away on July 24, 2020. This obviously put a pause on this book project.

In honor of my father's career and memory, I decided to resume the project. At this time, I was the Chairman of Otolaryngology-Head and Neck Surgery at the Southern Illinois University (SIU) School of Medicine, Springfield, IL. I reached out to the SIU Dental School on our sister campus (Edwardsville, IL) and was put in contact with Dr. Revathi Shekar who was faculty there at the time and has ably orchestrated the recruitment of and submissions from various members of the SIU Dental School of core concept chapters (Part I). She has now moved on to be faculty at the University of Pittsburgh School of Dentistry and contributed her own chapter. Dr. Anthony B. Sims, a practicing colleague of my father in the Washington, DC, area (Columbia, MD) and protegee, who collaborated extensively with my father and knew of the evolution of my father's practice and thinking, was able to contribute and recruit authors in a significant way to add advanced materials to this text (Part II). Thank you to Drs. Shekar and Sims for your support of this project.

This book has a broad application to the dental and medical professions. The book covers material related to patients presenting with craniofacial pain. The information contained within is of value to the frontline generalist (dentist or physician) as well as the specialist and even the academic/researcher. There has been much progress made in the understanding of the TMJ, its dysfunction, and its implications on overall health and well-being. It is hoped that this compilation will facilitate ongoing progress in areas of TMJ craniofacial pain and TMJ-related movement disorders. With the addition of online videos, readers will be able to see significant clinical demonstrations of TMJ therapeutics and its impact upon patients afflicted with movement disorders.

Springfield, IL, USA Brendan C. Stack Jr.

Acknowledgments

Brendan C. Stack, Sr., DDS, MS (1937–2020) (Fig. 1), was an orthodontist whose five decades of work helped clinicians better care for patients suffering from chronic craniofacial pain. Dr. Stack was expert at diagnosing the causes of chronic face and head pain and used orthodontic techniques, many of which he developed, to relieve pain, suffering, and associated symptoms.

Dr. Stack was born in New York, NY, to Eugene Francis Stack, Sr. (an attorney), and Catherine Loretta Curran (a high school teacher), second-generation Irish immigrants, and was raised in Great Neck (Long Island), NY (Figs. 2, 3 and 4). He graduated from St. Francis Xavier High School, a Jesuit Military School, in Manhattan, NY (Fig. 5). He continued his Jesuit education when he matriculated to Georgetown University in Washington, DC, where he obtained his bachelors and doctor of dental surgery degrees in 1958 and 1962, respectively (Fig. 6). While awaiting a place in an orthodontic residency, Dr. Stack served as a second lieutenant in the U.S. Public Health Service as a hospital dentist at the U.S. Public Health Hospital of New Orleans, LA. Upon completion of his intern year, he returned to Georgetown where he completed his residency and master's degree in orthodontics in 1965. He then set up several private practices in the Northern Virginia suburbs of Washington, DC.

Dr. Stack started to develop an interest in temporomandibular joint (TMJ) dysfunction in the late 1960s, before dysfunction in the joint had been widely recognized as a clinical entity, complication of previous orthodontic treatment, or a source for headaches, facial pain, imbalance, and gait disturbance among many other symptoms. In my father's own words from *My journey from orthodontics to craniofacial pain and TMJ to movement disorders*, "by 1967, I had begun to treat temporomandibular joint (TMJ) patients. A young man approximately 12 or 13 years old suffering with chronic headaches, repeated absences from school, clicking and locking of his jaw joints, and a myriad of typical TM joint symptoms came to my office. This was my first TMJ case and its successful treatment whetted my appetite for these types of patients, which continues to the present day." Dr. Stack explored his thoughts and impressions with many contemporary colleagues and advanced his and their knowledge. Such prominent pioneers in this field with whom he collaborated included Drs. Harold Gelb (1925–2022), Lawrence A. Funt (1925–2017), Bruce H. Kinnie (1932–2013), William Farrar (1927–1985), Jack Martini, and Jack L. Haden (1922–2022) among many others.

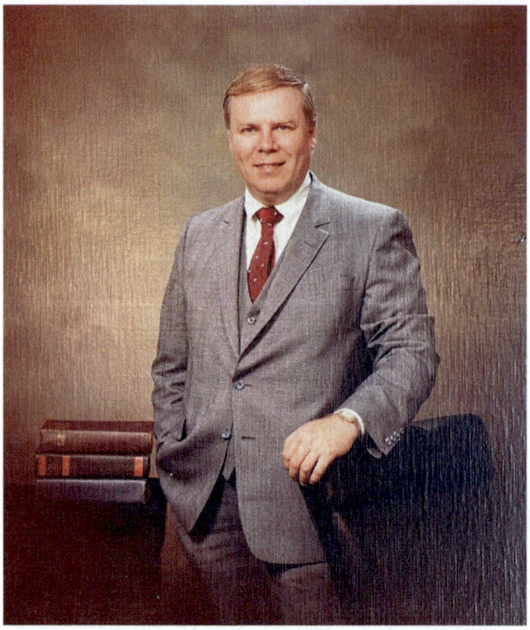

Fig. 1 Brendan C. Stack, Sr., pictured circa 1980s. (Courtesy of the Stack family trust)

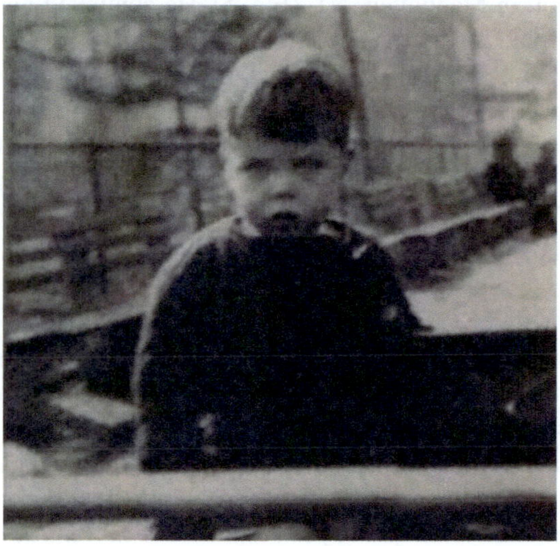

Fig. 2 Brendan C. Stack, Sr., pictured circa 1939. (Courtesy of the Stack family trust)

As a result of these early observations, he was a co-developer of the F–S (Funt–Stack) index and later the K–F–S (Kinnie–Funt–Stack) index of TMJ symptoms, which became standard diagnostic instruments (Fig. 7). This, combined with the care of thousands of patients, led Dr. Stack to lecture widely about his approaches and techniques for TMD-focused therapy. Consequently, he developed followings of like-minded colleagues in the United States, Europe, and Japan. Patients came from throughout the United States and abroad to be treated by Dr. Stack.

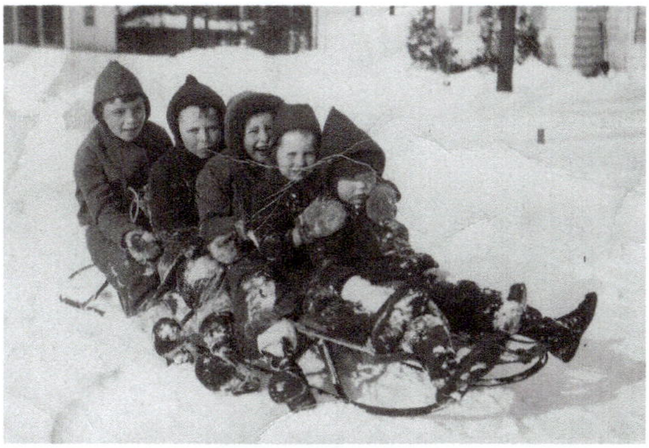

Fig. 3 Brendan C. Stack, Sr. (second from the left), with his siblings and neighbors circa 1940. (Courtesy of the Stack family trust)

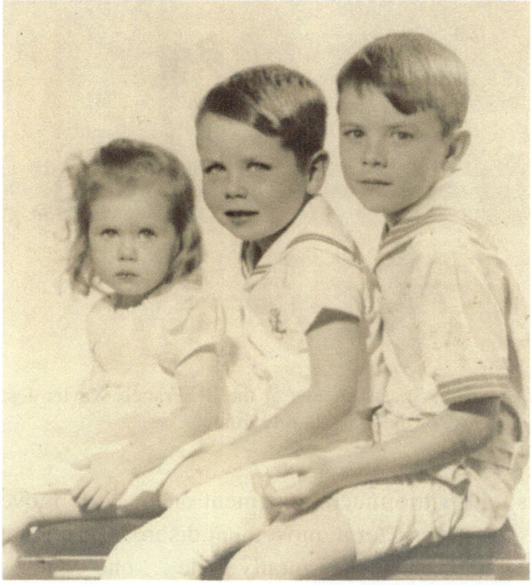

Fig. 4 The Eugene and "Loretta" Stack family children pictured circa 1940. The Stack siblings, seated left to right, Lorene Ann, Brendan Sr., and Eugene Francis, Jr. (Courtesy of the Stack family trust)

Over the years, Dr. Stack noticed that many facial pain patients had facial tics such as eye blinking, eyelid tics, mouth tics, head nodding, shoulder shrugging, and head tremors. Quoting my father, "I was asked to give a presentation on TMJ problems in children for a dental organization. This was at a time in the development of TMJ thinking where it was thought that TMJ was a middle-aged person's disease and that there was no such thing as TMJ dysfunction in children. Terms like pediatric headaches had not yet been used. In evenings subsequent to the request to give this presentation, I was viewing the slides of … patients whom I had treated, looking for children with TMJ problems. While perusing approximately 400 cases, I noticed in the records and photography that a high percentage of the patients had move-

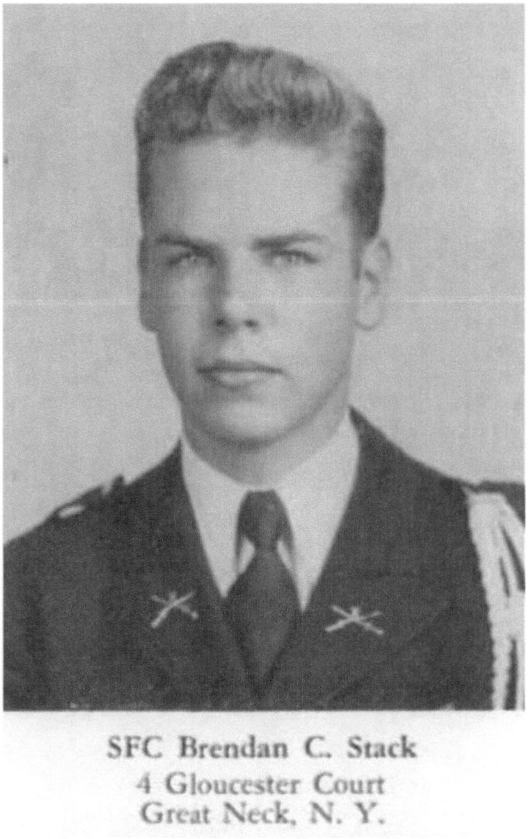

Fig. 5 Brendan C. Stack, Sr., as a cadet at the St. Francis Xavier Jesuit High School, New York, NY. (Courtesy of the Stack family trust)

ment disorders, either too much movement or too little movement … All I knew then was the generic term, movement disorders, and that by the end of my treatment most of these were totally gone … one young woman in particular stands out; she was a newly married 27-year-old who had just bought her first house. She had stated that she and her new husband made the mistake of buying a townhouse because she had to crawl up and down the stairs on her hands and knees and wished that she had bought a one level house … while I did not pay attention to it initially, I noticed … at the end of treatment she could go up and down the stairs normally. This was in addition to having eliminated her facial pain and her limited and deviated mouth opening."

"As the years went by, I continued to treat craniofacial pain and TMJ disorders with little thought to movement disorders. My underlying treatment philosophy evolved into the fact that many, but not all, movement disorder patients had an underlying internal derangement of the temporomandibular joints … which had not yet resulted in (typical) internal derangement of the TMJs but had resulted in an abnormal maxillomandibular relationship. It was this internal derangement or malrelationship that caused the movement disorders. I continued to treat patients with this philosophy with great success."

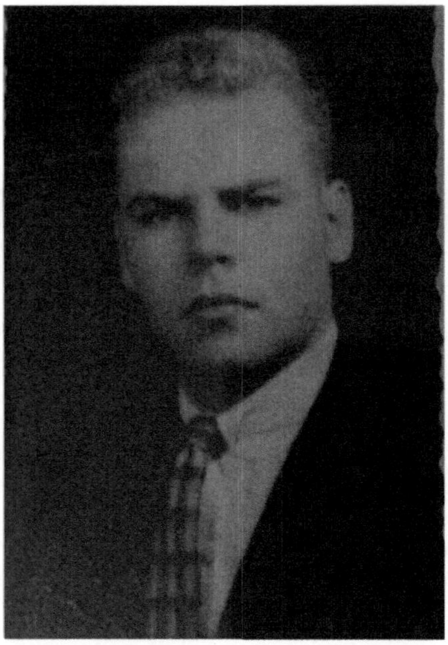

Fig. 6 Brendan C. Stack, Sr., as a student at Georgetown University, Washington, DC, 1954–1962. (Courtesy of the Stack family trust)

"What I accomplish with my appliances is the repositioning of the mandible into a new and different maxillomandibular relationship, decompressing the auriculotemporal nerve, and eliminating noxious input through the 5th cranial nerve into the central nervous system. To accelerate the patient's response, I frequently combine the use of these appliances with a very deep penetrating soft-tissue Lumix 2 (USA Laser Biotech, Inc., Richmond, VA)."

Dr. Stack considered tic patients as TMJ patients for their pain but also noticed tics dissipating at the same time. When word started spreading throughout the movement disorder patient community, Tourette's patients started coming to his practice. He was very successful in improving their symptoms and quality of life, and these techniques were accepted by some of his colleagues (Fig. 8).

The positive reception of Dr. Stack's presentations resulted in many continuing education lecture courses and the self-publication of many books and video presentations (http://www.orthodontic.ca/education/cemeetings/videos/stackofknowledge.pdf). He also had over 30 peer-reviewed articles published in the scientific literature, a significant amount for a private practitioner. Dr. Stack was responsible for mentoring, consulting, and training many TMJ-focused practitioners across the country. According to my father, "In January 2010, I was invited to be the keynote speaker at the National Meeting of the Parkinson's Research Association in Palm Springs, California. As a result of their referrals, I successfully treated a Parkinson's patient who was previously unsuccessfully treated with an implanted brain stimulator. All the foregoing led to my treatment of cervical torticollis and other types of movement disorders. My premise has always been the same: that the internal derangement and/or the resulting abnormal maxillomandibular relationship is the

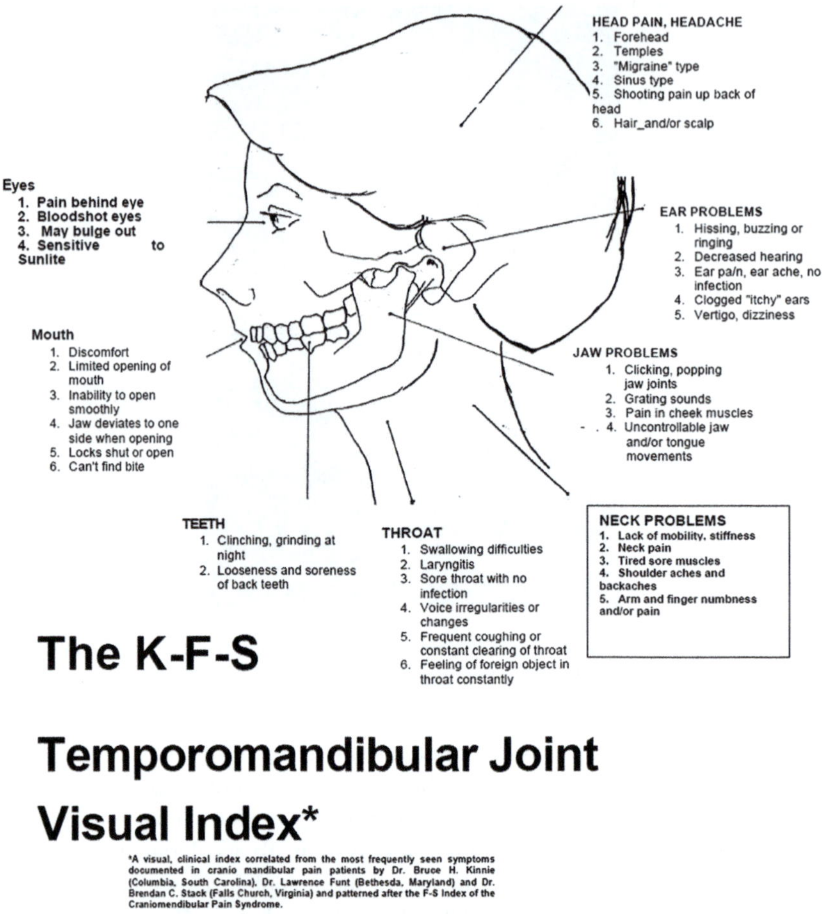

Fig. 7 The K–F–S temporomandibular joint visual index. **See Appendix**

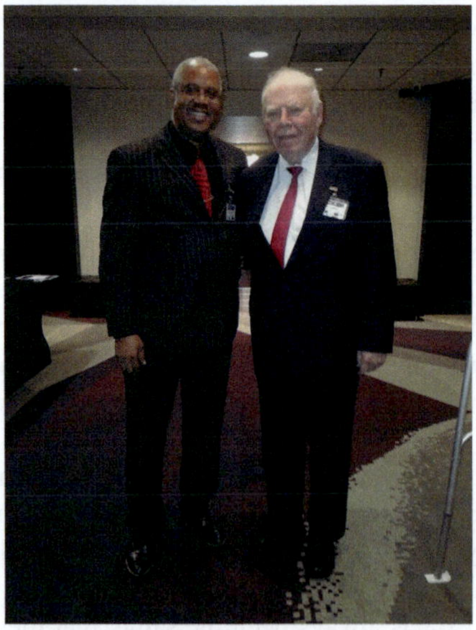

Fig. 8 Anthony B. Sims, DDS, ABCFP, IMD, DHS, close friend and student of Dr. Stack, pictured with him at a dental seminar event

underlying cause of the motor component of movement disorders. I do not think the treatment I stumbled upon treats anything other than the motor component of movement disorders. I leave the evaluation of various changes to the central nervous system (CNS) to others who are smarter than I."

"I have been on a journey. I had no idea where I would arrive when I started practicing in 1967. I also had no idea that along with treating TMJ and craniofacial pain patients, I would also treat patients with movement disorders. It's been a long journey, but one filled with learning and the personal satisfaction of having made a difference in the lives of my patients."

Dr. Stack was a co-founder and inaugural president (1985–1990) of the American Academy of Craniofacial Pain (www.aacfp.org), which was established to educate and certify practitioners that treat craniofacial pain. Later, the Jack L. Haden-Brendan C. Stack, Sr. (**Haden-Stack**), Award was established to recognize excellence among members of the AACP (Fig. 9). At the 1994 meeting of the AACP, Dr. Stack, Sr., invited his son, Brendan C. Stack, Jr., MD, to speak on mass lesions of the head and neck which could mimic TMD symptoms (Fig. 10). Dr. Stack was named "Clinician of the Year" in 1988 by the American Association of Functional Orthodontists (Fig. 11). He was the Tufts University's (Boston) 2003 recipient of the "Lifetime Achievement Award" for his years of contribution to the field of craniofacial pain. Dr. Stack's last practice was in Vienna, VA, where he had been located since 1980 (Fig. 12).

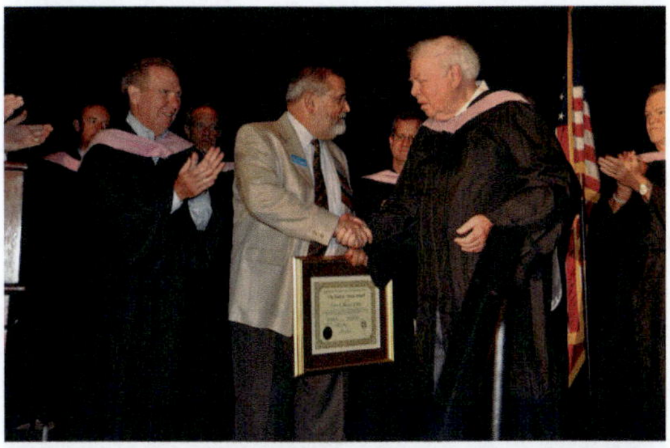

Fig. 9 Drs. Haden (left) and Stack (right) at the awarding of the Haden-Stack award to Dr. Allen J. Moses (center) at an annual AACP meeting

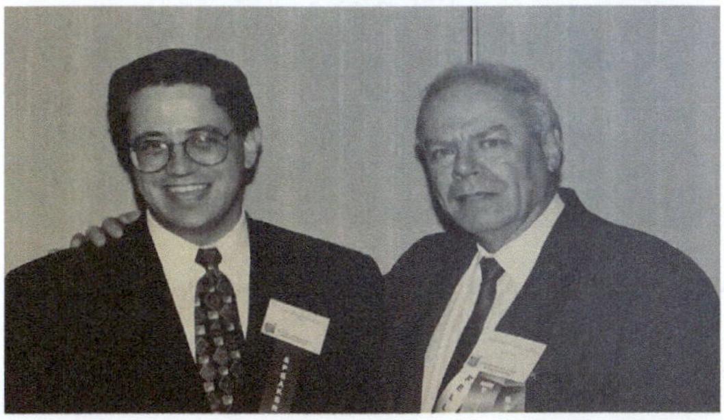

Fig. 10 Brendan C. Stack, Sr., pictured with his son Brendan C. Stack, Jr., (left) at the 1994 ACFP annual meeting, Arlington, VA. (Courtesy of the Stack family trust)

Upon his passing (Figs. 13 and 14), Dr. Stack left behind his children Brendan C. Stack, Jr., MD (Springfield, IL, and Roland, AR), Jennifer L. Wheeler (Phoenix, AZ), Maureen K. Stack (Medford, OR), Valerie A. Waite (North Salt Lake City, UT), Alexander J. Stack (Daly City, CA), Matthew A. Stack (Pasadena, MD), and Diana L. Milani (Highlands Ranch, CO) and 22 grandchildren.

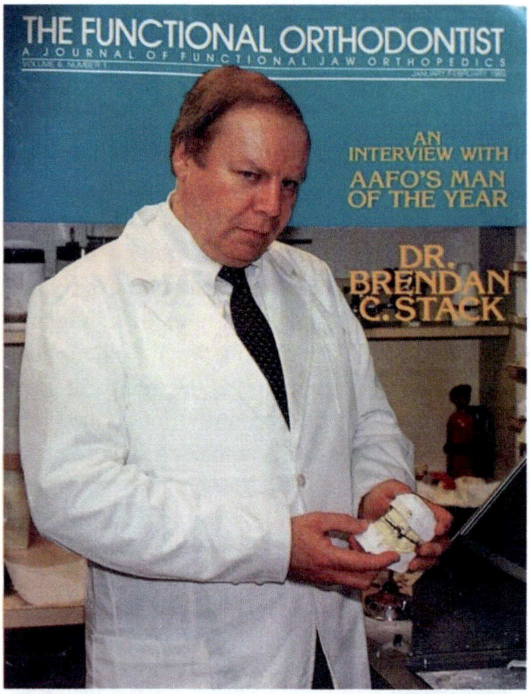

Fig. 11 Cover of the Functional Orthodontist, January/February 1989 issue

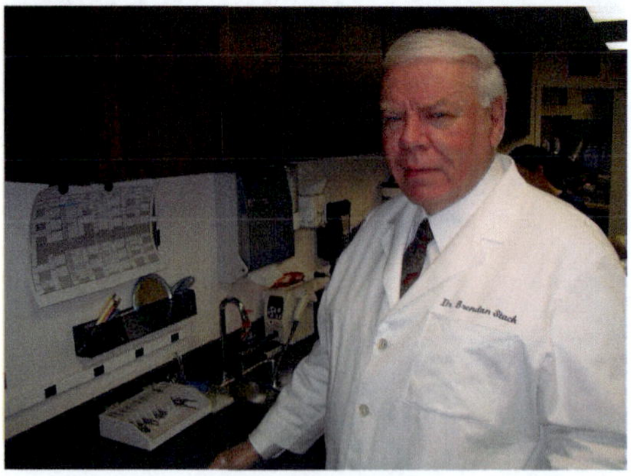

Fig. 12 Brendan C. Stack, Sr., at work in his office, Vienna, VA. (Courtesy of the Stack family trust)

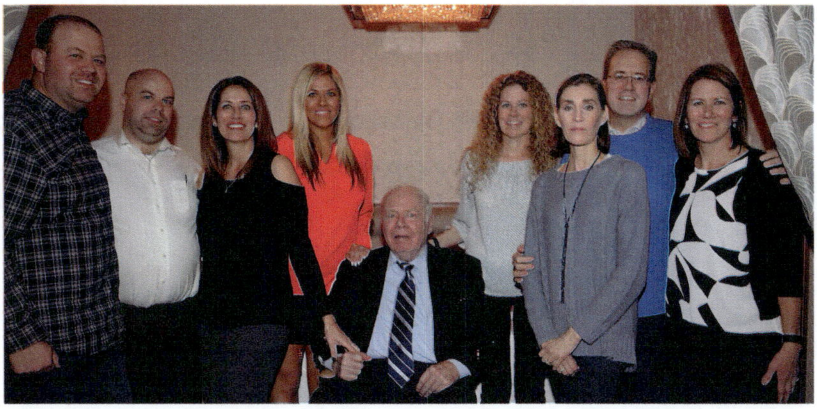

Fig. 13 Brendan C. Stack, Sr., on the occasion of his 80th birthday with his children, February 1, 2017, Tyson's Corners, VA. Pictured (L to R): Alexander J. "Alex" Stack, Matthew A. Stack, Maureen K. Stack, Diana L. Milani, Brendan C. Stack, Sr. (center), Jennifer L. Wheeler, Cynthia L. Stack (daughter-in-law), Brendan C. Stack, Jr., and Valerie A. Waite. (Courtesy of the Stack family trust)

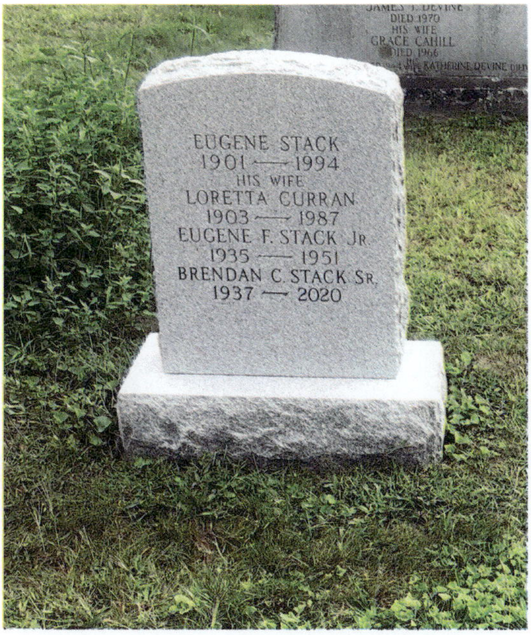
EUGENE STACK
1901 — 1994
HIS WIFE
LORETTA CURRAN
1903 — 1987
EUGENE F. STACK JR.
1935 — 1951
BRENDAN C. STACK SR.
1937 — 2020

Fig. 14 Grave marker of Brendan C. Stack, Sr., St. Jerome's Cemetery, Holyoke, MA, where he was interred with his father, mother, and elder brother. (Courtesy of the Stack family trust)

References

Stack BC. Dr. Brendan C. Stack: an interview with the 1988 AAFO Man of the Year. Interview by Craig Stoner. Funct Orthod. 1989;6(1):6–7, 9–19.

Stack BC. Journal of functional orthodontics interviews Dr. Brendan Stack on TMJ. Interview by Dr. Jimi Mehta. Funct Orthod. 1990;7(5):20–1, 24–5.

Stack BC. My journey from orthodontics to craniofacial pain and TMJ to movement disorders. Cranio. 2012;30(3):156–8. https://doi.org/10.1179/crn.2012.023.

Brown JL. Brendan C. Stack, The father of TMJ treatment. Cranio. 2020;38(6):357. https://doi.org/10.1080/08869634.2020.1823792.

Brendan C. Stack Jr.

Contents

Part I
Fundamentals

The Temporomandibular Joint: Form and Function

Anita R. Joy-Thomas and Robert D. Spears

1 Introduction

The temporomandibular joint (TMJ) is a specialized synovial joint that is essential for the full range of function of the mammalian jaw. It is a complex joint made up of various tissue types, including bone, cartilage, connective tissues, as well as associated muscles and tendons. The TMJ is described as a bilateral, diarthrodial, synovial joint that is located between the mandibular condyles and the temporal bones. Each TMJ is made up of the condylar head of the mandible, the glenoid fossa and articular eminence of the temporal bone, an articular disc, and a synovial membrane-lined fibrous capsule that encloses the entire joint (Fig. 1). The articulating surfaces of the joint are lined by fibrocartilage, rather than hyaline cartilage, in adults. The articular disc is another unique feature of the TMJ, which by its location divides the joint space into two chambers—superior and inferior (Fig. 2). This particular anatomical feature of the TMJ allows the joint to function as a unit in both hinge/axial/rotational (ginglymus) and gliding/translational (arthrodial) movements, thus also being described as a ginglymoarthrodial joint [1, 2].

As with any joint in the human body, the TMJ not only allows for a full range of motion associated with mastication, but it also reduces forces acting on the associated bones by dissipation or distribution of load-bearing from the associated bones to the surrounding soft tissues. TMJ dysfunction therefore affects not only the bony components of the joint, but also the soft tissue components. Therefore, from a functional standpoint and to better manage TMJ dysfunction, a thorough understanding of TMJ anatomy, both of the hard and soft tissue components, is essential.

A. R. Joy-Thomas (✉) · R. D. Spears
Department of Diagnostic and Biomedical Sciences, UTHealth Houston School of Dentistry, Houston, TX, USA
e-mail: Anita.JoyThomas@uth.tmc.edu; Robert.D.Spears@uth.tmc.edu

B. C. Stack Jr. et al. (eds.), *Craniofacial Pain*, https://doi.org/10.1007/978-3-031-57563-1_1

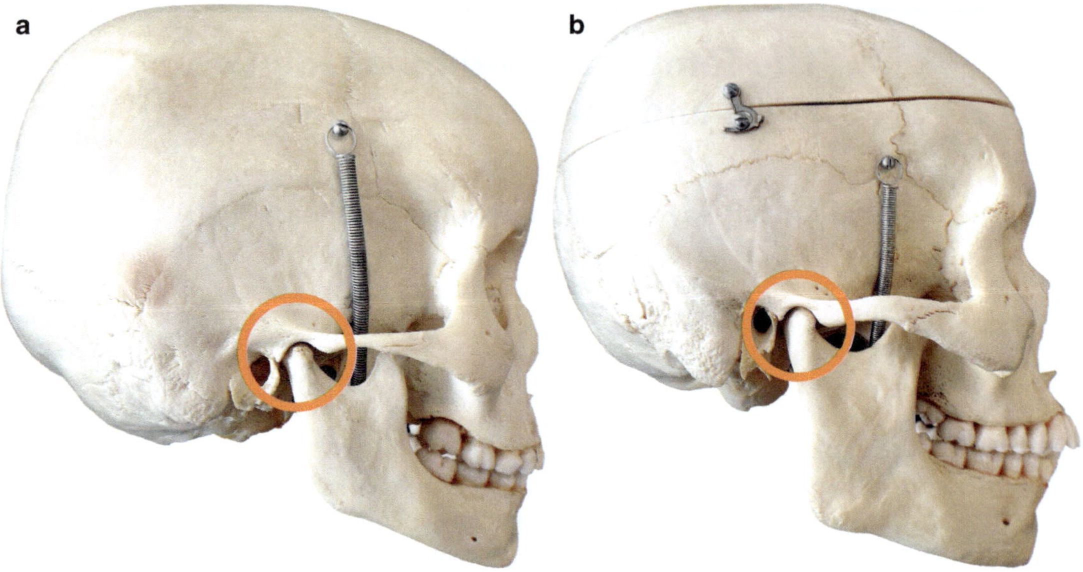

Fig. 1 Anatomy of the normal human temporomandibular joint. Photographs of human skulls from a young adolescent (**a**) and an adult (**b**) show the difference in size of the bony components of the temporomandibular joint. The circled area in both panels shows the condylar head of the mandible located posterior to the articular tubercle of the temporal bone. Note the difference in size of the articular tubercle between the adolescent skull and the adult skull. (*Anatomical specimen courtesy of Dr. Anita Joy-Thomas, UTHealth Houston School of Dentistry)*

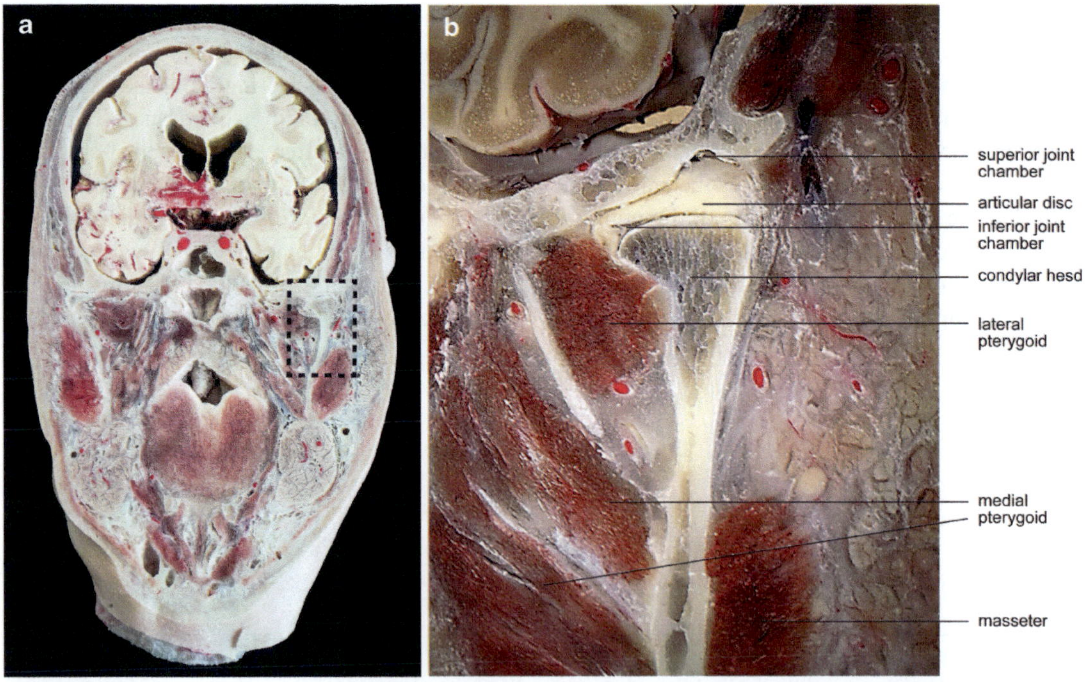

Fig. 2 Coronal section through the temporomandibular joint showing the articular disc and the two joint compartments. Image shows a coronal section through a plastinated anatomical specimen. The outlined area in panel **a** is enlarged in panel **b** and shows the articular disc situated in the joint space. The position of the articular disc divides the joint space into a superior and inferior chamber. Coronal sections through the condylar head of the mandible, and three muscles of mastication (masseter, inferior and superior heads of the lateral pterygoid, and superficial and deep heads of the medial pterygoid) are also visible. (*Plastinated anatomical specimen courtesy of the Anatomy Collection at the UTHealth Houston School of Dentistry)*

2 Embryology

The embryonic development of the human TMJ follows a similar process that is shared across various mammalian species. However, TMJ development is significantly different compared to other synovial joints in the body. In long bones, synovial joint formation occurs by cartilaginous differentiation at the locations of the joints, which then undergo cleavage or segmentation secondary to cartilage formation. This process occurs through the development of a noncartilaginous region known as the interzone, which serves as a critical signaling center, expressing bone morphogenetic proteins (BMPs), Wnt-14/beta-catenin, as well as BMP antagonists. The interplay between these signaling molecules allows for the interzone to maintain its nonchondrogenic nature. Interzone formation is followed by joint cavitation, which is regulated by the nonchondrogenic interzone cells secreting hyaluronan. The articular cartilage then continues to develop by appositional growth in the long bone [3–5]. In contrast, during TMJ development, there are two distinct and unconnected mesenchymal condensations or blastemas that grow toward each other while undergoing different ossification processes that ultimately result in the formation of the mandibular condyle and the glenoid fossa of the temporal bone. The condylar blastema arises from the secondary condyle cartilage of the mandible and forms bone through endochondral ossification. The glenoid fossa blastema arises from the otic capsule and undergoes intramembranous ossification [5–7]. The glenoid fossa blastema forms posterior and lateral to the developing condylar blastema. The condylar blastema then grows rapidly toward the glenoid fossa blastema, and during this growth, the intervening mesenchyme between the glenoid fossa and condylar blastemas is trapped, condenses, and differentiates into the lateral pterygoid muscle and the articular disc. This developmental sequence results in the superior belly of the lateral pterygoid muscle having an attachment on the medial aspect of the articular disc in the adult.

Early TMJ development includes the following stages—(1) blastematic stage (7–9 weeks in utero), (2) cavitation stage (9–11 weeks in utero), and (3) maturational stage (after 11 weeks in utero). During the blastematic stage is when mesenchymal condensation of cells occurs at the site of the future condylar cartilage. During this stage, intramembranous ossification of the squamous part of the temporal bone has also begun. During the cavitation stage, chondrocytes are clearly evident in the condylar blastema, and clefting occurs in the area that will form the future joint chambers, with the inferior cleft (future inferior joint chamber) forming first. Development of the TMJ occurs relatively later in utero (about 7–8 weeks) unlike most other synovial joints that have completed their initial cavity development by the seventh week in utero. In contrast, the TMJ has scarcely begun its development at this time and does not exhibit cavitation until approximately 9–11 weeks in utero. By week 13 in utero of the maturational stage, the area of the glenoid fossa acquires a clearly concave morphology. After week 14 in utero, a clear reduction in the size of Meckel's cartilage is also evident. It is only after about 18–20 weeks in utero that the TMJ is truly functional (i.e., with lateral pterygoid muscle attached to the condyle and the articular disc). After 18–20 weeks in utero, the TMJ takes over as the primary joint between the cranium and mandible. Later in the prenatal period, the condylar cartilage, which was originally carrot-shaped, gradually thins as birth approaches, and this is accompanied by the presence of vascular ingrowths into the condylar cartilage, a feature that is not seen in other cartilages.

2.1 Role of Meckel's Cartilage

In addition to these two mesenchymal condensations that contribute to TMJ development, the Meckel's cartilage, a primary cartilage derived from the first branchial arch, is critical in mandibular formation and growth. However, this cartilage has no part to play in the formation of the mandibular condyle. The cartilage that forms the condyles develops adjacent to the intramembra-

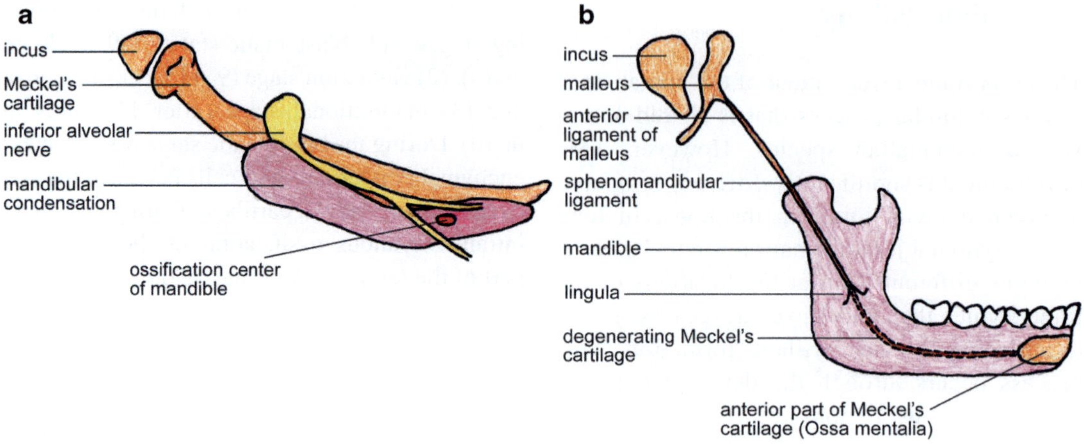

Fig. 3 Fate of Meckel's cartilage. Diagrammatic representation of the development of the mandible and the role of Meckel's cartilage. Panel **a** shows the Meckel's cartilage located lateral to the developing mandibular bone. Meckel's cartilage is continuous on its proximal end with the cartilage that will develop into the malleus and incus, two of the bones found in the middle ear. Panel **b** shows the mandible at birth. Remnants from the proximal/posterior part of Meckel's cartilage persist as the malleus and incus, the intermediate/central part of Meckel's cartilage persists as the anterior ligament of the malleus and the sphenomandibular ligament, while the distal/anterior part of Meckel's cartilage persists in the mandibular symphyseal area. *(Adapted and redrawn from Fawcett (1924). The Growth of the Jaws, Normal and Abnormal in Health and Disease)*

nous bone of the mandible; however, it is physically separate from and its development is chronologically later than Meckel's cartilage. Like other primary cartilages in the human, Meckel's cartilage is a rod of fetal cartilaginous skeleton in the mandible that begins with condensation of the cells to form a precartilaginous blastema very early in development (4–5 weeks of development) and forms the fetal template or anlagen of the developing mandible. Similar to primary limb cartilage, Meckel's cartilage arises from the mesenchyme of mesodermal origin via interaction with epithelial mesenchyme. This cartilage is located bilaterally and is positioned lateral to the developing mandibular bone but contributes little to mandibular bone formation [8]. This blastema extends as a solid hyaline cartilaginous rod surrounded by a fibrocellular capsule and extends from the developing ear region to the midline of the fused mandibular processes that forms the tip of the future chin. Along most of its length, Meckel's cartilage acts as a scaffold, lateral to which the mandible develops via intramembranous ossification. At its proximal end, Meckel's cartilage is continuous with the cartilage, which will form the malleus and incus bones of the middle ear. During the first 16–18 weeks of prenatal life, the synovial joint between the malleus and incus is thought to function as the (primary) jaw joint. Subsequently, portions of Meckel's cartilage differentiate into various tissues [8]. After it loses its function at 18–20 weeks (as the TMJ begins to function), Meckel's cartilage is gradually resorbed; in the adult, remnants of Meckel's cartilage exist as two ear ossicles, malleus and incus, and the sphenomandibular ligament (Fig. 3).

2.2 Development of the Condylar Cartilage and Mandibular Condyle

Once the mandibular ramus is formed using Meckel's cartilage as a scaffold, the condylar cartilage begins to develop from the periosteum of the mandibular ramus. A typical periosteum in the adult has two layers—an outer fibrous layer (protective in function) and an inner osteogenic layer (responsible for differentiation of cells during intramembranous bone formation). The perichondrium of the mandibular condylar cartilage is continuous with the periosteum of the mandibular ramus. During development of the condylar cartilage, the outer fibrous layer of the periosteum of the mandibular ramus continues to develop superiorly as the articular layer of the mandibular condylar cartilage (protective in function, and is in contact with the articular disc and the articular eminence of the temporal bone), while the inner osteogenic layer of the periosteum of the mandibular ramus develops superiorly to form the pre-chondroblastic layer of the developing mandibular condylar cartilage (responsible for differentiation and source of chondroprogenitor cells during intramembranous bone formation) (Fig. 4). Since the pre-chondroblastic layer originally develops from the osteogenic layer of the periosteum, it still retains the ability to differentiate not only into chondroblasts but also into bone-forming cells under the right stimulus, and they are therefore appropriately referred to as "skeletoblast" cells. These two most superficial layers of the condylar cartilage (articular and pre-chondroblastic layers) constitute the perichondrial articular envelope (Fig. 5). The articular layer is primarily made up of fibroblasts in a type I collagen matrix with some elastic fibers. This layer exhibits very low cell turnover. The pre-chondroblastic layer of the developing condylar cartilage is made up of multipotent mesenchymal cells in a sparse matrix containing type I collagen and proteoglycans. Immediately below the perichondrial artic-

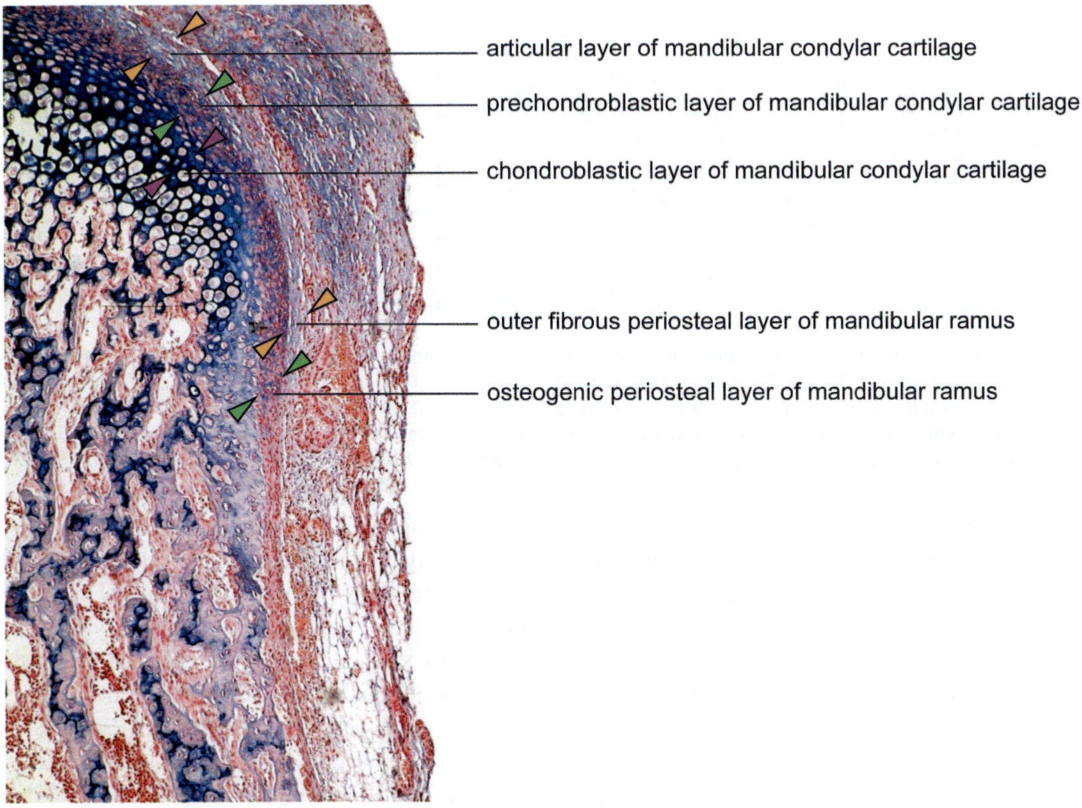

Fig. 4 Development of condylar cartilage. Alcian blue staining showing the layers in a developing mandibular condylar cartilage (MCC) of a rat. The outer fibrous layer of the periosteum of the developing mandibular ramus is continuous with and develops into the outer articular layer of the MCC (indicated by the orange arrowheads). The osteogenic layer of the periosteum develops into the pre-chondroblastic layer of the MCC (indicated by the green arrowheads). The histological image also shows the developing layer of chondroblasts (indicated by the pink arrowheads). (*Image adapted from Hinton, R.J. (2014), Genes that regulate morphogenesis and growth of the temporomandibular joint: A review. Dev. Dyn., 243: 864-874.* https://doi.org/10.1002/dvdy.24130*)*

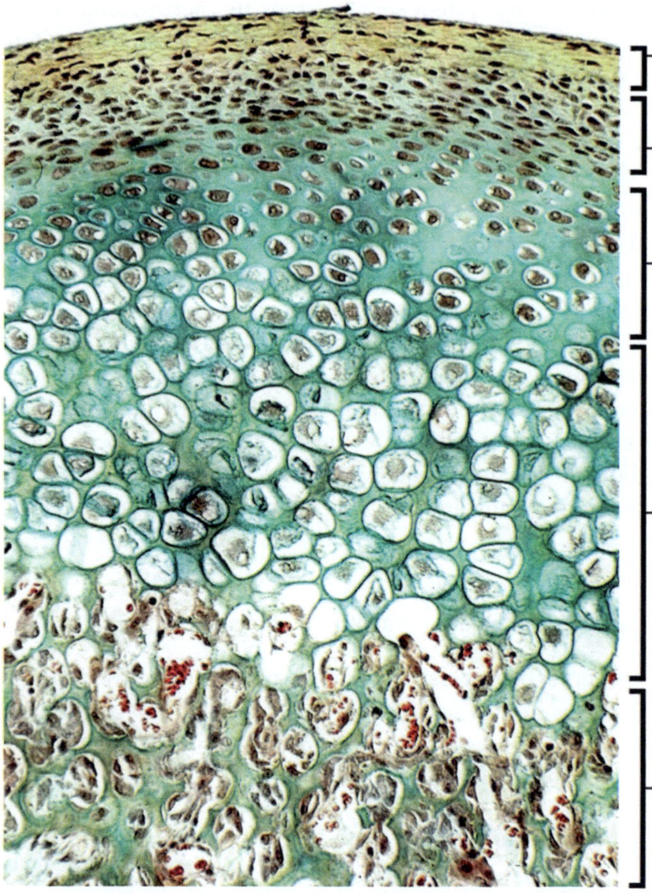

Fig. 5 Histological layers of condylar cartilage. Histological section with Attwood's staining showing the layers in a developing mandibular condylar cartilage (MCC) of a rat mandible. The layers from superior to inferior include an outer articular layer, a pre-chondroblastic layer, a chondroblastic layer, a hypertrophic layer, and a zone of mineralization or bone formation. (*Image adapted from Hinton RJ, Jing J, Feng JQ. Genetic Influences on Temporomandibular Joint Development and Growth. 2015. Curr. Tops. Dev. Biol., Vol. 115, p.85-109)*

ular envelope (articular layer and pre-chondroblastic layer) is the chondroblastic layer, which is made up of multiple layers of cells. Unlike the layers of chondroblasts seen in the growth plates of long bones or in the cranial base (anisotropic growth), these chondroblasts are not oriented in palisades or rows, but rather have no obvious directional orientation (isotropic growth). The chondroblastic layer begins with a zone of flattened cells and progresses to more rounded chondroblasts. These cells have considerably more matrix than seen in the pre-chondroblastic layer. The matrix is rich in type II collagen and aggrecan. The next layer of cells in the developing condylar cartilage is the hypertrophic layer wherein the cells enlarge greatly and eventually hypertrophy. The matrix contains both type I and type II collagen, with type I collagen more prevalent closer to the cartilage-bone interface. Type X collagen, a synthetic product specific to hypertrophic chondrocytes, is also present. The deeper layers show signs of mineralization as the next layer, i.e., the cartilage-bone interface, is approached (Fig. 5). At the cartilage-bone interface, blood vessels invade the developing tissue, bringing with them cells that help destroy the cartilage matrix. The hypertrophic chondrocytes undergo apoptosis or metaplastic change to transform into osteoblasts. New bone is deposited in and around the septa of the cartilage matrix (Fig. 5). Thus, the mandibular condyle forms with its articulating surface that will become a part of the future TMJ.

2.3 Development of the Articular Eminence and Mandibular Fossa

The articular eminence is virtually nonexistent at birth. It develops gradually until late adolescence as the masticatory forces on the joint increase with changes in diet during growth and development. This gradual growth eventually results in the mandibular fossa developing a deep concavity (Fig. 6). It develops gradually as dentition erupts.

The mandibular or glenoid fossa develops as the condyle develops. The fossa is a non-load-bearing area, directly inferior to the middle cranial fossa. The fossa is made up of relatively thin bone, covered superficially by a layer of periosteum. In mice, the mesenchymal condensation of the condyle, but not the glenoid fossa primordium, can be initially seen as early as embryonic day 13.5, followed soon after by mesenchymal condensation of the glenoid fossa [8]. In the absence of the condyle, the glenoid fossa condensation fails to sustain its development, leading to the lack of a definite glenoid fossa structure. Similar developmental defects are also observed in the glenoid fossa when the developing condyle is dislocated. Thus, the presence and proximity of the developing condyle, even if hypoplastic, are essential for the development of the glenoid fossa during TMJ formation [7]. It appears that the initial development of the glenoid fossa is independent of the condyle, but its continuous development relies on interaction with the condyle mediated by diffusible factors and not by direct tissue interaction. In contrast, development of the condyle continues independent of the glenoid fossa, since condylar cartilage development through intramembranous ossification is regulated by signaling from the developing mandibular ramus.

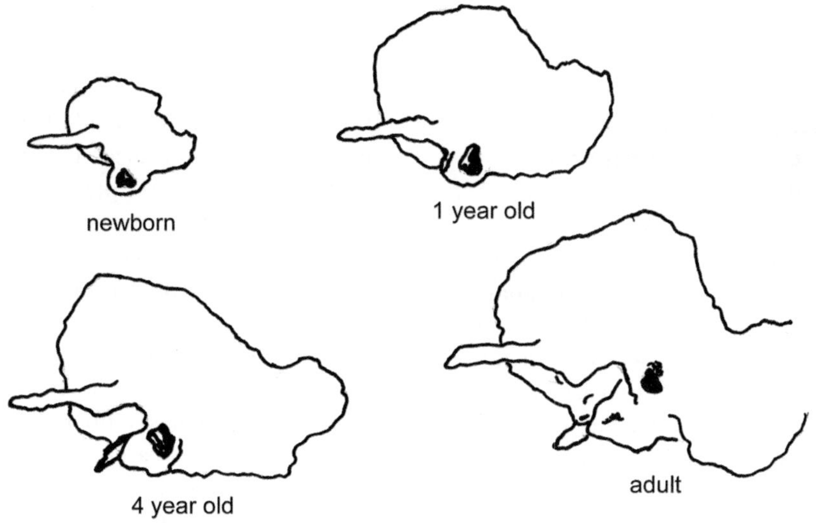

Fig. 6 Age changes of the articular eminence. Diagrammatic representation of the growth changes seen in the articular eminence and tubercle. With age, the eminence becomes larger, and the tubercle becomes more prominent and defined. Even in early childhood, the tubercle is not a very prominent structure. *(Adapted and drawn from anatomical specimens courtesy of the Anatomy Collection at the UTHealth Houston School of Dentistry)*

2.4 Development of the Articular Disc

The articular disc is a unique component of the TMJ that divides the joint into two chambers allowing for a wide range of motion (hinge and gliding). The articular disc forms from a third blastema of mesenchymal cells located between the condyle and the glenoid fossa. In mice studies, soon after a definitive condyle and glenoid fossa begin forming and assuming their positions and shapes, a disc becomes discernible as early as embryonic day 16.5. Almost immediately after, on embryonic day 17.5, synovial disc formation has been reported, which separates the superior and inferior joint chambers [8]. Several studies indicate appropriate signaling required for normal disc formation and suggest that the presence of the condyle is essential for the formation of a normal, functional disc [7, 9]. There is some evidence that Meckel's cartilage can substitute for the condyle to sustain glenoid fossa development to some extent in the absence of appropriate signaling. However, a functional TMJ with an articular disc cannot form without the condyle's full signaling influence [7].

3 Structure of the TMJ: Condyle, Glenoid Fossa, Articular Disc, Synovial Membrane

The TMJ is a continuum of anatomical structures that act as a unit to allow function. Anatomically, the TMJ is formed by the mandibular condyle and mandibular fossa. The bony landmarks around the joint include the articular tubercle, articular eminence, and tympanic plate (important for function of the joint, but not a structural part of the joint). With the condyle removed from the fossa, the sphenoid spine can be visualized, which reinforces the medial wall of the glenoid fossa and prevents the condyle from dislocating medially (Fig. 7). The condyle is the rounded headed of the mandibular ramus and is positioned in the glenoid fossa. It is tilted anteriorly at the neck of the condyle (Fig. 8). The condyle is about twice as long medial to lateral as it is anterior to posterior. It is angled perpendicular to the axis of the body of the mandible. The condyle has two poles—medial pole and lateral pole. The long axes of the condyles are not located perpendicular to the sagittal plane, but rather are tilted with the lateral poles located anterior to the medial poles (Figs. 7 and 8).

The glenoid fossa is concave to match the superior surface of the condyle. The space between the condyle and the fossa is divided by the articular disc into a superior and an inferior chamber. The disc is a biconcave structure and is made of three areas—an anterior band, an intermediate zone, and a posterior band, with the retrodiscal tissue connected posteriorly to the posterior band. The intermediate zone of the articular disc is completely avascular and aneural, while the anterior and posterior bands have a small number of blood vessels and nerve bundles in them. The entire articular disc is attached to the base of the skull, as well as to the head of the condyle, specifically to the medial and lateral poles, via discal or collateral ligaments. The disc exhibits a higher medial attachment compared to that on the lateral aspect, allowing the higher medial attachment to act as a stabilizing point with the lower lateral attachment providing a range of motion to allow the disc to move with the condyle as the mandible translates [10]. Anteriorly, the disc is also attached to the superior head of the lateral pterygoid muscle, and posteriorly the disc attaches to the retrodiscal tissue and joint capsule (Fig. 9). In younger individuals, the articular disc is made up of dense, irregular connective tissue that may be associated with chondrocytes and provides a smooth articulating surface. It consists largely of fibroblasts and elastic fibers in a collagenous matrix, similar to the articular layer of the condylar cartilage. With age and as the impact of masticatory forces on the disc increases, the tissue transforms into fibrocartilage, with collagen fibers oriented in such a way as to resist tensile forces in two directions—an outer concentric arrangement (attachment zone) and an inner anteroposterior arrangement (functional zone) of collagen fibers, with elastic fibers inter-

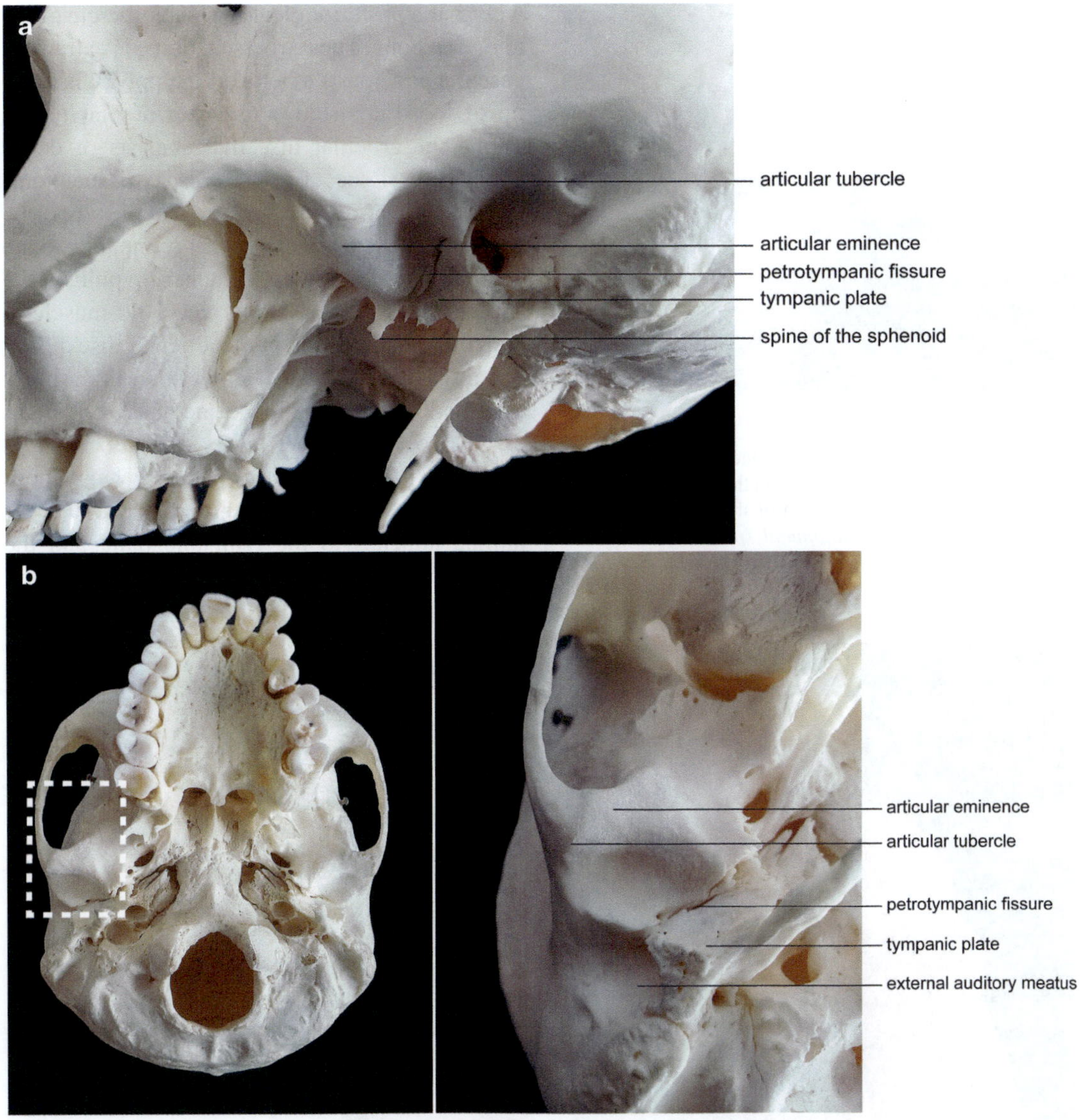

Fig. 7 Bony components of the temporomandibular joint. (**a**) Photograph of the lateral view of the human skull shows various skeletal landmarks associated with the temporomandibular joint. In addition to the articular eminence and tubercle, the petrotympanic fissure is seen dividing the glenoid/mandibular fossa. The spine of the sphenoid is also visible, which is an inferiorly projecting bony landmark located at the apex of the greater wing of the sphenoid. It serves as the origin of the sphenomandibular ligament. (**b**) Viewed from the inferior aspect of the skull, the same landmarks seen in panel **a** are seen. Note how broad the articular eminence is, extending mediolaterally. (*Anatomical specimen courtesy of Dr. Anita Joy-Thomas, UTHealth Houston School of Dentistry)*

spersed in an organized fashion [10–15]. Masticatory forces on the articular disc are not uniform, and the loaded areas are able to withstand tensile and compressive forces due to this very organized and dense arrangement of collagen fibers [11–15].

The retrodiscal tissue is an important part of the articular disc that is attached to the posterior band of the disc, divided into temporal, intermediate, and condylar regions [16] (Figs. 9 and 10). The retrodiscal tissue is attached to the posterior aspect of the neck of the mandibular condyle, as

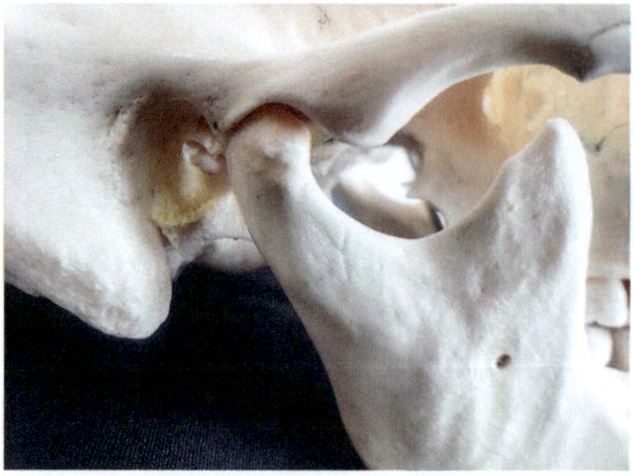

Fig. 8 Morphology of the condyle. Lateral view of the area around the right mandibular condyle shows the head of the condyle snugly located within the mandibular fossa/glenoid fossa. Note the location of the articular tubercle anterior to the fossa. (*Anatomical specimen courtesy of Dr. Anita Joy-Thomas, UTHealth Houston School of Dentistry*)

well as the posterior glenoid spine/tubercle of the temporal bone. The retrodiscal tissue is extremely vascular and boasts a rich nerve supply. It is made up of loose connective tissue or areolar tissue, unlike the articular disc that consists of dense connective tissue. The retrodiscal tissue nourishes the joint and acts as a cushion when the condyle presses against the tympanic plate [16–20]. It counteracts the anterior pull of the superior head of the lateral pterygoid muscle to help maintain position of the articular disc during opening and closing. The retrodiscal tissue is often called the bilaminar zone since it is organized into two distinct layers or laminae, separated by loose, highly vascularized, loose connective or areolar tissue [20, 21]. The superior lamina attaches to the tympanic plate and the posterior part of the glenoid fossa of the temporal

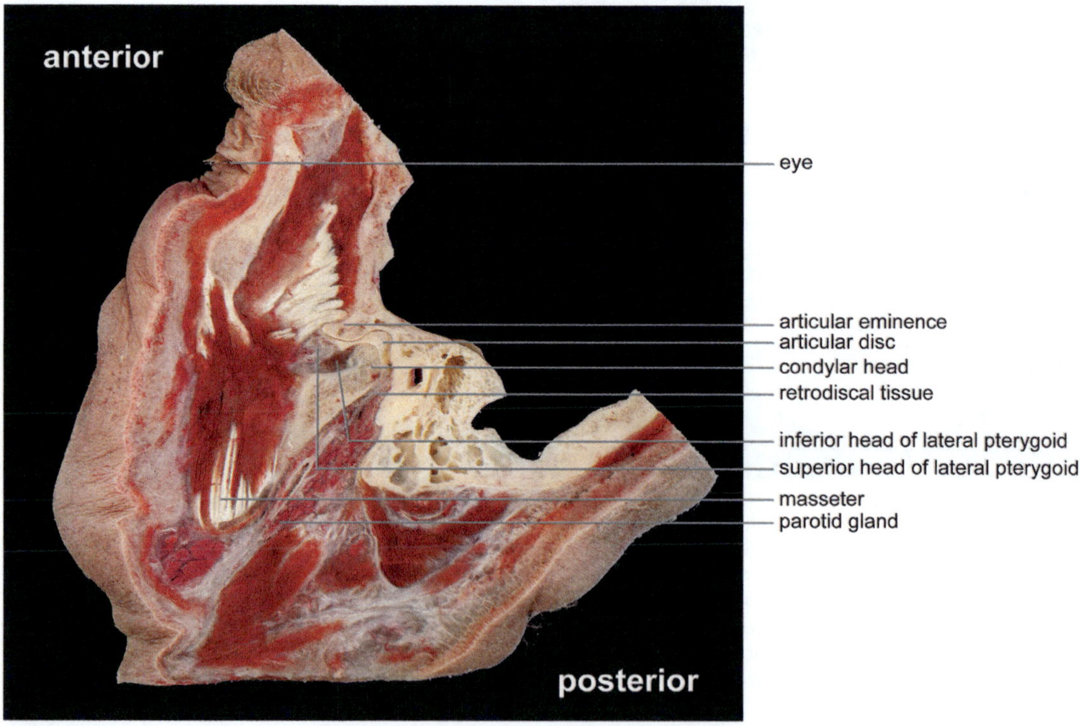

Fig. 9 Sagittal section through the temporomandibular joint showing the articular disc and retrodiscal tissue. A parasagittal view through the craniofacial area shows the articular disc located superior to the mandibular condyle in the joint space. Anteriorly, the disc can be seen attached to the superior head of the lateral pterygoid muscle, and posteriorly, it is continuous with the retrodiscal tissue. The section also shows parts of the inferior head of the lateral pterygoid and the masseter muscles. (*Plastinated anatomical specimen courtesy of the Anatomy Collection at the UTHealth Houston School of Dentistry*)

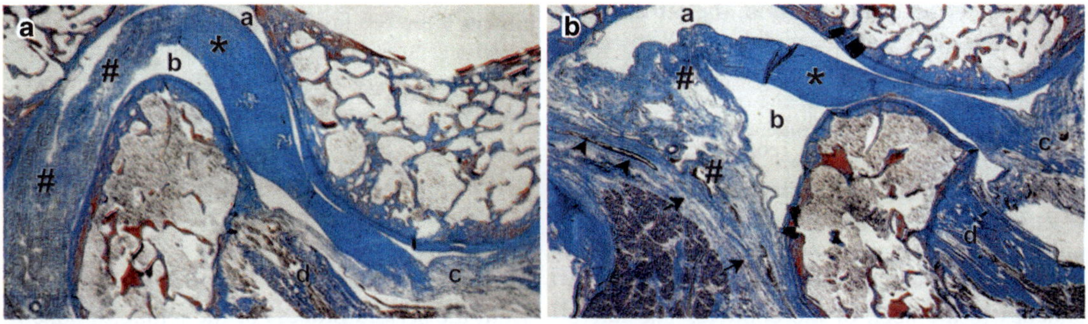

Fig. 10 Histology of the articular disc, retrodiscal tissue, and joint chambers. Sagittal section of the TMJ stained with Alcian blue shows details of the articular disc and related structures. Panel **a** shows the TMJ at rest, during which time, the articular disc (*) divides the joint space into a superior chamber (a) and an inferior chamber (b). Posteriorly, the articular disc can be seen continuing as the retrodiscal tissue (#). Panel **b** shows the TMJ in function, with the articular disc (*) moving anteriorly with the condylar head. This stretches the retrodiscal tissue (#) and causes distension of small blood vessels (black arrows). The superior (c) and inferior (d) heads of the lateral pterygoid are also seen inserting into the articular disc and the pterygoid fovea, respectively. *(Image adapted from Hinton RJ, Jing J, Feng JQ. Genetic Influences on Temporomandibular Joint Development and Growth. 2015. Curr. Tops. Dev. Biol., Vol.115, p.85-109)*

bone and is primarily made up of elastic fibers and a small amount of collagen fibers. Its elasticity allows the disc to move with the condyle during opening. The inferior lamina attaches to the posterior condylar neck, below the condylar cartilage, and is composed mostly of collagen fibers. It acts as an anchor to help prevent the articular disc from moving too far anteriorly during opening. Most of the blood supply and innervation to the joint enter through the retrodiscal tissue (Fig. 10). As the condyle translates forward during mandibular movements, the articular disc moves with the condyle. This translation of the disc with the condyle is possible due to the elastic fibers within the superior lamina of the retrodiscal tissue. The collagen fibers and the posterior attachments of the retrodiscal tissue prevent the disc from dislocating anteriorly during condylar movements [18, 21–24]. Excessive posterior movement of the mandible can cause the retrodiscal tissue to become compressed between the condyle and the tympanic plate. On the other hand, excessive anterior movement of the mandible can cause the retrodiscal tissue to become stretched. In both situations, pain, inflammation, and swelling can result [21–24].

The nonarticular surfaces of the TMJ are covered with a synovial membrane as a means to provide nutrition to and removal of metabolic waste products from the largely avascular joint. The synovial membrane has two layers—an intima and a subintima. The intimal layer is made up of cells called synoviocytes. Some synoviocytes produce synovial fluid, while other synoviocytes function as macrophages to clear cellular debris. The subintimal layer consists of fibroblasts and serves as supporting cells. This layer also contains collagen fibers and is very vascular. In the TMJ, the synovial membrane secretes synovial fluid that completely bathes the joint and provides the joint with nutrients. Synovial fluid contains a double glycoprotein called lubricin that lowers the coefficient of friction, thus allowing substantial lubrication of the articular surfaces. During mandibular movements, synovial fluid diffuses into the joint spaces and diffuses back from the joint spaces into the synovial membrane at rest [25].

4 Associated Structures of the TMJ: Ligaments, Muscles, and Neurovasculature

The TMJ does not function in isolation, rather the joint is influenced by several associated structures including joint ligaments, muscles of mastication, and associated neurovasculature. Several ligaments help control the forces asserted by and at the joint. These forces are perceived via proprioceptive afferents provided through the joint capsule, muscles of mastication, cutaneous receptors overlying the joint, stretch receptors within the joint, as well as receptors in the periodontal ligaments of teeth.

A fibrous joint capsule is attached to the articular tubercles, the squamotympanic suture, and the mandibular fossa. Inferiorly, the joint capsule attaches to the neck of the condyle. The lateral ligament or the temporomandibular ligament originates from the lower articular tubercle of the zygomatic arch and extends postero-inferiorly to attach to the lateral and posterior border of the neck of the mandible (Fig. 11). This ligament helps keep the condyle in the fossa while allowing the mandible to swing forward in protrusion. The lateral ligament also prevents the condyle from posterior displacement of the mandible, potentially causing injury to the retrodiscal tissue, and prevents the condyle from being driven upward into the base of the skull (as from an inferior blow to the jaw) [26, 27].

Two accessory ligaments help stabilize the joint, and these include the sphenomandibular and stylomandibular ligaments (Fig. 11). The sphenomandibular ligament is a remnant of Meckel's cartilage. It extends from the spine of the sphenoid bone to attach to the lingula of the mandible. As it extends inferiorly, fibers of this ligament may intertwine with fibers along the medial wall of the joint capsule. The mylohyoid nerve and several vessels cross the ligament. It lies superior and lateral to the lateral pterygoid muscle and the inferior alveolar nerve. Its main task is to protect the TMJ from an excessive translation of the condyle, after 10° of opening of the mouth. The stylomandibular ligament extends from the styloid process of the temporal bone to attach into the angle of the mandible. It functions to limit excessive protrusion of the mandible. In addition to these ligaments that control joint movements, the condyle also has two bundles of collateral ligaments or discal ligaments that originate from the articular disc and insert at the medial and lateral poles of the mandibular condyle. These ligaments serve to anchor the disc to the condyle [26, 27].

TMJ function is significantly influenced by function of the muscles of mastication, which move the mandible at the joints. The four bilaterally located muscles of mastication include the masseter, temporalis, medial pterygoid, and lateral pterygoid. The masseter muscle is the strongest and most powerful elevator of the mandible. It is a quadrangular muscle that covers the lateral aspect of the ramus of the mandible. It originates as two muscular heads from the zygomatic

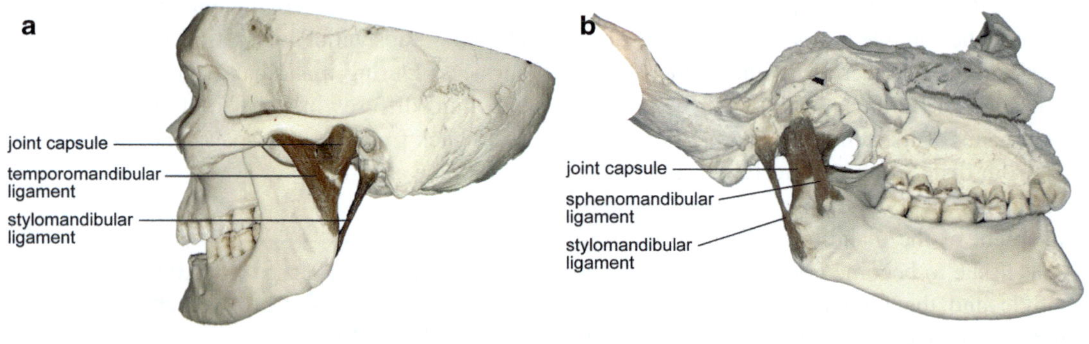

Fig. 11 Ligaments of the TMJ. Model of the ligaments associated with the TMJ is depicted in panels **a** and **b**. Panel **a** shows a left lateral view of the skull where the temporomandibular ligament is seen extending posteroinferiorly from the inferior aspect of the articular tubercle and surrounding areas and inserting into the lateral and posterior border of the neck of the mandible. The joint capsule is seen, which encloses the entire joint. The stylomandibular ligament, extending from the styloid process to the posterior aspect of the mandibular angle, is also seen. Panel **b** is a view of the ligaments from the interior aspect of a hemisected skull. In addition to the joint capsule and the stylomandibular ligament, the sphenomandibular ligament can also be seen. (*Anatomical specimen courtesy of Dr. Raymond Warner, UTHealth Houston School of Dentistry)*

arch—superficial head and deep head. The larger, superficial head originates from the maxillary process of the zygomatic bone and the anterior two-thirds of the zygomatic arch. These muscle fibers run inferiorly and posteriorly to attach to the lateral surface of the angle and lower half of the ramus of the mandible. The deep head of the masseter originates from the medial aspect and inferior margin of the zygomatic arch (note that its origin is partially covered by the superficial head). These fibers run vertically downwards to insert into the upper part of the ramus of the mandible and the coronoid process. Fibers of the superficial head are perpendicular to the Curve of Spee, resulting in maximum force applied on the occlusal plane when it contracts. In addition to elevation, the superficial head can also help protrude the mandible (Fig. 12). The innervation of the masseter muscle is via branches of the masseteric nerve, a branch of the mandibular nerve (cranial nerve V3), and it receives blood supply from the masseteric artery, a branch of the maxillary artery [8, 28–32].

The temporalis muscle is a large, flat muscle that lies in the confines of the temporal fossa of the skull. The muscle originates from the inferior temporal line, as well as the deep surface of the temporal fascia. The muscle fibers converge anteriorly to form a tendon which runs deep to the zygomatic arch and then inserts along the medial surface of the coronoid process and the anterior border of the ramus of mandible. The tendon of the temporalis exhibits two extensions—the superficial tendon inserts into the anterior crest and the deep tendon inserts into the temporal crest. If a denture is designed to overlap these tendons, when a patient laughs or coughs, it will displace the denture. The anterior fibers of the muscle are oriented in a more vertical direction resulting in elevation of the mandible when it contracts, while the posterior fibers are oriented in an almost horizontal direc-

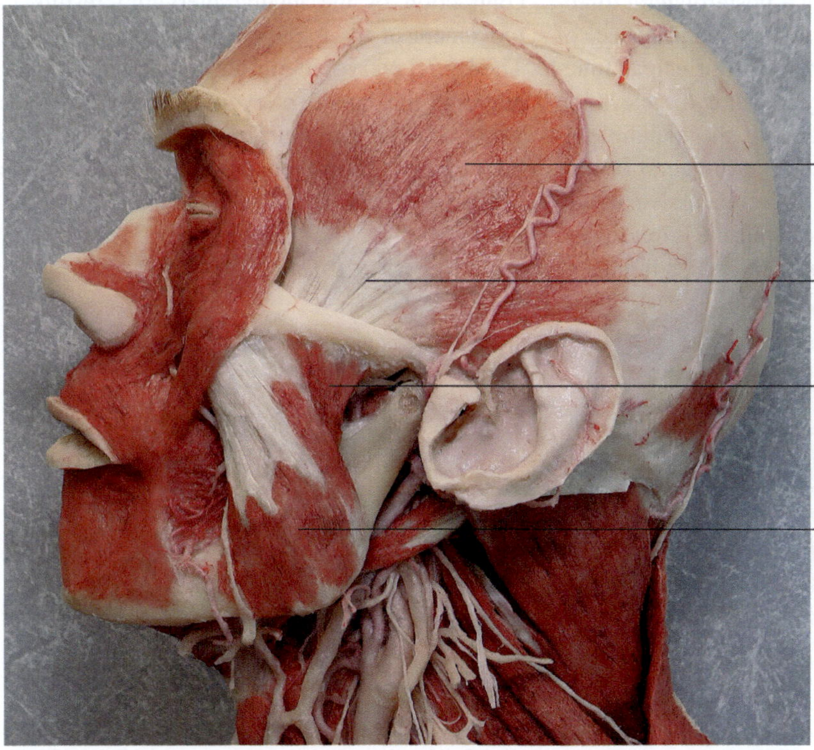

Fig. 12 Muscles of mastication—temporalis and masseter. Superficial dissection of the face shows the fan-shaped temporalis muscle and both heads of the masseter muscle. *(Plastinated anatomical specimen courtesy of the Anatomy Collection at the UTHealth Houston School of Dentistry)*

tion and allow retrusion of the mandible (this muscle is the most powerful retrudor of the mandible). The temporalis muscle also has a minor contribution to grinding movements by moving the mandible from side to side. The muscle is covered by the temporal fascia that originates from superior temporal line and inserts into the zygomatic arch, and the fascia helps support the zygomatic arch. The muscle is innervated by the deep temporal branches of the mandibular nerve and receives blood supply from the deep temporal branches of the maxillary artery and superficial temporal artery (Fig. 12) [8, 28, 29, 32–36].

The medial pterygoid muscle is a quadrangular muscle located in the infratemporal fossa. It has two muscular heads—superficial and deep. The larger deep head originates from the medial surface of the lateral pterygoid plate of the sphenoid bone and the adjacent pyramidal process of palatine bone. The smaller superficial head originates from the maxillary tuberosity. Both muscle heads converge and run in a posterolateral direction to eventually insert into the medial surface of the ramus of the mandible. The principal functions of the medial pterygoid are for elevation and side-to-side movements of the mandible. It can also protrude the mandible (bilateral or unilateral contraction) and allow excursive movements. The medial pterygoid muscle is innervated by the nerve to the medial pterygoid, a branch of the mandibular nerve (cranial nerve V3), and it receives blood supply from the pterygoid branches of the maxillary artery (Fig. 13) [8, 28, 29, 31, 32, 37].

The lateral pterygoid muscle is a triangular muscle with two heads, superior and inferior, that lies in the infratemporal fossa. The smaller, superior head originates from the inferior surface of the greater wing and infratemporal crest of the sphenoid bone, which form the roof of the infratemporal fossa. The larger, inferior head originates from the lateral surface of the lateral pterygoid plate of the sphenoid bone. The fibers from both heads merge and run posterolaterally to insert into the pterygoid fovea, a shallow bony depression located on the neck of the mandible. Additionally, some fibers of the superior head also insert into the joint capsule and articular disc. The lateral pterygoid muscle functions mainly to move the mandible anteriorly during opening. If there is bilateral contraction, the mandible is protruded and depressed, while unilateral contraction of the medial pterygoid results in movement of the mandible to the opposite side. The lateral pterygoid muscle is innervated by the nerve to the lateral pterygoid, a branch of the mandibular nerve (cranial nerve V3), and receives blood supply from the pterygoid branches of the maxillary artery (Fig. 13) [8, 28, 29, 31, 32, 38–41].

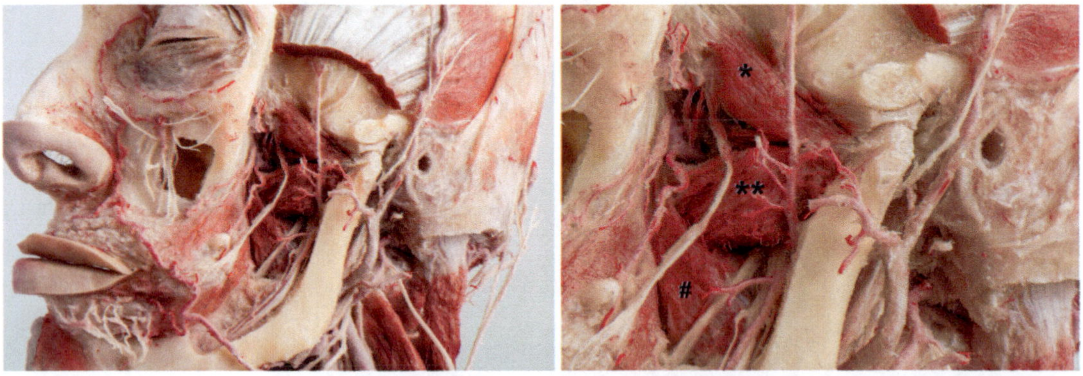

Fig. 13 Muscles of mastication—medial and lateral pterygoid. Deep dissection of the infratemporal fossa shows the medial and lateral pterygoid muscles. The area outlined in the image on the left is enlarged to show the superior (*) and inferior (**) heads of the lateral pterygoid muscle, as well as the medial pterygoid muscle (#). The superficial and deep heads are not separately seen in this specimen. (*Plastinated anatomical specimen courtesy of the Anatomy Collection at the UTHealth Houston School of Dentistry*)

The principal nerve responsible for sensation in the joint is the trigeminal nerve. The articular capsule in the anterolateral portion is innervated by branches of the masseteric nerve, which is derived from the mandibular nerve (V3). The lateral aspect of the joint capsule is innervated by the auriculotemporal nerve, also a branch of the mandibular nerve (V3). In some individuals, the joint is also innervated by the nerves to the masseter and the temporalis. The joint has several proprioceptive receptors, especially within the articular disc, including Golgi-Mazzoni corpuscles, Golgi tendon bodies, Pacinian corpuscles, and Ruffini endings, in addition to myelinated and unmyelinated nerve fibers. Arterial blood supply to the TMJ is provided primarily by the superficial temporal artery and the maxillary artery. The joint also receives arterial supply from branches of the masseteric artery, posterior auricular artery, ascending palatine artery, and ascending pharyngeal artery. Venous drainage is mainly via the pterygoid plexus located in the retrodiscal area [8, 28, 29, 31, 32].

5 Age-Related Changes in the TMJ

Multiple changes occur within the various components of the TMJ with aging, some as a result of increased forces at the joint and others as a result of the normal aging process.

5.1 Hard Tissue Components: Mandibular Condyle and Articular Eminence

Numerous changes are involved as the mandibular condyle ages. Histologically, an overall decrease in cellularity is observed. As the condyle shifts from a site of growth into a more functional role, the pre-chondroblastic layer shrinks in size and will eventually disappear. Similarly, the articular layer becomes more fibrocartilaginous, while the cartilage layer will see the disappearance of hypertrophic chondrocytes that play a vital role during growth until it ceases in late adolescence. Additionally, the histology of the condyle in older adults becomes one of predominately bony tissue underlying a thinner layer of cartilage that is still present at this stage. Changes are also observed within the extracellular matrix of the condyle as seen primarily in changes to the proteoglycan content. Similar changes are observed with the articular eminence during aging [42, 43].

5.2 Soft Tissue Components

Multiple changes are observed in the various soft tissue components of the TMJ, again in response to functional changes, as well as a part of the aging process. Similar to most areas of the body, a loss of cellularity with a concomitant increase in fiber content is observed. First, the articular disc is observed to transition from a dense connective structure to one that is much more fibrocartilaginous in composition [44, 45]. An observed decrease in cellularity in the retrodiscal tissues is seen with diminished vascularity and decreased presence of nerve fibers [45]. The synovial membrane becomes thinner and often is missing in regions it was normally located in, which can result in a loss of lubrication for the joint. Fewer synoviocytes can also mean a reduction in macrophage production and a diminished ability for joint tissues to clear away debris.

All of the above changes in both hard and soft tissues can contribute to the dysfunction that is often observed in the TMJ with aging.

6 Summary

A sound understanding of TMJ form, function, and embryology is essential for evaluation and treatment of patients suffering from TMD. The preceding chapter has outlined the development and form of the TMJ and described its relationships to its adjacent anatomy. This understanding sets the stage for a greater appreciation of the connections of TMD and a variety of symptomatic stigmata, many of which have no direct or obvious connection to the TMJ to the uninitiated clinician. Please relate your knowledge from this chapter to the content of chapters on the neurologic symptoms of TMD.

References

1. Hinton RJ. Genes that regulate morphogenesis and growth of the temporomandibular joint: a review. Dev Dyn. 2014;243(7):864–74. https://doi.org/10.1002/dvdy.24130. Epub 2014 Apr 16. PMID: 24668501.
2. Moskalewski S, Hyc A, Jankowska-Steifer E, Osiecka-Iwan A. Formation of synovial joints and articular cartilage. Folia Morphol (Warsz). 2013;72(3):181–7. https://doi.org/10.5603/fm.2013.0031. PMID: 24068678.
3. Archer CW, Dowthwaite GP, Francis-West P. Development of synovial joints. Birth Defects Res C Embryo Today. 2003;69(2):144–55. https://doi.org/10.1002/bdrc.10015. PMID: 12955858.
4. Mérida-Velasco JR, Rodríguez-Vázquez JF, Mérida-Velasco JA, Sánchez-Montesinos I, Espín-Ferra J, Jiménez-Collado J. Development of the human temporomandibular joint. Anat Rec. 1999;255(1):20–33. https://doi.org/10.1002/(SICI)1097-0185(19990501)255:1<20::AID-AR4>3.0.CO;2-N. PMID: 10321990.
5. Liang W, Li X, Gao B, Gan H, Lin X, Liao L, Li C. Observing the development of the temporomandibular joint in embryonic and post-natal mice using various staining methods. Exp Ther Med. 2016;11(2):481–9. https://doi.org/10.3892/etm.2015.2937. Epub 2015 Dec 16. PMID: 26893634; PMCID: PMC4734204.
6. Li X, Liang W, Ye H, Weng X, Liu F, Liu X. Overexpression of Shox2 leads to congenital dysplasia of the temporomandibular joint in mice. Int J Mol Sci. 2014;15(8):13135–50. https://doi.org/10.3390/ijms150813135. PMID: 25062348; PMCID: PMC4159784.
7. Wang Y, Liu C, Rohr J, Liu H, He F, Yu J, Sun C, Li L, Gu S, Chen Y. Tissue interaction is required for glenoid fossa development during temporomandibular joint formation. Dev Dyn. 2011;240(11):2466–73. https://doi.org/10.1002/dvdy.22748. Epub 2011 Sep 26. PMID: 21953591; PMCID: PMC3197963.
8. Nanci A. Ten Cate's oral histology-e-book: development, structure, and function. Elsevier Health Sciences; 2017.
9. Gu S, Wei N, Yu L, Fei J, Chen Y. Shox2-deficiency leads to dysplasia and ankylosis of the temporomandibular joint in mice. Mech Dev. 2008;125(8):729–42. https://doi.org/10.1016/j.mod.2008.04.003. Epub 2008 Apr 22. PMID: 18514492; PMCID: PMC3010750.
10. Loreto C, Leonardi R, Musumeci G, Pannone G, Castorina S. An ex vivo study on immunohistochemical localization of MMP-7 and MMP-9 in temporomandibular joint discs with internal derangement. Eur J Histochem. 2013;57:e12. https://doi.org/10.4081/ejh.2013.e12.
11. Scapino RP, Canham PB, Finlay HM, Mills DK. The behaviour of collagen fibres in stress relaxation and stress distribution in the jaw-joint disc of rabbits. Arch Oral Biol. 1996;41:1039–52. https://doi.org/10.1016/S0003-9969(96)00079-9.
12. Shengyi T, Yinghua X. Biomechanical properties and collagen fiber orientation of TMJ discs in dogs: part 1. Gross anatomy and collagen fiber orientation of the discs. J Craniomandib Disord. 1991;5:28–34.
13. Detamore MS, Orfanos JG, Almarza AJ, French MM, Wong ME, Athanasiou KA. Quantitative analysis and comparative regional investigation of the extracellular matrix of the porcine temporomandibular joint disc. Matrix Biol. 2005;24:45–57. https://doi.org/10.1016/j.matbio.2004.11.006.
14. Gage J, Shaw R, Moloney F. Collagen type in dysfunctional temporomandibular joint disks. J Prosthet Dent. 1995;74:517–20. https://doi.org/10.1016/S0022-3913(05)80355-5.
15. Runci AM, Cascone P, Anastasi GP, Santoro G, Nicita F, Picciolo G, Favaloro A, Rizzo G, Cutroneo G. Articular disc of a human temporomandibular joint: evaluation through light microscopy, immunofluorescence and scanning electron microscopy. J Funct Morphol Kinesiol. 2021;6(1):22. https://doi.org/10.3390/jfmk6010022. PMID: 33669061; PMCID: PMC8006253.
16. Rees LA. The structure and function of the mandibular joint. Br Dent J. 1954;96(6):125–33.
17. Scapino RP. Histopathology associated with malposition of the human temporomandibular joint disc. Oral Surg Oral Med Oral Pathol. 1983;55(4):382–97.
18. Scapino RP. The posterior attachment: its structure, function, and appearance in TMJ imaging studies. Part 1. J Craniomandib Disord. 1991;5(2):83–95.
19. Kino K, Ohmura Y, Amagasa T. Reconsideration of the bilaminar zone in the retrodiskal area of the temporomandibular joint. Oral Surg Oral Med Oral Pathol. 1993;75(4):410–21.
20. Piette E. Anatomy of the human temporomandibular joint. An updated comprehensive review. Acta Stomatol Belg. 1993;90(2):103–27.
21. Wilkinson TM, Crowley CM. A histologic study of retrodiscal tissues of the human temporomandibular joint in the open and closed position. J Orofac Pain. 1994;8(1):7–17.
22. Christo JE, Bennett S, Wilkinson TM, Townsend GC. Discal attachments of the human temporomandibular joint. Aust Dent J. 2005;50(3):152–60.
23. Osborn JW. The disc of the human temporomandibular joint: design, function and failure. J Oral Rehabil. 1985;12(4):279–93.
24. Scapino RP. Morphology and mechanism of the jaw joint. In: McNeill C, editor. Science and practice of occlusion. Quintessence: Chicago; 1997. p. 23–40.
25. Kayoko NI, Norio A, Nobuyuki I, Akiko S, Yoshiro K, Takeyasu M. Synovial membrane in the temporoman-

dibular joint—Its morphology, function and development. Arch Histol Cytol. 2003;66(4):289–306.
26. Veronica I, Thomas B, Nicol V. Temporomandibular joint: review of anatomy and clinical implications. Dent Clin N Am. 2023;67(2):199–209. https://doi.org/10.1016/j.cden.2022.11.003.
27. Alomar X, Medrano J, Cabratosa J, Clavero JA, Lorente M, Serra I, Monill JM, Salvador A. Anatomy of the temporomandibular joint. Semin Ultrasound CT MRI. 2007;28(3):170–83. https://doi.org/10.1053/j.sult.2007.02.002.
28. Drake RL, Vogl AW, Mitchell AWM. Gray's anatomy for students. VitalSource bookshelf, 3rd ed. Elsevier Health Sciences (US); 2014.
29. Leperchey F. [Embryogeny of facial, mastication, tongue, palate and neck muscles (author's transl)]. Rev Stomatol Chir Maxillofac. 1979;80(2):45–67.
30. Arnold F. Handbuch der Anatomie des Menschen, mit Rücksicht auf Physiologie und praktische Medicin. Freiburg im Breisgau: Herder'sche Verlagshandlung; 1845.
31. Terminologia Anatomica: International Anatomical Terminology. New York: Thieme Medical Publishers; 1998.
32. Waschke J, Böckers TM, Paulsen F, editors. Sobotta anatomy textbook, 1st ed. Munich: Elsevier; 2019.
33. Yu SK, Kim TH, Yang KY, Bae CJ, Kim HJ. Morphology of the temporalis muscle focusing on the tendinous attachment onto the coronoid process. Anat Cell Biol. 2021;54(3):308–14. https://doi.org/10.5115/acb.21.074. PMID: 34353976; PMCID: PMC8493017.
34. Geers C, Nyssen-Behets C, Cosnard G, Lengelé B. The deep belly of the temporalis muscle: an anatomical, histological and MRI study. Surg Radiol Anat. 2005;27:184–91. https://doi.org/10.1007/s00276-004-0306-3.
35. Sedlmayr JC, Kirsch CF, Wisco JJ. The human temporalis muscle: superficial, deep, and zygomatic parts comprise one structural unit. Clin Anat. 2009;22:655–64. https://doi.org/10.1002/ca.20837.
36. Gaudy JF, Zouaoui A, Bravetti P, Charrier JL, Laison F. Functional anatomy of the human temporal muscle. Surg Radiol Anat. 2001;23:389–98. https://doi.org/10.1007/s00276-001-0389-z.
37. El Haddioui A, Bravetti P, Gaudy JF. Anatomical study of the arrangement and attachments of the human medial pterygoid muscle. Surg Radiol Anat. 2007;29:115–24.
38. Stöckle M, Fanghänel J, Knüttel H, Alamanos C, Behr M. The morphological variations of the lateral pterygoid muscle: a systematic review. Ann Anat. 2019;222:79–87.
39. Desmons S, Graux F, Atassi M, Libersa P, Dupas PH. The lateral pterygoid muscle, a heterogeneous unit implicated in temporomandibular disorder: a literature review. Cranio. 2007;25(4):283–91.
40. Usui A, Akita K, Yamaguchi K. An anatomic study of the divisions of the lateral pterygoid muscle based on the findings of the origins and insertions. Surg Radiol Anat. 2008;30(4):327–33.
41. El Haddioui A, Laison F, Zouaoui A, Bravetti P, Gaudy JF. Functional anatomy of the human lateral pterygoid muscle. Surg Radiol Anat. 2005;27(4):271–86.
42. Richards LC, Brown T. Dental attrition and degenerative arthritis of the temporomandibular joint. J Oral Rehabil. 1981;8:293–307. https://doi.org/10.1111/j.1365-2842.1981.tb00504.x.
43. Moffett BC, Johnson LC, MaCabe JB, et al. Articular remodeling in the adult human temporomandibular joint. Am J Anat. 1964;115:119.
44. Chen PJ, Dutra EH, Mehta S, O'Brien MH, Yadav S. Age-related changes in the cartilage of the temporomandibular joint. Geroscience. 2020;42(3):995–1004. https://doi.org/10.1007/s11357-020-00160-w. Epub 2020 Jan 28. PMID: 31993924; PMCID: PMC7287006.
45. Blackwood HJJ. Cellular remodeling in articular tissue. J Dent Res. 1966;45:480.

The Etiology of Temporomandibular Disorders

Feras Al Khatib and Achint Utreja

1 Introduction

Temporomandibular disorder (TMD) is an umbrella term referring to the dysfunction and pathologic conditions of the musculoskeletal and neuromuscular elements of the temporomandibular joint (TMJ), masticatory muscles, and adjacent structures [1]. TMD is the most frequent pathology in the orofacial complex. Its biomechanics and anatomy are quite complex (Figs. 1 and 2). The most common clinical manifestations of TMD are masticatory muscle pain, limited range of mouth opening, noise from the TMJ, and chronic myofascial pain [2]. Other symptoms can also be present including headache, neuralgias, toothache(s), and earache [3].

The dental profession is divided over the etiology and treatment of the TMD. Almost every discipline in dentistry played some role in the development of this topic. For the most part, these contributions depended on poorly conducted research, experience, personal opinions, and treatment philosophies, which created some confusion in understanding the etiology and treatment approaches [4]. Each dental specialty looked at TMD from their own perspective and biases using their own terminology to describe the problems and suggest their treatment plans. Some prosthodontists believed that full mouth rehabilitation in centric relation (CR) by itself can relieve TMD symptoms. On the other hand, some orthodontists suggest that finishing their orthodontic treatment in ideal occlusion can treat TMD symptoms.

The etiology of TMD has always been a controversial topic. Our understanding of the etiology has evolved over the last few years. For decades, it was believed that TMDs were caused mainly by occlusal factors. Thus, changing the patients' occlusion was a common practice in dentistry to treat patients with TMD. As the profession demanded more evidence-based research and practice, it became clear that there were more factors involved in the onset of TMD [5]. Recent research from the fields of behavioral sciences, psychology, genetics, pain pathophysiology, neurophysiology, and endocrinology has significantly revolutionized our understanding of TMDs and how they should be managed [4]. In fact, more recent research suggests that TMD is a multifactorial complex disorder with overlapping comorbidities of physical signs and symptoms associated with changes in emotional status, behavior, and social interaction as a manifestation of the central nervous system. TMDs are no longer believed to be caused by a single factor only [2, 6]. More recently, there has been a grad-

F. Al Khatib (✉) · A. Utreja
Section of Orthodontics, Southern Illinois University School of Dental Medicine, Alton, IL, USA
e-mail: falkhat@siue.edu; autreja@siue.edu

B. C. Stack Jr. et al. (eds.), *Craniofacial Pain*, https://doi.org/10.1007/978-3-031-57563-1_2

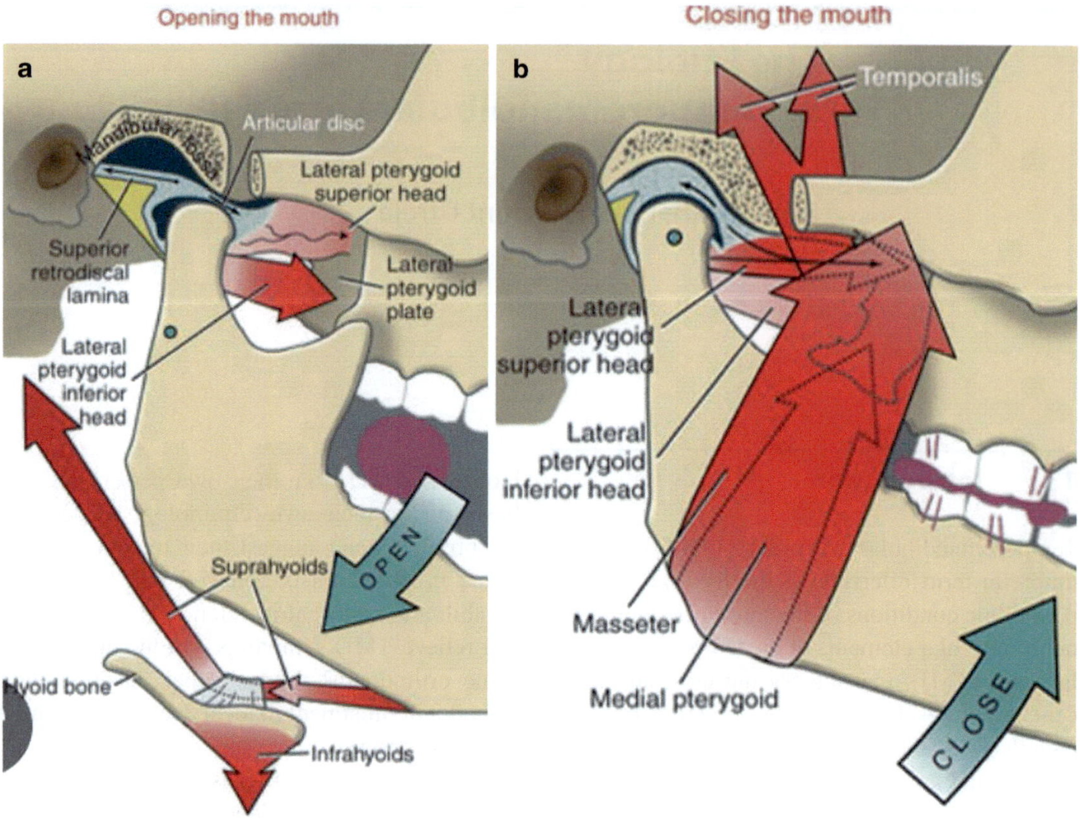

Fig. 1 The biomechanical operation of the TMJ and associated structures

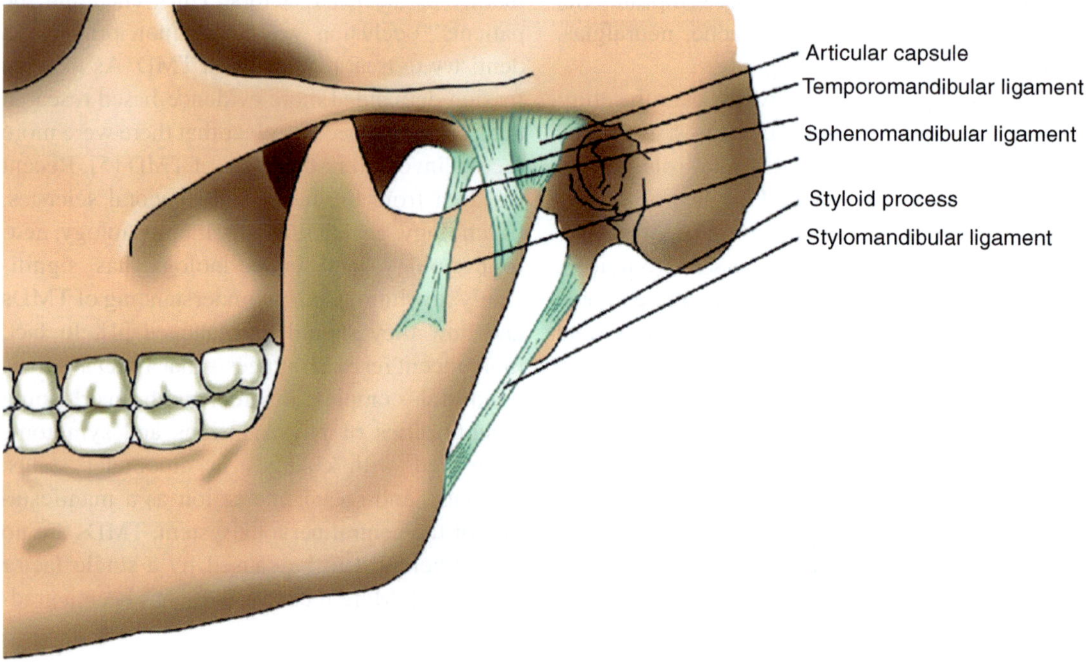

Fig. 2 The ligamentous anatomy supporting the TMJ

ual shift from the dental-based and mechanical model to a biopsychosocial medical model for the diagnosis and treatment of TMDs.

Factors such as increased joint friction, functional shift, occlusal overloading, trauma, hypermobility of the joints, bruxism, sleep apnea, stress, anxiety, and depression could all play a role in the onset of, or coexist with, TMD. These factors can contribute independently or collectively. In this chapter, we will discuss the role of the different factors that are believed to be involved in the etiology of TMD.

2 The Role of Occlusion

The relationship between occlusion and temporomandibular disorders (TMDs) is probably one of the most controversial topics in the scientific literature. For many decades, occlusion was believed to be the main reason for patients to develop TMD. This was mainly based on the clinical observation and higher prevalence of TMD in individuals with dental malocclusion compared with the general population [7]. In 1934, the otolaryngologist Costin observed 11 patients whom their TMD symptoms were improved after undergoing occlusal corrections involving their overbites and vertical dimension. He hypothesized that their malocclusion influenced their TMJ and by consequence caused their TMD. Since then, malocclusion and TMD were connected.

Later studies suggested that occlusal equilibration to normalize the interocclusal dental contacts could help in relieving the TMD symptoms [8]. Thompson assumed that malocclusion might cause the posterior and superior displacement of the condyle within its fossa and suggested that correcting dental malocclusion would alleviate TMD symptoms [9]. Since then, the association between malocclusion and TMD has been extensively assessed in the literature, frequently with inconsistent results [10]. Many recent published papers could not establish a direct cause-effect relationship between the occlusion and TMD [8, 11–16].

2.1 Dental and Skeletal Malocclusion

2.1.1 Malocclusion in the Transverse Plane

It was widely believed that patients with unilateral posterior crossbite (UPCB) present an asymmetric activation of the masticatory muscles due to the altered dental contacts between the right and the left sides, overloading one side over the other. In addition, the abnormal occlusal contacts might alter the relationship between the condyle and fossa [17]. Because of these anatomic and functional modifications, it has been hypothesized that patients with UPCB might present increased risk to develop myofascial pain and TMJ clicking. However, the literature showed conflicting findings. In their systemic review, Iodice et al. [18] could not establish an association between posterior crossbite, muscle pain, and disc displacement because the distribution of the studies supporting or not supporting the association was similar. In a 10-year follow-up for the same group of patients, the authors did not find an association between UPCB and TMJ clicking in the first assessment during adolescence [18]. An association was later reported after 10 years along with self-reports of TMJ clicking [19].

Orthodontic treatment for these individuals did not reduce the risk of reporting TMJ noises, questioning the role of occlusal factors. This led to a potential contribution of anatomic factors, such as asymmetries in the glenoid fossa and condylar head, that might influence joint function in patients with UPCB. These findings were confirmed by a prospective study with a 30-year follow-up on 903 individuals investigating the association between posterior crossbite, overjet, overbite, and clicking of TMJ. No greater risk of TMD clicking was reported in the presence of posterior crossbite and abnormal overjet or overbite [20]. On the other hand, in a recent study on 1019 adolescents, a significant association was found between posterior crossbite and TMD diagnosis, but no association was found between deep bite and TMD [21] (Fig. 3).

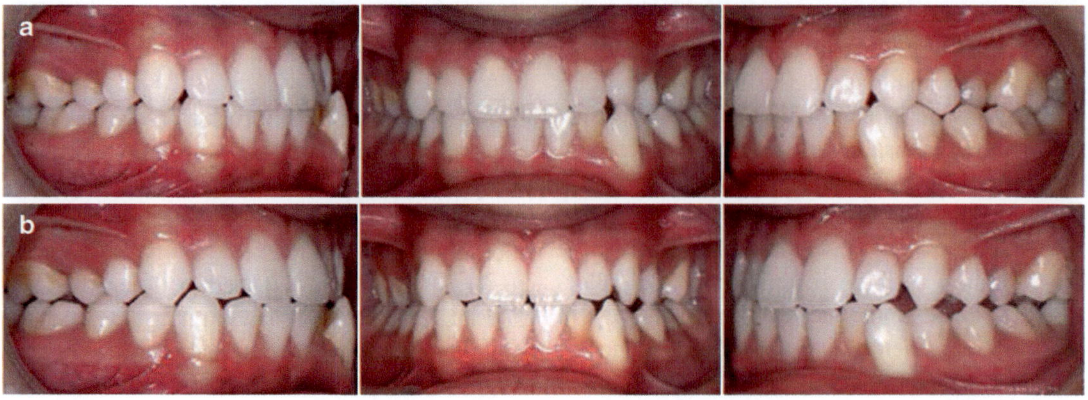

Fig. 3 Some studies linked the unilateral posterior crossbite (UPCB) to TMD, especially if they were associated with a functional shift. (**a**) Photos are taken in maximum intercuspation position. Note the unilateral crossbite on the left side and the midline deviation. (**b**) Photos of the same patient taken in centric relation. Note the premature interference between the upper and lower premolars on the left side causing the mandible to shift to the left upon full closure

The association between masticatory muscle pain and UPCB has also been investigated. To evaluate if the occlusal alteration results in an asymmetrical muscle function and overloading of the muscles, muscular activity was assessed in children with and without UPCB using a standardized electromyographic protocol. The results showed that UPCB did not contribute to an asymmetric activation of the temporalis and masseter muscles during their function. These findings were different in the adults where individuals with severe malocclusions presented asymmetrical muscular activity [22], unlike the group with normal occlusion who presented more symmetrical and balanced muscular activation [23]. These findings suggest that in growing subjects, an asymmetrical muscular activity is commonly experienced without signs and symptoms of TMD. Adults with asymmetric masticatory muscle activity might be related to the presence of muscular pain and chronic myalgia [10, 24].

2.1.2 Sagittal and Vertical Malocclusions

In a recent systemic review, Manfredini et al. [25] tried to assess the association between TMD and the features of dental occlusion including the vertical and sagittal malocclusions. They found no cause-effect relation between the TMD and dental malocclusion. Thus, they encouraged all clinicians to abandon the gnathological paradigm in their TMD practice. However, in their other systemic review, they tried to link the facial morphology to the TMDs. They found an association between the skeletal class II profile and hyperdivergent growth pattern with the development of disc displacements and degenerative TMD [26]. This might be due to the joint's instability in these individuals and the potential risk of developing disc position abnormalities. This instability can be caused by the poor reciprocal fitting of the articular surfaces (small condyle and wide glenoid fossa) [27].

On the other hand, the development of an anterior open bite or a unilateral posterior open bite can be a sign of an idiopathic resorption of the condyle or a bilateral or unilateral condylar degenerative osteoarthritis [28, 29]. In such case, malocclusion is the sign of the development of the TMD rather than being the cause (Fig. 4).

2.2 A Sudden Change in the Occlusion

Adaptation within the masticatory system is possible within certain biological limits whenever the occlusion is altered for most individuals. However,

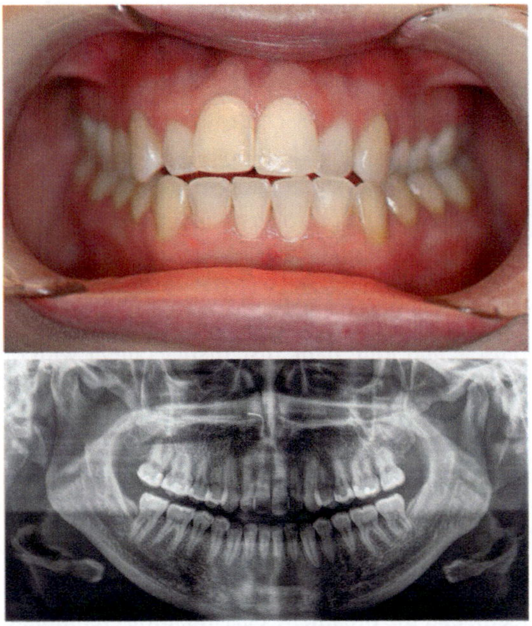

Fig. 4 Unilateral idiopathic condylar resorption of the left condyle, resulting in changes in the patient's occlusion. Anterior open bite and lower midline shift toward the affected condyle (Left) are the most common occlusal changes

changing the occlusion can affect the muscular activity, which can cause TMD symptoms [5, 30, 31]. Although it was widely believed that introducing occlusal contacts can increase bruxism, recent studies do not support this belief [32–34].

In a very-well-designed study, Le Bell et al. [35] placed artificial occlusal interferences in healthy individuals and another group with a past history of TMD symptoms reporting no symptoms at the time the interferences were placed. The interferences were removed after 2 weeks for both groups. The normal subjects reported some initial symptoms, which resolved in a few days, whereas the group with a history of TMD reported significantly higher symptoms. Their findings suggest that the normal group has higher adaptability and therefore less vulnerability to develop TMD symptoms. The difference in adaptability could explain the great variation in the results of studies that investigate the relationship between occlusion and TMD [5] and suggest that other factors such as genetics and stress contribute together with the occlusal factors to the onset of TMD symptoms.

In two different studies, Bucci et al. evaluated the occlusal tactile acuity (OTA) which is the ability to detect and recognize fine objects between antagonist teeth during maximal intercuspation. In the first study, they compared adults reporting a high or low frequency of awake oral parafunctional behaviors [36]. In the second, they compared the sensitivity of the TMD patients to a control group [37]. They found that TMD patients and the group reporting high frequency of awake oral parafunction reported significantly higher OTA. These findings suggest that individuals with parafunctional habits and those presenting with TMD pain might be more vulnerable to occlusal changes following dental therapies, and so more at risk to develop maladaptive behaviors [10].

The way the brain interprets the OTA stimulus can probably explain the different adaptability of individuals [10]. The neurological signaling originating in the masticatory system originates from a complex specialized system of receptors in the periodontium, the tooth, and the soft tissues. This influx of information is continuously analyzed by the central nervous system (CNS), which would adjust the movements and position of the jaw accordingly [38]. Therefore, the sensorimotor neuroplasticity (CNS changes) is an important factor which determines how well an individual adapts to the occlusal alteration that can result from any dental treatment. This might be explained by the fact that the somatosensory function is strongly influenced by the psychosocial domains, which are often impaired in some TMD subjects [10].

2.3 Orthopedic Instability

The theory of orthopedic stability is based on the belief that a harmony should exist between the position of the condyles in their articular eminences with the discs correctly positioned between the articulating surfaces and the intercuspal position of the teeth [5, 15]. The orthopedic instability occurs when such harmony does not exist leading one or both condyles to unstable position with the disc and articular fossa. The condyle on the affected side seeks a more stable relation with the disc by moving superiorly.

Juniper suggests that an occlusal interference can result from a change in the relationship between the upper and lower teeth following a displacement of the condyle and the disc. He also suggested that the condyle might be displaced because of a spasm in the masticatory muscles causing an occlusal interference. In this case, the interferences become the consequence rather than being the cause [39].

Although there are not many studies in the literature to support the theory of orthopedic stability, Okesson [5] believes that the missing element in these studies is the dynamics of loading. For him, the lack of orthopedic stability between the stable occlusion and stable joint position is just a risk factor and does not by itself cause TMD unless coupled with excessive loading of the TMJ. Continued loading in activities such as heavy chewing, biting, and bruxism can lead to changes in the TMJ structure including clicking, locking, pain, and bony degeneration, if the joints are not in a stable position during these activities [5]. The amount of loading and degree of orthopedic instability are two important factors that determine whether an intracapsular disorder will develop. A discrepancy of less than 2 mm is not likely to create any problems [40, 41].

In a recent cohort study, Nicot et al. [42]. found an association between the craniofacial asymmetry, abnormal pattern of condylar modeling, and TMD. The signs and symptoms of TMD are more likely to occur when condylar asymmetry and ramus asymmetry do not match. The TMD sign reported the most was the masticatory muscle myalgia, which they suggested is the result of the unequal force distribution and condylar unitability. Similar results were found by Klobas et al. [43] who followed 29 TMD patients 5 years after they had surgery to correct a retruded position of the mandible focusing on the condylar asymmetry. They reported a significant decrease in static and dynamic facial pain and significant increase in the active mouth opening capacity for these patients. Individuals with condylar asymmetry showed the greatest improvement after oral stability was achieved [42].

2.4 Why the Controversy?

In their systemic review, De Kanter et al. [44] aimed to clarify this controversy by reviewing 2419 published papers about TMD and occlusion. They suggested that a possible explanation for the ongoing controversy about occlusion and TMD is definition based.

Malocclusions and TMDs are two broad terms. Currently, the term TMD might include muscle and joint pain, disc displacement with or without joint noises, and pathologies that bring to an osseous remodeling of the TMJ [45]. Occlusion is used to describe four different entities in the dental field: the Angle classification: to classify the dental and skeletal relationship; the static contact between the upper and lower teeth; the dynamic contact between the upper and lower teeth; and the prosthetic classifications (complete dentition versus incomplete and the presence of fixed/removable prosthetics). In addition, the dental relationship and the disharmonies can be evaluated in three different planes, the sagittal, transverse, and vertical planes. Thus, considering the etiology, the cause and effect relation, and vice versa, there are almost unlimited possibilities to research [44].

Another systemic review aimed to explore why the link between occlusal factors, TMD, and dysfunction has not been clearly evident in the dental literature was done by Cordray [46]. He concluded that inaccuracies in the methodology, small sample size, lack of proper instrumentation, inaccurate diagnosis, and improper technique to accurately register the condyle position are all possible factors that can invalidate the findings . He emphasized the role of eliminating the influence of the neuromusculature on condylar position in the three dimensions and the resulting inter-arch relationship. When there is a change in the condylar position between centric relation (CR) and maximum intercuspation of teeth (MI), the muscles, due to the repetitive closure, might develop a memory to guide the mandible during closure. This neuromusculature guidance deviates the mandible to close in maximum intercuspation (MI) to avoid any interferences regardless of the condylar seated position

[47–49]. He found that researchers have not routinely used neuromuscular deprogramming to achieve neuromuscular release before conducting occlusal and condylar position evaluation [46].

For future research, he suggests using a lager sample size to prove statistical significance. He proposes to use a simple and universally accepted system to diagnose and assess TMD symptoms and differential diagnosis of the pain. Accurate registration of condylar position requires experienced clinicians or researchers to avoid invalid or flawed conclusion. He recommends the use of an accurate and reproducible method to guide the condyles to their seated position and the use of proper instrumentation for the registration. He also emphasizes that neuromusculature deprogramming should be performed routinely on the sample individuals to eliminate the influence of the neuromusculature guidance of the mandible to accurately register the condylar position [46].

2.5 Conclusion

The role of occlusion in the etiology of TMD is still unclear. The fact that many studies did not find a strong relation between condylar position, occlusal factors, and TMD does not mean that such a relation does not exist. The way the occlusion contributes to the onset of TMD should be revisited. The recent studies did not find a relation between the static occlusion (Angle classification) and TMD. However, the dynamic occlusion seems to play a role in the onset of TMD. Thus, more methodologically well-designed research, including larger samples, will be needed to clarify the role of occlusion, keeping in mind that the occlusal changes and interferences can be the consequence of a TMD rather than being its cause.

3 Emotional Stress and Psychosocial Factors

Stress is described by Hans Selye [50] as "the non-specific response of the body to any demand made upon it." Stress is an emotion that all human beings experience; it can be a motivational force driving individuals to accomplish and succeed. Thus, stress is not always bad. Stress is generated by stressors which are defined as the factors or experiences triggering the stress. The body reacts to pleasant stressors (preparing for a wedding) and unpleasant stressors (divorce) by creating certain demands for adaptation or readjustment (the fight/flight response), which are related in degree to the intensity of the stressor [50]. Measuring the intensity of a stressor on a certain individual is almost impossible because the perception of the intensity and the type of the stressor vary greatly between individuals. Stress can be released by the individuals either externally (hitting, shouting, breaking objects, or physical exercise) or internally developing a psychophysiological disorder (increased blood pressure, irritable bowel syndrome, asthma, or increased tonicity of the head and neck musculature) [5].

The acute response to a sudden stressor is necessary for survival. The problems arise from the ones causing prolonged emotional stressors without the ability to change them (bullying, unhappy marriage) [5]. These prolonged exposures upregulate the autonomic nervous system on a chronic basis, which can compromise the individual's ability to adapt and even fight diseases [51–55]; if the stress is prolonged, the muscle may show signs of fatigue, tightness, and pain. The central nervous system can play an active role in maintaining the pain condition, making management more difficult [5].

An abundance of evidence exists explaining the role that emotional stress plays in TMD onset and chronicity. Mood disorders and personality disorders are significantly linked to muscle disorders, as opposed to disc or joint disorders [56]. Studies also show that emotional stress is associated with greater severity and persistence of TMD-related clinical symptoms. Moreover, emotional stress and depression levels were found to be higher in individuals with chronic TMDs [57–61]. Recent studies found an association between stressful life experiences such as SARS-CoV-2 pandemic [62–64], renal failure patients and patients undergoing hemodialysis [65], and increased TMD and bruxism symptoms.

Another study found a substantial adverse effect of the smartphone on TMD symptoms [66].

There is increasing evidence that the emotional stress the individual undergoes can influence the masticatory function. The emotional state of the individual is controlled by the hypothalamus, the reticular system, and particularly the limbic system. The hypothalamus-pituitary-adrenal axis (HPA axis) is activated when the body is under stress and prepares the autonomic nervous system to respond [5]. The HPA axis increases the activity of the gamma efferents, which leads to the contraction of intrafusal fibers of the muscle spindles. This sensitizes the spindle in a way that any slight stretching of the muscle will cause a reflex contraction. The overall effect is an increase in tonicity of the muscle [51]. This can also increase the levels of nonfunctional muscle activity such as bruxism or tooth clenching [67]. Emotional stress can also influence the individual's sympathetic activity, which can increase muscle tone [68, 69], thereby producing a painful muscle condition. Increased sympathetic activity or tone therefore represents an etiologic factor that can influence TMD symptoms [70].

Studies showed that individuals with chronic TMD pain exhibit greater psychological maladjustment compared to healthy controls [71, 72]. They also reported higher mean levels of somatic awareness, pain catastrophizing, psychosocial stress, and affective distress when compared to pain-free individuals [51, 73–76]. Psychological dysfunction is associated with greater severity and persistence of TMD-related clinical symptoms. Studies showed that scores on measures of psychological distress were positively correlated with reported TMD pain and pain-related disability [75, 77, 78]. Pain was also related to depression in painful TMD patients [79].

Between 2006 and 2008, the Orofacial Pain Prospective Evaluation and Risk Assessment (OPPERA) study aimed to discover the etiologic influences on TMD pain. The prospective cohort study included 2737 individuals who did not have TMD when they enrolled and were followed for up to 5.2 years to identify those who developed TMD. The primary aim of the study was to identify psychological characteristics at enrollment that were associated with the development of first-onset TMD. The study found that TMD cases reported higher levels of psychological symptoms, affective distress, somatic symptoms, and pain catastrophizing compared to TMD-free controls [80]. Other studies involving patients with existing TMD found that psychological factors, such as somatic symptoms and depression, predict long-term persistence of TMD pain [81, 82].

4 Trauma

Trauma to the orofacial structures can contribute to functional disturbances to the masticatory system. The association between trauma and TMD was well elaborated in the literature specially after a direct blow to the face in a car or a motorcycle accident [1, 83–101]. It is expected that trauma to facial structures would result in more intracapsular disorders than muscular disorders. Kim et al. [83]. reported that TMD patients with trauma history displayed more severe subjective, objective, and psychological dysfunction than those without trauma history. Another study found that TMD patients with a history of whiplash trauma reported more TMD symptoms, such as limited jaw opening, more TMD pain, more headaches, and stress symptoms compared with non-TMD controls [101].

There are two different types of traumas that can affect the facial area: macrotrauma which can be defined as any sudden force that can cause any structural changes (car accident) and microtrauma which refers to repeatedly small forces applied to the facial structures over a long period of time (bruxism) [102]. Macrotrauma can be either direct or indirect in relation to the mandible and TMJ.

4.1 Indirect Trauma

This refers to injury that may occur to the TMJ secondary to a sudden force, but not one that occurs directly to the mandible. The whiplash injury (cervical flexion or extension) is the most common type of indirect trauma associated with TMD reported in the literature [101, 103–105]. The precise relation of this association is still unknown [100, 106, 107]. Okeson believes that the constant deep pain input originating in the cervical spine commonly creates heterotopic symptoms in the face, which might be sensory referred pain and/or co-contraction of masticatory muscles [5].

4.2 Direct Trauma

This refers to any direct injuries to the TMJ or mandible. If these injuries lead to elongation of the discal ligaments or thinning of the disc, they can cause derangements of the condyle-disc complex disorders. A direct blow to the chin can instantly create an intracapsular disorder. Open-mouth trauma (teeth are separated when trauma occurs) can lead to discal displacement and to the symptoms of clicking and catching. This can be explained by the sudden displacement of the condyle from its fossa following the trauma. This displacement is resisted by the ligament which can become elongated if the forces are great, resulting in an increased looseness of the ligament. This compromises the normal condyle-disc mechanics, which may lead to discal displacement with and without reduction [86, 103, 108–113]. Usually, the joint opposite to the site of the trauma receives the most injury. This can be explained because the condyle in the side of the trauma is supported by the medial wall of the fossa. This prevents the condyle from displacement and the ligaments on that side from elongating. However, on the opposite side, the condyle is only supported laterally by the ligament without any bony support. This can quickly force the condyle to be displaced laterally and suddenly elongate the ligament resulting in disc displacement on that side [5].

The incidence of the injury to the condyle-disc complex seems to be less in a closed-mouth trauma. The intercuspation of the teeth maintains the jaw position, resisting joint displacement. This observation is supported when examining the incidence of injury associated with athletic activity. Athletes who wear soft protective mouth appliances significantly have fewer jaw-related injuries than those that do not [114–116]. Therefore, it is recommended to wear a soft appliance holding the teeth tightly in intercuspal position in activities where traumas to the face are expected.

Direct trauma may also be iatrogenic. It is important to mention that dental and medical professionals can cause a disc derangement problem that might last the patient's lifetime. Any procedure that overextends the jaw (long dental appointments, third molar extractions [117], intubation procedures [118, 119]) can lead to ligament elongations. The risk is higher if the patient is sedated because the jaw would be no longer stabilized by the muscles [120, 121].

5 Parafunctional Activities

Parafunctional activities, also known as nonfunctional activities, include clenching or grinding of the teeth (bruxism) and other oral habits (gum chewing, nail biting, biting foreign objects, ice crushing) that result in muscle hyperactivity, which can be defined as any increase in the muscular activity over and above that necessary for function. Muscle hyperactivity also includes any general increase in the level of muscle tonus even if it does not involve jaw movement or tooth contact. Muscle hyperactivity might be linked to the onset of TMD [87, 122].

Both diurnal (parafunction that occurs through the day) and nocturnal (which occurs at night) are often performed at a subconscious level without the individual even being aware of them [123, 124]. Thus, questioning the patients is not a reliable method to confirm the existence of the parafunction [125]. The masseter muscle contracts periodically when individuals place their teeth together and apply force when concentrating in their daily activities [126, 127]. These contractions might be relevant to the task they are performing (playing certain musical instruments [128], biting on the mouthpiece while diving [129]) or irrelevant to the task (working out, reading, practicing dentistry). Nocturnal activities are more common between individuals compared with diurnal activities [130–132]. Most of the normal individuals present a certain amount of nocturnal activities [133–135]. Nocturnal activities can be in the form of single episodes (clenching) or rhythmic contractions (bruxing). Both can occur on the same individual, and it is not known if they are different presentation to the same phenomenon or if they have completely different etiologies [5]. Bruxism is "a repetitive jaw-muscle activity characterized by clenching or grinding of the teeth and/or by bracing or thrusting of the mandible. Bruxism has two distinct circadian manifestations: it can occur during sleep (indicated as sleep bruxism [SB]) or during wakefulness (indicated as awake bruxism [AB])" [136].

The role of bruxism in TMD is controversial. Studies showed an association between self-reported/questionnaire-diagnosed bruxism and TMD symptoms [137–139]. These findings were consistent with studies of clinically diagnosed bruxism [16, 61, 140–142]. A study by Sierrwald et al. [143]. found that both awake bruxism and sleep bruxism are significant risk factors for TMD pain. This risk is even higher in cases of simultaneous presence. These findings were confirmed by other studies [144, 145]. On the other hand, no association with TMD was found in the studies that looked at tooth wear as the potential result of bruxism (Fig. 5) [146]. Also, experimental studies of forced, voluntary bruxism-like muscle activities elicited only transient muscle pain [147, 148]. Polysomnography (PSG) or electromyography (EMG) sleep studies to measure muscle activities provided inconsistent findings [149–151].

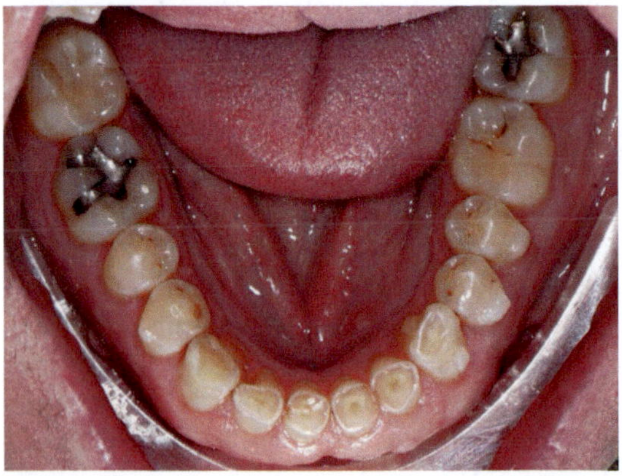

Fig. 5 Tooth wear is a common finding in sleep bruxism (SB)

5.1 Etiology of Bruxism

The etiology of bruxism and of TMD seems to share many things in common. They both have a lot of controversy about their real cause. Interestingly, in the early years, occlusal interferences were suspected to play an important role in the onset of bruxism. Therefore, clinicians attempted to correct the occlusion to treat the bruxism [47, 152]. However, recent studies did not find any role for occlusion in the etiology of bruxism [32, 145, 153, 154]. Similar to the etiology of TMD, emotional stress seems to influence bruxing activity [155]. Studies that monitored levels of nocturnal bruxing activity recorded a temporal pattern linked to stressful events [130–132]. A recent study, conducted in two culturally different countries, aimed to evaluate the effect of the SARS-CoV-2 pandemic on the possible prevalence and worsening of TMD and bruxism symptoms. The study found that the coronavirus pandemic has caused significant adverse effects on the psychoemotional status of both countries' populations, resulting in the intensification of their bruxism and TMD symptoms [62]. These findings were similar to those of another study that surveyed 506 individuals; half the subjects in the study reported an increase in bruxism behaviors, while up to one-third reported an increase in their symptoms involving the TMJ and jaw muscles [63]. Another study concluded that, because of the increased levels of anxiety and depression, renal failure patients and patients undergoing hemodialysis patients are more sensitive to TMD and sleep bruxism than healthy people [65]. A recent study showed that although awake bruxers have larger levels of anxiety, somatization, and neuroticism, they displayed more adapted coping strategies. They concluded that awake bruxism may play a positive role in stress coping, which would be compatible with the hypothesis of mastication as a means of relieving psychological tension [156].

Many studies linked bruxism events to certain medications [157–160] although no strong link was evident [161]. However, some studies and case reports found an increase in bruxism activities with the use of certain antidepressants (selective serotonin reuptake inhibitors, SSRIs) [162, 163]. It was recommended to avoid this class of antidepressants in TMD patients as it might aggravate their symptoms, suggesting alternative classes of medications [164]. Other studies fund that caffeine, alcohol, tobacco, and drug abuse can increase bruxism [165]. There is an increased evidence that there is a genetic predisposition to bruxism [166–168].

5.2 Stages of Sleep and Bruxism

Studies that investigated the stages of sleep during which bruxism occurred were not conclusive. While some studies found that bruxing events occurred during the rapid eye movement (REM) stage [169], other studies did not report any activities during this stage (Fig. 5) [170]. Other studies found that bruxing events occur during both REM and non-REM sleep stages [133, 171] with higher sustained contraction during REM compared to non-REM phases of sleep [172]. However, some studies showed that bruxing is linked to the arousal phases of sleep [173, 174]. Tooth grinding was induced following sonic and tactical stimulation or after directing a flashing light toward a sleeping person's face [170]. Lower sleep efficiency was reported in patients with sleep bruxism caused by a higher number of bruxism episodes. Morning headaches were associated with the severity of sleep bruxism during REM phase [175].

5.3 Bruxism and Muscular Pain and Activity

Studies that used polysomnography (PSG) for the diagnosis of sleep bruxism found contradictory results regarding its association with TMD pain. Some studies reported positive association [176], while others reported either no association [136] or even a negative one [149, 177].

In their experiment, Muzalev et al. [178] reported reduced sleep bruxism activity after the experimental TMD pain was provoked in nine individuals with clinical signs of sleep bruxism. They concluded that these findings are in accordance with the Pain Adaptation Model [179]. The muscle pain leads to a reduction in muscle activity of the painful muscles, aiming to protect it from further injury and, therefore, promote healing [178].

5.4 Bruxing Events and Masticatory Symptoms

Patients with pain scored a higher number of bruxing events during REM sleep than patients who did not report any pain. Both groups had more bruxing events compared to the control group [172]. Interestingly, in another study, the group without pain actually had more bruxing events per night than the ones with pain [149]. This can be explained by the muscular adaptation. Patients who brux regularly might develop stronger and larger mastication muscles with more tooth wear to their dentition. Patients who awake with muscle pain probably do not frequently brux, and therefore their muscles are not conditioned to this activity [5].

Parafunctional activities do not always lead to problems, but there are some factors that can determine whether parafunction activities can result in TMD symptoms.

- **The intensity of bruxing events**: A study by Clarke et al. [169] found that an average bruxing event involved 60% of the maximum clenching power before the person went to sleep, which is a significant amount of force when compared to the forces generated during functional activities.
- **The duration of bruxing events**: The number and duration of bruxing events vary greatly between individuals. A study by Kydd and Daly [180] found that patients clenched their teeth for a total mean duration of 11.4 min per night in single episodes ranging from 20 to 40 s per episode. Okeson et al. [133–135] found that bruxing events averaged from 5 to 6 s. Clarke et al. [181] found that bruxers spent 38.7 min with their teeth together during an 8-h period compared to 5.4 min for the control group. In their study, the average of bruxing events was only five times during an entire sleep period. The number and duration of bruxing events that

can create muscle symptoms vary from patient to patient [182]. Patients can start feeling pain in their masticatory muscles after 20–60 s of voluntary clenching [183–185].

- **Direction of applied forces**: During functional movements of the mandible (chewing, swallowing), the mandible primarily moves in a vertical direction and forces are also applied to the teeth in a vertical direction. Supportive structures of the teeth are designed to tolerate vertical forces. However, during parafunctional activities, the mandible shifts from side to side, and forces are applied to the teeth horizontally. Tooth wear patterns suggest that most parafunctional activity occurs in eccentric positions [186]. These forces are not well accepted by the surrounding structures and increase the likelihood of damage to the teeth and supportive structures. Often, the condyles are translated far from a stable position. Thus, there is an increased likelihood of pathologic effects to the teeth and joints.
- **Type of muscle contraction**: Muscle contraction during parafunction activities is sustained over a long period of time, inhibiting normal blood flow within the muscle tissues. This increases the metabolic products within the muscle tissues, creating the symptoms of fatigue, pain, and spasms [184, 187].

Most individuals have some type of parafunctional activity that never results in any major consequence. In some individuals, parafunctional activities can be the major etiology of TMD. In other cases, it might contribute with other major etiologies in the onset of TMD symptoms. Controlling parafunctional activities does not always result in controlling TMD. It is crucial to be able to understand and differentiate when parafunctional activity is important to the patient's symptoms and when it is only an accompanying condition [5]. Performing irreversible occlusal changes including prostheses and occlusal adjustments to relief TMD or treat bruxism is not an acceptable strategy yet based on the best available evidence [34, 188].

6 Sleep Apnea and TMD

Obstructive sleep apnea (OSA) is characterized by upper airway obstruction causing respiratory hypopneas (reductions) or apneas (pauses), and airway patency is restored by central nervous system arousal (Fig. 6) [189]. Untreated OSA can result in serious consequences including diabetes, depression, cardiovascular diseases, oxyhemoglobin desaturation, hypertension, sleep fragmentation, snoring, arousals, and increased risk of mortality [190–196]. Musculoskeletal pain, increased pain sensitivity, and decreased pain thresholds were reported when total sleep was experimentally reduced and slow-wave and rapid eye movement stages of sleep were disturbed [197]. Nasal continuous positive airway pressure (CPAP) and oral appliances that hold the jaw in a forward position are effective in maintaining airway patency in OSA [189]. Reduced blood pressure [198] increasing pain tolerance [199] and decreased pain sensitivity [194] were noticed in treatment with both appliances.

There is emerging evidence in the literature that OSA is associated with chronic pain disorders including temporomandibular disorder (TMD). Cunali et al. [200] found that the prevalence of TMD in OSA patients referred to have oral appliances was 75%. Smith et al. [201] reported that 28% of their 53 myofascial TMD patients were diagnosed with sleep apnea. Benetti et al. [202] found that the prevalence of TMD signs and symptoms is significantly higher in untreated patients with OSA (51%) compared to healthy controls (32%). The Orofacial Pain Prospective Evaluation and Risk Assessment (OPPERA) study supported these findings reporting a significant association of OSA symptoms and TMD, with prospective cohort evidence finding that OSA symptoms preceded first-onset TMD. In the case-control study, chronic TMD was more than three times as frequent among adults with low relative to high likelihood of OSA [189].

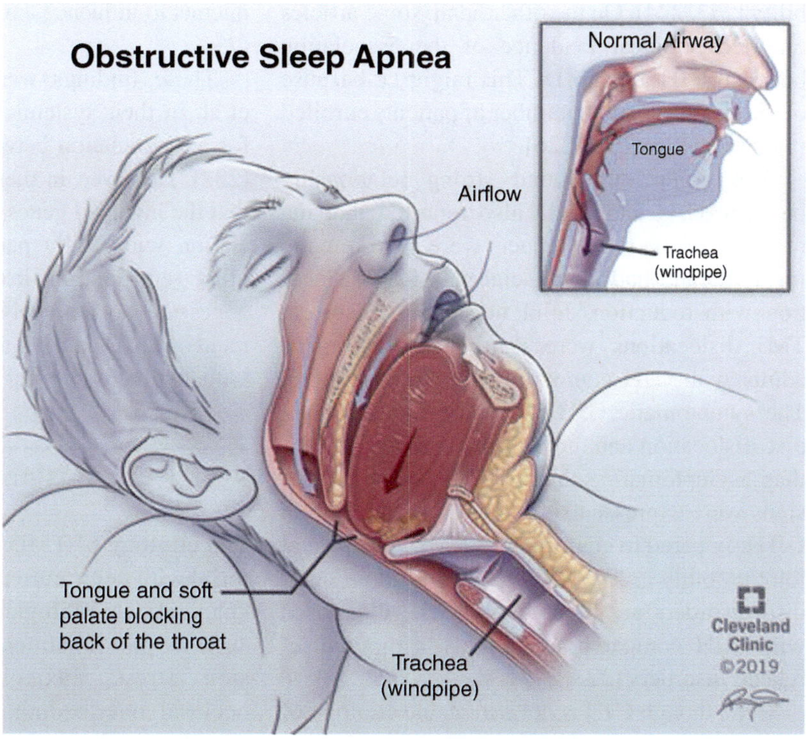

Fig. 6 Collapse of jaw and soft tissue of the airway during sleep apnea

In a nationwide cohort study on the Taiwanese nationals, Wu et al. [203] identified a total of 10,408 suspected sleep apnea (SA) patients, after excluding individuals who were diagnosed with TMD prior to SA. Their aim was to understand the association between SA and TMD. In their study, they confirmed an increased TMD incidence in the SA patients. They concluded that several mechanics might explain this association. OSA patients are more sensitive to pain because of the sleep disturbance [204]. They postulated that TMD might be caused by a systemic inflammation as OSA patients display intermittent hypoxemia, which increases the levels of inflammatory cytokines leading to a systemic inflammation [205, 206]. OSA patients may have craniofacial configurations and/or muscle dysfunction that predispose them to the development of TMD. Finally, mandibular advancement oral appliances as a treatment modality for OSA may also cause TMD. Several other studies reported the potential role of mandibular advancement appliances in the onset of TMD in OSA patients [207–215].

7 Generalized Joint Hypermobility

Generalized joint hypermobility (GJH) is a hereditary condition in which the joints have a range of motion that exceeds the normal [216]. GJH has been found to be associated with musculoskeletal injuries [217], fibromyalgia [218], anxiety [219], and musculoskeletal pain [220]. GJH can be asymptomatic or symptomatic [221]. It may also be non-syndromic or syndromic. The collagen metabolism is affected in Ehlers-Danlos syndrome (EDS), which would affect not only the skin, but also the joints, muscles, and cardiovascular and gastrointestinal systems. EDS might also have dental implications including poor wound healing, mucosal fragility, prolonged bleeding, temporomandibular joint dislocation, and, in some forms, periodontal disease [222].

Numerous studies have suggested that GJH is a risk factor positively associated with TMDs. They found that the prevalence of TMDs is higher in subjects with symptoms of articular hypermobility [223, 224]. On the other hand, some articles reported no clear evidence of the association between GJH and TMD. This might be because of the relatively small number of patients enrolled in these studies [225, 226].

The group that found strong relationship between GJH and TMD also reported that the majority of the GJH subjects were symptomatic for TMD and had myofascial pain disc dislocation with reduction. Joint noises and recurrent TMJ dislocations were a frequent finding in adults with GJH compared to control samples. The symptomatic GJH subjects presented more disc dislocation and more prolonged dislocations than asymptomatic subjects. TMJ hypermobility signs were expressed significantly more often in GJH compared to controls with TMD and normal joint mobility [227]. TMD patients with articular disc disorders are more likely to be diagnosed with GJH compared to patients without disc-related disorders [228].

Even though GJH is not a treatable etiology of the TMD, understanding its role is very important in the patient education and in avoiding unnecessary local treatment procedures of displaced discs in the TMD hypermobile individuals [223, 229]. It also indicates the importance of evaluating the TMD patients in an interdisciplinary approach as the underlying systematic condition might eventually affect the prognosis of both conditions [228].

8 Genetics

Increasing evidence suggests that genetic factors contribute significantly to individual differences in response to both experimental and clinical pain [230]. In the prospective cohort project, OPPERA [6] explored genetic risk factors for TMD pain. It assessed 358 candidate pain genes using a candidate gene panel. The study found an association between TMD and two genes: catechol-*O*-methyltransferase (COMT) and 5-hydroxytryptamine (serotonin) receptor 2A (HTR2A). It also proposed the biological pathways through which genetic variations could causally interact to influence the development of TMD pain [231].

These findings were supported by Visscher et al. in their systemic review showing evidence for an association between TMD pain and genes [232]. However, in their conclusion, they believe that the involved genes seem to have a small association with TMD pain only and interact with other genes and environmental influences. These genes are not uniquely involved in the development of TMD pain but are associated with the individual vulnerability for pain in general [2, 232].

9 Conclusion

The etiology of TMD is complex and multifactorial with neuromuscular, psychosocial, biomechanical, and biological origins. Several factors such as parafunctional habits, trauma, depression, stress, anxiety, psychosocial distress, occlusal overloading, increased joint friction, multifactorial somatic symptoms, functional shift, sleep apnea, and genetics can independently or collectively play a role in the onset of TMD symptoms. More recently, there has been a gradual shift from the dental-based and mechanical model to a biopsychosocial medical model for the diagnosis and treatment of TMDs. The ability to identify the etiology and to accurately diagnose the TMD symptoms is crucial to make the proper treatment plan for each patient. Irreversible occlusal changes in TMD patients to treat their TMD symptoms should be avoided as it is not backed up by any currently accepted evidence.

References

1. Okeson JP. Management of temporomandibular disorders and occlusion. 8th ed. St. Louis: Elsevier; 2020.
2. Gauer RL, Semidey MJ. Diagnosis and treatment of temporomandibular disorders. Am Fam Physician. 2015;91(6):378–86.
3. List T, Jensen RH. Temporomandibular disorders: old ideas and new concepts. Cephalalgia. 2017;37(7):692–704.

4. Karkazi F, Ozdemir F. Temporomandibular disorders: fundamental questions and answers. Turk J Orthod. 2020;33(4):246–52.
5. Kandasamy S, Greene CS. The evolution of temporomandibular disorders: a shift from experience to evidence. J Oral Pathol Med. 2020;49(6):461–9.
6. Slade GD, Ohrbach R, Greenspan JD, et al. Painful temporomandibular disorder. J Dent Res. 2016;95(10):1084–92.
7. Lai YC, Yap AU, Turp JC. Prevalence of temporomandibular disorders in patients seeking orthodontic treatment: a systematic review. J Oral Rehabil. 2020;47(2):270–80.
8. Shroff B. Malocclusion as a cause for temporomandibular disorders and orthodontics as a treatment. Oral Maxillofac Surg Clin North Am. 2018;30(3):299–302.
9. JR T. Temporomandibular disorders: diagnosis and treatment. In: Sarnat BG, editor. The temporomandibular joint. 1964. p. 146–82.
10. Michelotti A, Rongo R, D'Anto V, Bucci R. Occlusion, orthodontics, and temporomandibular disorders: cutting edge of the current evidence. J World Fed Orthod. 2020;9(3S):S15–8.
11. McNamara JA Jr, Seligman DA, Okeson JP. Occlusion, orthodontic treatment, and temporomandibular disorders: a review. J Orofac Pain. 1995;9(1):73–90.
12. Luther F. TMD and occlusion part I. Damned if we do? Occlusion: the interface of dentistry and orthodontics. Br Dent J. 2007;202(1):E2; discussion 38–9.
13. Luther F. TMD and occlusion part II. Damned if we don't? Functional occlusal problems: TMD epidemiology in a wider context. Br Dent J. 2007;202(1):E3; discussion 38–9.
14. Stone JC, Hannah A, Nagar N. Dental occlusion and temporomandibular disorders. Evid Based Dent. 2017;18(3):86–7.
15. Al-Ani Z. Occlusion and temporomandibular disorders: a long-standing controversy in dentistry. Prim Dent J. 2020;9(1):43–8.
16. Ebadian B, Abbasi M, Nazarifar AM. Frequency distribution of temporomandibular disorders according to occlusal factors: a cross-sectional study. Dent Res J (Isfahan). 2020;17(3):186–92.
17. Sonnesen L, Bakke M, Solow B. Bite force in pre-orthodontic children with unilateral crossbite. Eur J Orthod. 2001;23(6):741–9.
18. Iodice G, Danzi G, Cimino R, Paduano S, Michelotti A. Association between posterior crossbite, masticatory muscle pain, and disc displacement: a systematic review. Eur J Orthod. 2013;35(6):737–44.
19. Michelotti A, Iodice G, Piergentili M, Farella M, Martina R. Incidence of temporomandibular joint clicking in adolescents with and without unilateral posterior cross-bite: a 10-year follow-up study. J Oral Rehabil. 2016;43(1):16–22.
20. Olliver SJ, Broadbent JM, Thomson WM, Farella M. Occlusal features and TMJ clicking: a 30-year evaluation from a cohort study. J Dent Res. 2020;99(11):1245–51.
21. Khayat NAR, Shpack N, Perelman AE, et al. Association between posterior crossbite and/or deep bite and temporomandibular disorders among Palestinian adolescents: a sex comparison. Cranio. 2021;39(1):29–34.
22. Farronato G, Giannini L, Galbiati G, Sesso G, Maspero C. Orthodontic-surgical treatment: neuromuscular evaluation in skeletal class II and class III patients. Prog Orthod. 2012;13(3):226–36.
23. De Felicio CM, Sidequersky FV, Tartaglia GM, Sforza C. Electromyographic standardized indices in healthy Brazilian young adults and data reproducibility. J Oral Rehabil. 2009;36(8):577–83.
24. Valentino R, Cioffi I, Vollaro S, et al. Jaw muscle activity patterns in women with chronic TMD myalgia during standardized clenching and chewing tasks. Cranio. 2021;39(2):157–63.
25. Manfredini D, Lombardo L, Siciliani G. Temporomandibular disorders and dental occlusion. A systematic review of association studies: end of an era? J Oral Rehabil. 2017;44(11):908–23.
26. Paduano S, Rongo R, Bucci R, et al. Is there an association between various aspects of oral health in southern Italy children? An epidemiological study assessing dental decays, periodontal status, malocclusions and temporomandibular joint function. Eur J Paediatr Dent. 2018;19(3):176–80.
27. Peretta RM. Future perspectives in TMD pathophysiology. Current concepts on temporomandibular disorders. Berlin: Quintessence Publishing; 2010. p. 153–70.
28. Chen YJ, Shih TT, Wang JS, Wang HY, Shiau YY. Magnetic resonance images of the temporomandibular joints of patients with acquired open bite. Oral Surg Oral Med Oral Pathol Oral Radiol Endod. 2005;99(6):734–42.
29. Caldas W, Conti ACDCF, Janson G, Conti PCR. Occlusal changes secondary to temporomandibular joint conditions: a critical review and implications for clinical practice. J Appl Oral Sci. 2016;24(4):411–9.
30. Ingervall B, Carlsson GE. Masticatory muscle activity before and after elimination of balancing side occlusal interference. J Oral Rehabil. 1982;9(3):183–92.
31. Kirveskari P, Alanen P, Jamsa T. Association between craniomandibular disorders and occlusal interferences. J Prosthet Dent. 1989;62(1):66–9.
32. Rugh JD, Barghi N, Drago CJ. Experimental occlusal discrepancies and nocturnal bruxism. J Prosthet Dent. 1984;51(4):548–53.
33. Lobbezoo F, Ahlberg J, Manfredini D, Winocur E. Are bruxism and the bite causally related? J Oral Rehabil. 2012;39(7):489–501.
34. Manfredini D, Poggio CE. Prosthodontic planning in patients with temporomandibular disorders and/or bruxism: a systematic review. J Prosthet Dent. 2017;117(5):606–13.

35. Le Bell Y, Jamsa T, Korri S, Niemi PM, Alanen P. Effect of artificial occlusal interferences depends on previous experience of temporomandibular disorders. Acta Odontol Scand. 2002;60(4):219–22.
36. Bucci R, Koutris M, Lobbezoo F, Michelotti A. Occlusal sensitivity in individuals with different frequencies of oral parafunction. J Prosthet Dent. 2019;122(2):119–22.
37. Bucci R, Koutris M, Palla S, et al. Occlusal tactile acuity in temporomandibular disorder pain patients: a case-control study. J Oral Rehabil. 2020;47(8):923–9.
38. Svensson P, Graven-Nielsen T. Craniofacial muscle pain: review of mechanisms and clinical manifestations. J Orofac Pain. 2001;15(2):117–45.
39. Juniper RP. Temporomandibular joint dysfunction: a theory based upon electromyographic studies of the lateral pterygoid muscle. Br J Oral Maxillofac Surg. 1984;22(1):1–8.
40. Padala S, Padmanabhan S, Chithranjan AB. Comparative evaluation of condylar position in symptomatic (TMJ dysfunction) and asymptomatic individuals. Indian J Dent Res. 2012;23(1):122.
41. Pullinger AG, Seligman DA. Quantification and validation of predictive values of occlusal variables in temporomandibular disorders using a multifactorial analysis. J Prosthet Dent. 2000;83(1):66–75.
42. Nicot R, Chung K, Vieira AR, et al. Condyle modeling stability, craniofacial asymmetry and ACTN3 genotypes: contribution to TMD prevalence in a cohort of dentofacial deformities. PLoS One. 2020;15(7):e0236425.
43. Klobas L, Gambardella U, Hansson TL. A 5-year follow-up of temporomandibular disorder treatment emphasizing condylar asymmetry. Cranio. 2006;24(4):265–73.
44. De Kanter RJAM, Battistuzzi PGFCM, Truin G-J. Temporomandibular disorders: "occlusion" matters! Pain Res Manag. 2018;2018:8746858.
45. Schiffman E, Ohrbach R, Truelove E, et al. Diagnostic criteria for temporomandibular disorders (DC/TMD) for clinical and research applications: recommendations of the International RDC/TMD Consortium Network* and Orofacial Pain Special Interest Groupdagger. J Oral Facial Pain Headache. 2014;28(1):6–27.
46. Cordray FE. The relationship between occlusion and TMD. Open J Stomatol. 2017;7(1):35–80.
47. Ramfjord SP. Bruxism, a clinical and electromyographic study. J Am Dent Assoc. 1961;62:21–44.
48. Girardot A. The nature of condylar displacement in patients with temporomandibular pain-dysfunction. Orthod Rev. 1987;1(1):16–23.
49. Beard CC, Clayton JA. Effects of occlusal splint therapy on TMJ dysfunction. J Prosthet Dent. 1980;44(3):324–35.
50. Selye H. Stress without distress. 1st ed. Philadelphia: J. B. Lippincott; 1974.
51. Carlson CR, Okeson JP, Falace DA, et al. Comparison of psychologic and physiologic functioning between patients with masticatory muscle pain and matched controls. J Orofac Pain. 1993;7(1):15–22.
52. Afari N, Ahumada SM, Wright LJ, et al. Psychological trauma and functional somatic syndromes: a systematic review and meta-analysis. Psychosom Med. 2014;76(1):2–11.
53. Schmidt JE, Carlson CR. A controlled comparison of emotional reactivity and physiological response in masticatory muscle pain patients. J Orofac Pain. 2009;23(3):230–42.
54. Sherman JJ, Carlson CR, Wilson JF, Okeson JP, McCubbin JA. Post-traumatic stress disorder among patients with orofacial pain. J Orofac Pain. 2005;19(4):309–17.
55. Carlson CR, Reid KI, Curran SL, et al. Psychological and physiological parameters of masticatory muscle pain. Pain. 1998;76(3):297–307.
56. Kight M, Gatchel RJ, Wesley L. Temporomandibular disorders: evidence for significant overlap with psychopathology. Health Psychol. 1999;18(2):177–82.
57. Dworkin SF, Huggins KH, LeResche L, et al. Epidemiology of signs and symptoms in temporomandibular disorders: clinical signs in cases and controls. J Am Dent Assoc. 1990;120(3):273–81.
58. Gatchel RJ, Peng YB, Peters ML, Fuchs PN, Turk DC. The biopsychosocial approach to chronic pain: scientific advances and future directions. Psychol Bull. 2007;133(4):581–624.
59. Keefe FJ, Rumble ME, Scipio CD, Giordano LA, Perri LM. Psychological aspects of persistent pain: current state of the science. J Pain. 2004;5(4):195–211.
60. Yadav U, Ahmed J, Ongole R, et al. Influence of psychosocial factors and parafunctional habits in temporomandibular disorders: a cross-sectional study. Perm J. 2020;24.
61. Wu J, Huang Z, Chen Y, et al. Temporomandibular disorders among medical students in China: prevalence, biological and psychological risk factors. BMC Oral Health. 2021;21(1):549.
62. Emodi-Perlman A, Eli I, Smardz J, et al. Temporomandibular disorders and bruxism outbreak as a possible factor of orofacial pain worsening during the COVID-19 pandemic-concomitant research in two countries. J Clin Med. 2020;9(10):3250.
63. Colonna A, Guarda-Nardini L, Ferrari M, Manfredini D. COVID-19 pandemic and the psyche, bruxism, temporomandibular disorders triangle. Cranio. 2021:1–6.
64. Di Giacomo P, Serritella E, Imondi F, Di Paolo C. Psychological impact of COVID-19 pandemic on TMD subjects. Eur Rev Med Pharmacol Sci. 2021;25(13):4616–26.
65. Somay E, Tekkarismaz N. Evaluation of sleep bruxism and temporomandibular disorders in patients undergoing hemodialysis. Niger J Clin Pract. 2020;23(10):1375–80.
66. Emodi-Perlman A, Hochhauser T, Winocur P, Friedman-Rubin P, Eli I. The effect of smartphones on daytime sleepiness, temporomandibular disor-

ders, and bruxism among young adults. Quintessence Int. 2021;52(6):548–59.
67. Rugh JD, Montgomery GT. Physiological reactions of patients with TM disorders vs symptom-free controls on a physical stress task. J Craniomandib Disord. 1987;1(4):243–50.
68. Grassi C, Passatore M. Action of the sympathetic system on skeletal muscle. Ital J Neurol Sci. 1988;9(1):23–8.
69. Passatore M, Grassi C, Filippi GM. Sympathetically-induced development of tension in jaw muscles: the possible contraction of intrafusal muscle fibres. Pflugers Arch. 1985;405(4):297–304.
70. Bertoli E, de Leeuw R, Schmidt JE, Okeson JP, Carlson CR. Prevalence and impact of post-traumatic stress disorder symptoms in patients with masticatory muscle or temporomandibular joint pain: differences and similarities. J Orofac Pain. 2007;21(2):107–19.
71. Eli I. Psychosocial factors in the etiology, diagnosis and management of temporomandibular disorders. Alpha Omegan. 2003;96(2):20–3.
72. Rollman GB, Gillespie JM. The role of psychosocial factors in temporomandibular disorders. Curr Rev Pain. 2000;4(1):71–81.
73. Fillingim RB, Ohrbach R, Greenspan JD, et al. Potential psychosocial risk factors for chronic TMD: descriptive data and empirically identified domains from the OPPERA case-control study. J Pain. 2011;12(11 Suppl):T46–60.
74. Macfarlane TV, Gray RJM, Kincey J, Worthington HV. Factors associated with the temporomandibular disorder, pain dysfunction syndrome (PDS): Manchester case-control study. Oral Dis. 2001;7(6):321–30.
75. Manfredini D, Winocur E, Ahlberg J, Guarda-Nardini L, Lobbezoo F. Psychosocial impairment in temporomandibular disorders patients. RDC/TMD axis II findings from a multicentre study. J Dent. 2010;38(10):765–72.
76. Quartana PJ, Buenaver LF, Edwards RR, et al. Pain catastrophizing and salivary cortisol responses to laboratory pain testing in temporomandibular disorder and healthy participants. J Pain. 2010;11(2):186–94.
77. Boyce PM, Koloski NA, Talley NJ. Irritable bowel syndrome according to varying diagnostic criteria: are the new Rome II criteria unnecessarily restrictive for research and practice? Am J Gastroenterol. 2000;95(11):3176–83.
78. Yatani H, Studts J, Cordova M, Carlson CR, Okeson JP. Comparison of sleep quality and clinical and psychologic characteristics in patients with temporomandibular disorders. J Orofac Pain. 2002;16(3):221–8.
79. Osiewicz M, Lobbezoo F, Ciapala B, Pytko-Polonczyk J, Manfredini D. Pain predictors in a population of temporomandibular disorders patients. J Clin Med. 2020;9(2):452.
80. Fillingim RB, Ohrbach R, Greenspan JD, et al. Psychological factors associated with development of TMD: the OPPERA prospective cohort study. J Pain. 2013;14(12 Suppl):T75–90.
81. Epker J, Gatchel RJ. Coping profile differences in the biopsychosocial functioning of patients with temporomandibular disorder. Psychosom Med. 2000;62(1):69–75.
82. Garofalo JP, Gatchel RJ, Wesley AL, Ellis E 3rd. Predicting chronicity in acute temporomandibular joint disorders using the research diagnostic criteria. J Am Dent Assoc. 1998;129(4):438–47.
83. Kim HI, Lee JY, Kim YK, Kho HS. Clinical and psychological characteristics of TMD patients with trauma history. Oral Dis. 2010;16(2):188–92.
84. Howard RP, Hatsell CP, Guzman HM. Temporomandibular joint injury potential imposed by the low-velocity extension-flexion maneuver. J Oral Maxillofac Surg. 1995;53(3):256–62; discussion 63.
85. Melugin MB, Indresano AT, Clemens SP. Glenoid fossa fracture and condylar penetration into the middle cranial fossa: report of a case and review of the literature. J Oral Maxillofac Surg. 1997;55(11):1342–7.
86. Yun PY, Kim YK. The role of facial trauma as a possible etiologic factor in temporomandibular joint disorder. J Oral Maxillofac Surg. 2005;63(11):1576–83.
87. Ohrbach R, Fillingim RB, Mulkey F, et al. Clinical findings and pain symptoms as potential risk factors for chronic TMD: descriptive data and empirically identified domains from the OPPERA case-control study. J Pain. 2011;12(11 Suppl):T27–45.
88. De Boever JA, Keersmaekers K. Trauma in patients with temporomandibular disorders: frequency and treatment outcome. J Oral Rehabil. 1996;23(2):91–6.
89. Probert TC, Wiesenfeld D, Reade PC. Temporomandibular pain dysfunction disorder resulting from road traffic accidents—an Australian study. Int J Oral Maxillofac Surg. 1994;23(6 Pt 1):338–41.
90. Ferrari R, Leonard MS. Whiplash and temporomandibular disorders: a critical review. J Am Dent Assoc. 1998;129(12):1739–45.
91. Brown CR. TMJ injuries from direct trauma. Pract Periodontics Aesthet Dent. 1997;9(5):581–2.
92. Hlawitschka M, Loukota R, Eckelt U. Functional and radiological results of open and closed treatment of intracapsular (diacapitular) condylar fractures of the mandible. Int J Oral Maxillofac Surg. 2005;34(6):597–604.
93. Levy Y, Hasson O, Zeltser R, Nahlieli O. Temporomandibular joint derangement after air bag deployment: report of two cases. J Oral Maxillofac Surg. 1998;56(8):1000–3.
94. O'Connor RC, Shakib K, Brennan PA. Recent advances in the management of oral and maxillofacial trauma. Br J Oral Maxillofac Surg. 2015;53(10):913–21.
95. Kolbinson DA, Epstein JB, Burgess JA. Temporomandibular disorders, headaches, and neck pain following motor vehicle accidents and the

effect of litigation: review of the literature. J Orofac Pain. 1996;10(2):101–25.
96. Thoren H, Iizuka T, Hallikainen D, Nurminen M, Lindqvist C. An epidemiological study of patterns of condylar fractures in children. Br J Oral Maxillofac Surg. 1997;35(5):306–11.
97. Brooke RI, Stenn PG. Postinjury myofascial pain dysfunction syndrome: its etiology and prognosis. Oral Surg Oral Med Oral Pathol. 1978;45(6):846–50.
98. Burgess JA, Kolbinson DA, Lee PT, Epstein JB. Motor vehicle accidents and TMDS: assessing the relationship. J Am Dent Assoc. 1996;127(12):1767–72; quiz 85.
99. Kolbinson DA, Epstein JB, Senthilselvan A, Burgess JA. A comparison of TMD patients with or without prior motor vehicle accident involvement: initial signs, symptoms, and diagnostic characteristics. J Orofac Pain. 1997;11(3):206–14.
100. Klobas L, Tegelberg A, Axelsson S. Symptoms and signs of temporomandibular disorders in individuals with chronic whiplash-associated disorders. Swed Dent J. 2004;28(1):29–36.
101. Haggman-Henrikson B, Rezvani M, List T. Prevalence of whiplash trauma in TMD patients: a systematic review. J Oral Rehabil. 2014;41(1):59–68.
102. Zhang ZK, Ma XC, Gao S, Gu ZY, Fu KY. Studies on contributing factors in temporomandibular disorders. Chin J Dent Res. 1999;2(3–4):7–20.
103. Weinberg S, Lapointe H. Cervical extension-flexion injury (whiplash) and internal derangement of the temporomandibular joint. J Oral Maxillofac Surg. 1987;45(8):653–6.
104. Barnsley L, Lord S, Bogduk N. Whiplash injury. Pain. 1994;58(3):283–307.
105. Kronn E. The incidence of TMJ dysfunction in patients who have suffered a cervical whiplash injury following a traffic accident. J Orofac Pain. 1993;7(2):209–13.
106. McKay DC, Christensen LV. Whiplash injuries of the temporomandibular joint in motor vehicle accidents: speculations and facts. J Oral Rehabil. 1998;25(10):731–46.
107. Kasch H, Hjorth T, Svensson P, Nyhuus L, Jensen TS. Temporomandibular disorders after whiplash injury: a controlled, prospective study. J Orofac Pain. 2002;16(2):118–28.
108. Harkins SJ, Marteney JL. Extrinsic trauma: a significant precipitating factor in temporomandibular dysfunction. J Prosthet Dent. 1985;54(2):271–2.
109. Pullinger AG, Monteiro AA. History factors associated with symptoms of temporomandibular disorders. J Oral Rehabil. 1988;15(2):117–24.
110. Burgess J. Symptom characteristics in TMD patients reporting blunt trauma and/or whiplash injury. J Craniomandib Disord. 1991;5(4):251–7.
111. Moloney F, Howard JA. Internal derangements of the temporomandibular joint. III. Anterior repositioning splint therapy. Aust Dent J. 1986;31(1):30–9.
112. Westling L, Carlsson GE, Helkimo M. Background factors in craniomandibular disorders with special reference to general joint hypermobility, parafunction, and trauma. J Craniomandib Disord. 1990;4(2):89–98.
113. Pullinger AG, Seligman DA. Trauma history in diagnostic groups of temporomandibular disorders. Oral Surg Oral Med Oral Pathol. 1991;71(5):529–34.
114. Seals RR Jr, Morrow RM, Kuebker WA, Farney WD. An evaluation of mouthguard programs in Texas high school football. J Am Dent Assoc. 1985;110(6):904–9.
115. Garon MW, Merkle A, Wright JT. Mouth protectors and oral trauma: a study of adolescent football players. J Am Dent Assoc. 1986;112(5):663–5.
116. Singh GD, Maher GJ, Padilla RR. Customized mandibular orthotics in the prevention of concussion/mild traumatic brain injury in football players: a preliminary study. Dent Traumatol. 2009;25(5):515–21.
117. Akhter R, Hassan NM, Ohkubo R, et al. The relationship between jaw injury, third molar removal, and orthodontic treatment and TMD symptoms in university students in Japan. J Orofac Pain. 2008;22(1):50–6.
118. Gould DB, Banes CH. Iatrogenic disruptions of right temporomandibular joints during orotracheal intubation causing permanent closed lock of the jaw. Anesth Analg. 1995;81(1):191–4.
119. Oofuvong M. Bilateral temporomandibular joint dislocations during induction of anesthesia and orotracheal intubation. J Med Assoc Thail. 2005;88(5):695–7.
120. Knibbe MA, Carter JB, Frokjer GM. Postanesthetic temporomandibular joint dysfunction. Anesth Prog. 1989;36(1):21–5.
121. Mangi Q, Ridgway PF, Ibrahim Z, Evoy D. Dislocation of the mandible. Surg Endosc. 2004;18(3):554–6.
122. Gavish A, Halachmi M, Winocur E, Gazit E. Oral habits and their association with signs and symptoms of temporomandibular disorders in adolescent girls. J Oral Rehabil. 2000;27(1):22–32.
123. Dutra KM, Pereira FJ Jr, Rompre PH, et al. Orofacial activities in sleep bruxism patients and in normal subjects: a controlled polygraphic and audio-video study. J Oral Rehabil. 2009;36(2):86–92.
124. Yachida W, Arima T, Castrillon EE, et al. Diagnostic validity of self-reported measures of sleep bruxism using an ambulatory single-channel EMG device. J Prosthodont Res. 2016;60(4):250–7.
125. Marbach JJ, Raphael KG, Dohrenwend BP, Lennon MC. The validity of tooth grinding measures: etiology of pain dysfunction syndrome revisited. J Am Dent Assoc. 1990;120(3):327–33.
126. Kobs G, Bernhardt O, Kocher T, Meyer G. Oral parafunctions and positive clinical examination findings. Stomatologija. 2005;7(3):81–3.
127. Harness DM, Donlon WC, Eversole LR. Comparison of clinical characteristics in myogenic, TMJ internal derangement and atypical facial pain patients. Clin J Pain. 1990;6(1):4–17.
128. Taddey JJ. Musicians and temporomandibular disorders: prevalence and occupational etiologic considerations. Cranio. 1992;10(3):241–4.

129. Koob A, Ohlmann B, Gabbert O, et al. Temporomandibular disorders in association with scuba diving. Clin J Sport Med. 2005;15(5):359–63.
130. Rugh JD, Solberg WK. Electromyographic studies of bruxist behavior before and during treatment. J Calif Dent Assoc. 1975;3(9):56–9.
131. Solberg WK, Clark GT, Rugh JD. Nocturnal electromyographic evaluation of bruxism patients undergoing short term splint therapy. J Oral Rehabil. 1975;2(3):215–23.
132. Clark GT, Beemsterboer PL, Solberg WK, Rugh JD. Nocturnal electromyographic evaluation of myofascial pain dysfunction in patients undergoing occlusal splint therapy. J Am Dent Assoc. 1979;99(4):607–11.
133. Okeson JP, Phillips BA, Berry DT, et al. Nocturnal bruxing events in healthy geriatric subjects. J Oral Rehabil. 1990;17(5):411–8.
134. Okeson JP, Phillips BA, Berry DT, Cook YR, Cabelka JF. Nocturnal bruxing events in subjects with sleep-disordered breathing and control subjects. J Craniomandib Disord. 1991;5(4):258–64.
135. Okeson JP, Phillips BA, Berry DT, Baldwin RM. Nocturnal bruxing events: a report of normative data and cardiovascular response. J Oral Rehabil. 1994;21(6):623–30.
136. Lobbezoo F, Ahlberg J, Glaros A, et al. Bruxism defined and graded: an international consensus. J Oral Rehabil. 2013;40(1):2–4.
137. Ciancaglini R, Gherlone EF, Radaelli G. The relationship of bruxism with craniofacial pain and symptoms from the masticatory system in the adult population. J Oral Rehabil. 2001;28(9):842–8.
138. Johansson A, Unell L, Carlsson GE, Söderfeldt B, Halling A. Risk factors associated with symptoms of temporomandibular disorders in a population of 50-and 60-year-old subjects. J Oral Rehabil. 2006;33(7):473–81.
139. Ekman A, Rousu J, Napankangas R, et al. Association of self-reported bruxism with temporomandibular disorders—Northern Finland Birth Cohort (NFBC) 1966 study. Cranio. 2020, 41:1–6.
140. Israel HA, Diamond B, Saed-Nejad F, Ratcliffe A. The relationship between parafunctional masticatory activity and arthroscopically diagnosed temporomandibular joint pathology. J Oral Maxillofac Surg. 1999;57(9):1034–9.
141. Manfredini D, Cantini E, Romagnoli M, Bosco M. Prevalence of bruxism in patients with different research diagnostic criteria for temporomandibular disorders (RDC/TMD) diagnoses. Cranio. 2003;21(4):279–85.
142. Chien YC, Seferovic D, Holland JN, Walji MF, Adibi SS. When should sleep bruxism be considered in the diagnosis of temporomandibular disorders? Oral Surg Oral Med Oral Pathol Oral Radiol. 2020;130(6):645–50.
143. Sierwald I, John MT, Schierz O, et al. Association of temporomandibular disorder pain with awake and sleep bruxism in adults. J Orofac Orthop/Fortschr Kieferorthop. 2015;76(4):305–17.
144. Khayat N, Winocur E, Emodi Perelman A, et al. The prevalence of posterior crossbite, deep bite, and sleep or awake bruxism in temporomandibular disorder (TMD) patients compared to a non-TMD population: a retrospective study. Cranio. 2021;39(5):398–404.
145. Boscato N, Nascimento GG, Leite FRM, et al. Role of occlusal factors on probable bruxism and orofacial pain: data from the 1982 Pelotas birth cohort study. J Dent. 2021;113:103788.
146. John MT, Frank H, Lobbezoo F, Drangsholt M, Dette K-E. No association between incisal tooth wear and temporomandibular disorders. J Prosthet Dent. 2002;87(2):197–203.
147. Arima T, Svensson P, Arendt-Nielsen L. Experimental grinding in healthy subjects: a model for postexercise jaw muscle soreness? J Orofac Pain. 1999;13(2):104.
148. Svensson P, Burgaard A, Schlosser S. Fatigue and pain in human jaw muscles during a sustained, low-intensity clenching task. Arch Oral Biol. 2001;46(8):773–7.
149. Rompré P, Daigle-Landry D, Guitard F, Montplaisir J, Lavigne G. Identification of a sleep bruxism subgroup with a higher risk of pain. J Dent Res. 2007;86(9):837–42.
150. Rossetti LMN, de Araujo CDRP, Rossetti PHO, Conti PCR. Association between rhythmic masticatory muscle activity during sleep and masticatory myofascial pain: a polysomnographic study. J Orofac Pain. 2008;22(3):190.
151. Sinclair A, Wieckiewicz M, Ettlin D, et al. Temporomandibular disorders in patients with polysomnographic diagnosis of sleep bruxism: a case-control study. Sleep Breath. 2021;26:941.
152. Ramfjord SP. Dysfunctional temporomandibular joint and muscle pain. J Prosthet Dent. 1961;11(2):353–74.
153. Kardachi BJ, Bailey JO, Ash MM. A comparison of biofeedback and occlusal adjustment on bruxism. J Periodontol. 1978;49(7):367–72.
154. Castroflorio T, Bargellini A, Rossini G, Cugliari G, Deregibus A. Sleep bruxism in adolescents: a systematic literature review of related risk factors. Eur J Orthod. 2017;39(1):61–8.
155. Schiffman EL, Fricton JR, Haley D. The relationship of occlusion, parafunctional habits and recent life events to mandibular dysfunction in a non-patient population. J Oral Rehabil. 1992;19(3):201–23.
156. Soto-Goni XA, Alen F, Buiza-Gonzalez L, et al. Adaptive stress coping in awake bruxism. Front Neurol. 2020;11:564431.
157. Ashcroft GW, Eccleston D, Waddell JL. Recognition of amphetamine addicts. Br Med J. 1965;1(5426):57.
158. Magee KR. Bruxism related to levodopa therapy. JAMA. 1970;214(1):147.

159. Brandon S. Unusual effect of fenfluramine. Br Med J. 1969;4(5682):557–8.
160. Malki GA, Zawawi KH, Melis M, Hughes CV. Prevalence of bruxism in children receiving treatment for attention deficit hyperactivity disorder: a pilot study. J Clin Pediatr Dent. 2004;29(1):63–7.
161. Winocur E, Gavish A, Voikovitch M, Emodi-Perlman A, Eli I. Drugs and bruxism: a critical review. J Orofac Pain. 2003;17(2):99–111.
162. Ellison JM, Stanziani P. SSRI-associated nocturnal bruxism in four patients. J Clin Psychiatry. 1993;54(11):432–4.
163. Lobbezoo F, van Denderen RJ, Verheij JG, Naeije M. Reports of SSRI-associated bruxism in the family physician's office. J Orofac Pain. 2001;15(4):340–6.
164. Rajan R, Sun YM. Reevaluating antidepressant selection in patients with bruxism and temporomandibular joint disorder. J Psychiatr Pract. 2017;23(3):173–9.
165. Bertazzo-Silveira E, Kruger CM, Porto De Toledo I, et al. Association between sleep bruxism and alcohol, caffeine, tobacco, and drug abuse: a systematic review. J Am Dent Assoc. 2016;147(11):859–66.e4.
166. Abe K, Shimakawa M. Genetic and developmental aspects of sleep talking and teeth-grinding. Acta Paedopsychiatr. 1966;33(11):339–44.
167. Hublin C, Kaprio J. Genetic aspects and genetic epidemiology of parasomnias. Sleep Med Rev. 2003;7(5):413–21.
168. Hublin C, Kaprio J, Partinen M, Koskenvu M. Parasomnias: co-occurrence and genetics. Psychiatr Genet. 2001;11(2):65–70.
169. Clarke NG, Townsend GC, Carey SE. Bruxing patterns in man during sleep. J Oral Rehabil. 1984;11(2):123–7.
170. Sato T, Harada Y. Tooth-grinding during sleep as an arousal reaction. Experientia. 1971;27(7):785–6.
171. Bader GG, Kampe T, Tagdae T, Karlsson S, Blomqvist M. Descriptive physiological data on a sleep bruxism population. Sleep. 1997;20(11):982–90.
172. Ware JC, Rugh JD. Destructive bruxism: sleep stage relationship. Sleep. 1988;11(2):172–81.
173. Macaluso GM, Guerra P, Di Giovanni G, et al. Sleep bruxism is a disorder related to periodic arousals during sleep. J Dent Res. 1998;77(4):565–73.
174. Lavigne GJ, Huynh N, Kato T, et al. Genesis of sleep bruxism: motor and autonomic-cardiac interactions. Arch Oral Biol. 2007;52(4):381–4.
175. Ahci S, Bal B, Benbir-Senel G, Karadeniz D, Oral K. Polysomnographic characteristics of sleep-related bruxism: what are the determinant factors for temporomandibular disorders? Cranio. 2021:1–7.
176. Rossetti LMN, Rossetti PHO, Conti PCR, dos Reis Pereira de Araujo C. Association between sleep bruxism and temporomandibular disorders: a polysomnographic pilot study. Cranio. 2008;26(1):16–24.
177. Lavigne GJ, Rompré PH, Montplaisir JY, Lobbezoo F. Short communication motor activity in sleep bruxism with concomitant jaw muscle pain. A retrospective pilot study. Eur J Oral Sci. 1997;105(1):92–5.
178. Muzalev K, Visscher CM, Koutris M, Lobbezoo F. Effect of experimental temporomandibular disorder pain on sleep bruxism: a pilot study in males. Clin Oral Investig. 2020;24(1):103–11.
179. Lund JP, Donga R, Widmer CG, Stohler CS. The pain-adaptation model: a discussion of the relationship between chronic musculoskeletal pain and motor activity. Can J Physiol Pharmacol. 1991;69(5):683–94.
180. Kydd WL, Daly C. Duration of nocturnal tooth contacts during bruxing. J Prosthet Dent. 1985;53(5):717–21.
181. Clarke NG, Townsend GC. Distribution of nocturnal bruxing patterns in man. J Oral Rehabil. 1984;11(6):529–34.
182. Baba K, Haketa T, Sasaki Y, Ohyama T, Clark GT. Association between masseter muscle activity levels recorded during sleep and signs and symptoms of temporomandibular disorders in healthy young adults. J Orofac Pain. 2005;19(3):226–31.
183. Christensen LV. Facial pain from experimental tooth clenching. Tandlaegebladet. 1970;74(2):175–82.
184. Christensen LV, Mohamed SE. Contractile activity of the masseter muscle in experimental clenching and grinding of the teeth in man. J Oral Rehabil. 1984;11(2):191–9.
185. Christensen LV. Some subjective-experiential parameters in experimental tooth clenching in man. J Oral Rehabil. 1979;6(2):119–36.
186. Christensen LV, Mohamed SE, Harrison JD. Delayed onset of masseter muscle pain in experimental tooth clenching. J Prosthet Dent. 1982;48(5):579–84.
187. Christensen LV. Facial pain and internal pressure of masseter muscle in experimental bruxism in man. Arch Oral Biol. 1971;16(9):1021–31.
188. Delgado-Delgado R, Iriarte-Alvarez N, Valera-Calero JA, et al. Association between temporomandibular disorders with clinical and sociodemographic features: an observational study. Int J Clin Pract. 2021;75(5):e13961.
189. Sanders AE, Essick GK, Fillingim R, et al. Sleep apnea symptoms and risk of temporomandibular disorder: OPPERA cohort. J Dent Res. 2013;92(7 Suppl):70S–7S.
190. Senaratna CV, Perret JL, Lodge CJ, et al. Prevalence of obstructive sleep apnea in the general population: a systematic review. Sleep Med Rev. 2017;34:70–81.
191. Sánchez-de-la-Torre M, Campos-Rodriguez F, Barbé F. Obstructive sleep apnoea and cardiovascular disease. Lancet Respir Med. 2013;1(1):61–72.
192. Young T, Finn L, Peppard PE, et al. Sleep disordered breathing and mortality: eighteen-year follow-up of the Wisconsin sleep cohort. Sleep. 2008;31(8):1071–8.
193. Peppard PE, Young T, Palta M, Skatrud J. Prospective study of the association between sleep-disordered breathing and hypertension. N Engl J Med. 2000;342(19):1378–84.
194. Khalid I, Roehrs TA, Hudgel DW, Roth T. Continuous positive airway pressure in severe

obstructive sleep apnea reduces pain sensitivity. Sleep. 2011;34(12):1687–91.
195. Goldstein C, Zee PC. Obstructive sleep apnea-hypopnea and incident stroke: the sleep heart health study. Am J Respir Crit Care Med. 2010;182(10):1332; author reply 32–3.
196. Redline S, Yenokyan G, Gottlieb DJ, et al. Obstructive sleep apnea-hypopnea and incident stroke: the sleep heart health study. Am J Respir Crit Care Med. 2010;182(2):269–77.
197. Moldofsky H. The significance of the sleeping-waking brain for the understanding of widespread musculoskeletal pain and fatigue in fibromyalgia syndrome and allied syndromes. Joint Bone Spine. 2008;75(4):397–402.
198. Gotsopoulos H, Chen C, Qian J, Cistulli PA. Oral appliance therapy improves symptoms in obstructive sleep apnea: a randomized, controlled trial. Am J Respir Crit Care Med. 2002;166(5):743–8.
199. Onen SH, Onen F, Albrand G, et al. Pain tolerance and obstructive sleep apnea in the elderly. J Am Med Dir Assoc. 2010;11(9):612–6.
200. Cunali PA, Almeida FR, Santos CD, et al. Prevalence of temporomandibular disorders in obstructive sleep apnea patients referred for oral appliance therapy. J Orofac Pain. 2009;23(4):339–44.
201. Smith MT, Wickwire EM, Grace EG, et al. Sleep disorders and their association with laboratory pain sensitivity in temporomandibular joint disorder. Sleep. 2009;32(6):779–90.
202. Alessandri-Bonetti A, Scarano E, Fiorita A, Cordaro M, Gallenzi P. Prevalence of signs and symptoms of temporo-mandibular disorder in patients with sleep apnea. Sleep Breath. 2021;25(4):2001–6.
203. Wu JH, Lee KT, Kuo CY, et al. The association between temporomandibular disorder and sleep apnea—a nationwide population-based cohort study. Int J Environ Res Public Health. 2020;17(17):6311.
204. Bair E, Gaynor S, Slade GD, et al. Identification of clusters of individuals relevant to temporomandibular disorders and other chronic pain conditions: the OPPERA study. Pain. 2016;157(6):1266–78.
205. Park JW, Chung JW. Inflammatory cytokines and sleep disturbance in patients with temporomandibular disorders. J Oral Facial Pain Headache. 2016;30(1):27–33.
206. Doufas AG, Tian L, Padrez KA, et al. Experimental pain and opioid analgesia in volunteers at high risk for obstructive sleep apnea. PLoS One. 2013;8(1):e54807.
207. Randerath WJ, Verbraecken J, Andreas S, et al. Non-CPAP therapies in obstructive sleep apnoea. Eur Respir J. 2011;37(5):1000–28.
208. Marklund M. Subjective versus objective dental side effects from oral sleep apnea appliances. Sleep Breath. 2020;24(1):111–7.
209. Merrill RL. Temporomandibular disorder pain and dental treatment of obstructive sleep apnea. Dent Clin North Am. 2012;56(2):415–31.
210. Spencer J, Patel M, Mehta N, et al. Special consideration regarding the assessment and management of patients being treated with mandibular advancement oral appliance therapy for snoring and obstructive sleep apnea. Cranio. 2013;31(1):10–3.
211. Starcich R. [Cultural and scientific realities of internal medicine studies]. Recenti Prog Med. 1990;81(7–8):549–550.
212. Doff MH, Veldhuis SK, Hoekema A, et al. Long-term oral appliance therapy in obstructive sleep apnea syndrome: a controlled study on temporomandibular side effects. Clin Oral Investig. 2012;16(3):689–97.
213. Perez CV, de Leeuw R, Okeson JP, et al. The incidence and prevalence of temporomandibular disorders and posterior open bite in patients receiving mandibular advancement device therapy for obstructive sleep apnea. Sleep Breath. 2013;17(1):323–32.
214. Ishiyama H, Inukai S, Nishiyama A, et al. Effect of jaw-opening exercise on prevention of temporomandibular disorders pain associated with oral appliance therapy in obstructive sleep apnea patients: a randomized, double-blind, placebo-controlled trial. J Prosthodont Res. 2017;61(3):259–67.
215. Cunali PA, Almeida FR, Santos CD, et al. Mandibular exercises improve mandibular advancement device therapy for obstructive sleep apnea. Sleep Breath. 2011;15(4):717–27.
216. Juul-Kristensen B, Ostengaard L, Hansen S, et al. Generalised joint hypermobility and shoulder joint hypermobility,—risk of upper body musculoskeletal symptoms and reduced quality of life in the general population. BMC Musculoskelet Disord. 2017;18(1):226.
217. Pacey V, Nicholson LL, Adams RD, Munn J, Munns CF. Generalized joint hypermobility and risk of lower limb joint injury during sport: a systematic review with meta-analysis. Am J Sports Med. 2010;38(7):1487–97.
218. Acasuso-Diaz M, Collantes-Estevez E. Joint hypermobility in patients with fibromyalgia syndrome. Arthritis Care Res. 1998;11(1):39–42.
219. Bulbena A, Gago J, Pailhez G, et al. Joint hypermobility syndrome is a risk factor trait for anxiety disorders: a 15-year follow-up cohort study. Gen Hosp Psychiatry. 2011;33(4):363–70.
220. Remvig L, Jensen DV, Ward RC. Epidemiology of general joint hypermobility and basis for the proposed criteria for benign joint hypermobility syndrome: review of the literature. J Rheumatol. 2007;34(4):804–9.
221. Tinkle BT. Symptomatic joint hypermobility. Best Pract Res Clin Rheumatol. 2020;34(3):101508.
222. Nayani S, Dick J, Curl C. Ehlers-Danlos syndrome: a review. Dent Update. 2019;46(7):634–44.
223. Hirsch C, John MT, Stang A. Association between generalized joint hypermobility and signs and diagnoses of temporomandibular disorders. Eur J Oral Sci. 2008;116(6):525–30.
224. Buckingham RB, Braun T, Harinstein DA, et al. Temporomandibular joint dysfunction syndrome:

a close association with systemic joint laxity (the hypermobile joint syndrome). Oral Surg Oral Med Oral Pathol. 1991;72(5):514–9.
225. Conti PC, Miranda JE, Araujo CR. Relationship between systemic joint laxity, TMJ hypertranslation, and intra-articular disorders. Cranio. 2000;18(3):192–7.
226. Dijkstra PU, Kropmans TJ, Stegenga B. The association between generalized joint hypermobility and temporomandibular joint disorders: a systematic review. J Dent Res. 2002;81(3):158–63.
227. De Coster PJ, Van den Berghe LI, Martens LC. Generalized joint hypermobility and temporomandibular disorders: inherited connective tissue disease as a model with maximum expression. J Orofac Pain. 2005;19(1):47–57.
228. Chang TH, Yuh DY, Wu YT, et al. The association between temporomandibular disorders and joint hypermobility syndrome: a nationwide population-based study. Clin Oral Investig. 2015;19(8):2123–32.
229. Seckin U, Tur BS, Yilmaz O, et al. The prevalence of joint hypermobility among high school students. Rheumatol Int. 2005;25(4):260–3.
230. Fillingim RB, Wallace MR, Herbstman DM, Ribeiro-Dasilva M, Staud R. Genetic contributions to pain: a review of findings in humans. Oral Dis. 2008;14(8):673–82.
231. Smith SB, Mir E, Bair E, et al. Genetic variants associated with development of TMD and its intermediate phenotypes: the genetic architecture of TMD in the OPPERA prospective cohort study. J Pain. 2013;14(12 Suppl):T91–101, e1–3.
232. Visscher CM, Lobbezoo F. TMD pain is partly heritable. A systematic review of family studies and genetic association studies. J Oral Rehabil. 2015;42(5):386–99.

Orthodontics and Temporomandibular Disorders

Achint Utreja and Feras Al Khatib

1 Introduction

The temporomandibular joint (TMJ) is a complex structure that connects two rigid components of the craniofacial skeleton: the temporal and mandibular bones. The extensive range of motion provided by the joint to the lower jaw is made possible by the constitutive bones, cartilage, ligaments, and muscles. All of these connective tissues work in tandem to maintain the structural and functional integrity of the TMJ. Consequently, changes and/or perturbations in any of the joint components, such as those resulting from dental treatment, can potentially affect the joint. Although their definition has evolved over the years, temporomandibular joint disorders (TMDs) are categorized as musculoskeletal conditions that involve not only the TMJ but also the masticatory muscles and adjoining soft tissue structures. This chapter analyzes the historical and contemporary perspectives on temporomandibular disorders (TMDs) and orthodontics.

The specialty of orthodontics and dentofacial orthopedics is founded on the tenets of achieving a balanced and harmonious occlusion in patients with malocclusion. Traditionally, orthodontic correction of a developing malocclusion was thought to result in a stable condylar position. However, an often-cited lawsuit against an orthodontist in 1987 challenged this notion and led to extensive research on the relationship between orthodontic treatment and TMDs [1]. In this case, the orthodontist was blamed and held responsible for causing TMD in a 16-year-old female patient who was treated with fixed orthodontic appliances. It was alleged that tooth extractions and excessive pressure applied from an extraoral appliance (headgear) led to internal derangements of the TMJ. Although there was no scientific evidence to support this claim, the jury returned a "guilty" verdict for not just the orthodontist on trial but also the specialty of orthodontics in general!

2 Historical Perspective

Clinical diagnosis plays a pivotal role in dental treatment planning. TMD patients frequently present with increased overjet, deep overbite, and occlusal interferences. These findings were precluded by the identification of Costen's syndrome in the medical literature in 1934 [2]. This syndrome, affecting the TMJs and ears, is associated with joint pain and sounds, headache, limited mandibular opening, myofascial pain and tenderness, and otologic symptoms. Due to the anatomical proximity of the TMJ to the external auditory meatus, the similarity in the clinical observations is not surprising. From an orthodontic standpoint,

A. Utreja (✉) · F. Al Khatib
Section of Orthodontics, Department of Growth, Development and Structure, Southern Illinois University School of Dental Medicine, Alton, IL, USA
e-mail: autreja@siue.edu; falkhat@siue.edu

B. C. Stack Jr. et al. (eds.), *Craniofacial Pain*, https://doi.org/10.1007/978-3-031-57563-1_3

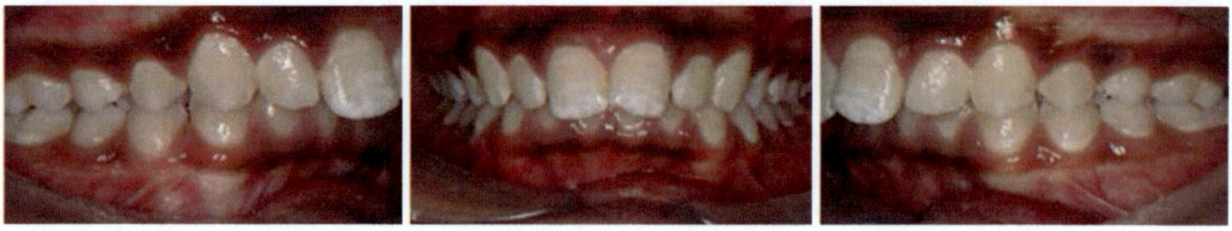

Fig. 1 A class II malocclusion is clinically associated with increased overjet due to either excessive maxillary growth or deficient mandibular growth. Functional appliances reposition the mandible anteriorly in an effort to redirect mandibular growth

most of these findings pointed towards a skeletal class II division 1 malocclusion with insufficient mandibular growth [3]. Posterior and superior displacement of the mandibular condyle in the glenoid fossa was assumed to be responsible for the malocclusion-related TMD symptoms [4]. Subsequently, various designs of oral appliances that raised the vertical dimension were proposed to address both TMJ and ear symptoms [5, 6]. Based on the early clinical evidence, orthodontic and dental educators advocated a detailed examination of TMJ function as an integral part of orthodontic clinical diagnosis.

Gnathology, defined as the study of the masticatory system, is closely related to understanding TMJ function during health and disease. The Gnathological Society, founded in 1926, stressed the importance of jaw kinematics and intraoral telemetry to achieve both a balanced and harmonious occlusion as well as optimum TMJ function [7]. Establishment of canine-guided occlusion and ensuring coincidence of maximum intercuspation with centric relation of the mandible were believed to be important for preventing and treating TMDs [8–10]. In situations where these gnathologic "goals" were not achieved with orthodontic treatment, custom-fabricated oral appliances were prescribed for TMDs. Various designs of these occlusal splints to treat TMDs have been proposed over the years, but scientific evidence for their efficacy is lacking [11].

In the 1970s, a gnathologic-prosthodontic concept of occlusion was introduced to the specialty of orthodontics by Ronald Roth. He believed that orthodontic treatment could modify the occlusion similar to full-mouth prosthodontic rehabilitation [12, 13]. This was consistent with the preexisting view that occlusal disharmonies and improper condyle position caused TMD [14]. According to Roth, the attainment of tooth and condyle positions recommended by the Gnathological Society was crucial for a stable orthodontic outcome as well as to prevent and/or cure TMD. Further, he stated that by ignoring gnathologic concepts, orthodontists could contribute to the development of TMDs. Although there was no evidence to support these claims, they sought to establish a relationship between orthodontic treatment and TMDs by placing the onus on orthodontists.

In the 1980s, the specialty of orthodontics witnessed another conflict in the ongoing debate about TMDs. This decade saw increasing numbers of "functional" orthodontic appliances being introduced to correct skeletal class II malocclusions (Fig. 1). Although their designs vary, most of these appliances aim to redirect growth by repositioning it more anteriorly. A group of orthodontists promoted functional appliances as more effective and less likely to cause TMDs compared to traditional orthodontic appliances such as elastics, headgears, chin cups, and treatment plans that required extraction of teeth. Unfortunately, these claims were not backed by scientific evidence either until the landmark lawsuit mentioned previously in this chapter changed all that [1].

3 Evidence-Based Perspective

3.1 Malocclusion and TMD

The term "malocclusion" in orthodontics is a rather broad categorization that encompasses both skeletal and dental discrepancies between the maxilla and mandible. Additionally, the relationship between the jaws may be affected in the sagittal, transverse, or vertical planes [15], thus further complicating a direct analysis between TMD and malocclusion.

3.2 Malocclusions in the Transverse Plane

In the transverse dimension, posterior crossbites of skeletal or dental origin are the primary concerns. A bilateral posterior crossbite results from a small maxilla or a large mandible and may be associated with TMD symptoms such as headache, muscle pain, and clicking [16]. As these are mostly attributable to an aberrant path of closure of the mandible, orthodontic correction of the crossbite can alleviate some of the TMD symptoms.

A unilateral posterior crossbite, on the other hand, is more challenging to treat orthodontically (Fig. 2). This is due to the underlying asymmetric muscular activity and the resulting altered condyle position in the glenoid fossa between the crossbite and non-crossbite sides. Unilateral posterior crossbites are prevalent in young individuals and directly affect the masticatory system, leading to abnormal occlusal contacts [17, 18] and overloading the masticatory muscles asymmetrically [19] (Fig. 2). These in turn have been implicated in causing myofascial pain and TMJ clicking.

A 10-year follow-up study was conducted to analyze the relationship between unilateral posterior crossbite and TMJ clicking [20]. During the initial observation period of adolescents, there was no association between the crossbite and joint clicking [17]. However, this changed after 10 years when an association was seen and the study participants self-reported joint clicking [20]. Orthodontic treatment in these subjects did not decrease the likelihood of self-reporting TMJ clicking, suggesting that occlusal factors are not the primary determinants of the reported symptoms. Instead, anatomic factors such as asymmetries in the glenoid fossa and/or mandibular condyle could be related to joint symptoms either concomitant to or resulting from a unilateral posterior crossbite.

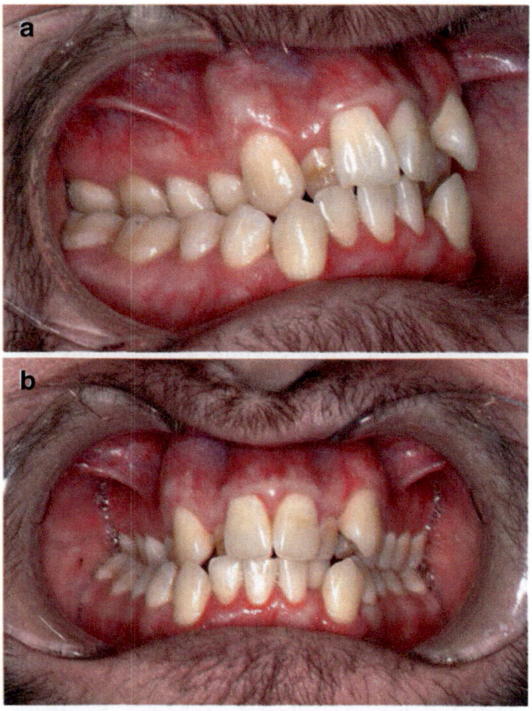

Fig. 2 (**a**) A unilateral posterior crossbite seen on the patient's right side. This transverse malocclusion is associated with deviation of the mandible to one side during jaw closure. (**b**) A common clinical finding is premature contact (during jaw closure) on a tooth or a group of teeth that are out of alignment compared to the other teeth

A prospective study evaluated the association (if any) between malocclusion characteristics during adolescence and TMJ clicking later in life [21]. Posterior crossbite, overbite, and overjet measured in subjects at age 15 years were compared against self-reported TMJ clicking at age 45 years. Results showed that neither the malocclusion variables that were analyzed nor a history of orthodontic treatment was associated with TMJ clicking. Overall, there is insufficient scientific evidence to establish a direct link between posterior crossbite and TMJ clicking.

The activity of the masticatory muscles has been investigated in relation to posterior crossbite and TMD. A systematic review concluded that there is no evidence to establish a relationship between posterior crossbite, masticatory muscle pain, and TMJ disc displacement [18]. Specifically, with a unilateral posterior crossbite, it could be speculated that unbalanced activation of the masticatory muscles can predispose to TMD. A study found that unilateral posterior crossbite and asymmetric muscle activity are not always related as children can present with asymmetric muscle activity even in the absence of a crossbite [22]. In adults, asymmetric activity of the anterior temporalis and masseter muscles is associated with severe malocclusions [23]. Thus, it appears that although deviations in the function of masticatory muscles are asymptomatic in children, these become symptomatic with TMD signs in adults.

3.3 Malocclusions in the Sagittal and Vertical Planes

Over the past few decades, multiple clinical studies and literature reviews have analyzed various malocclusion traits and TMD. A systematic review asked if there was an association between sagittal and vertical dental occlusion discrepancies and TMD [24]. Similar to previous reports on this topic, this study reiterated that there is no evidence of an association between dental occlusion and the pathophysiology of TMD [24]. The authors also pointed out that although occlusal interferences are noted in patients with TMD, it is unclear if the interferences are due to TMD or vice versa (Fig. 3).

3.3.1 Class II Treatment

Orthodontic treatment mechanics such as intermaxillary elastics and headgears that are used in patients with or without extractions of permanent teeth have been highlighted over the years as the leading causes of TMD. However, multiple clinical studies and scientific reviews have shown that orthodontic treatment with fixed appliances to retract the maxillary anterior teeth does not distally position the mandibular condyles in the glenoid fossa and/or lead to anterior displacement of the TMJ disc [25–30].

3.3.2 Class III Treatment

A skeletal class III malocclusion can be due to a small maxilla, large mandible, or a combination of both (Fig. 4). In patients with excessive mandibular growth, an orthodontic appliance known as the chin cup is used to exert a growth-restrictive force on the mandible. As the force vector from this appliance passes either directly through or close to the mandibular condyle, its use is believed to predispose patients to developing

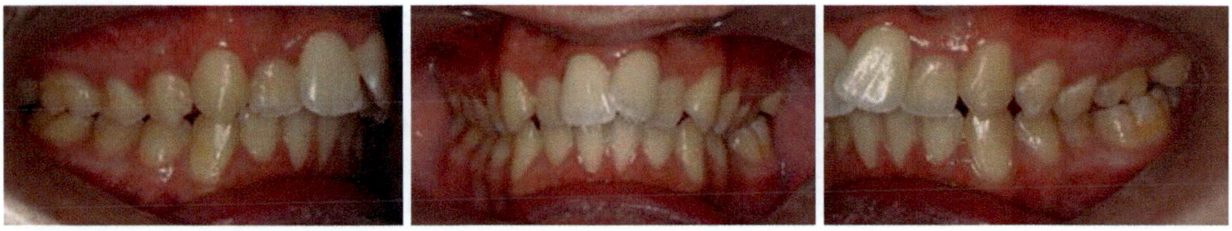

Fig. 3 A class II malocclusion associated with a unilateral posterior crossbite can be challenging to treat orthodontically. Occlusal interference in these cases is associated with TMDs

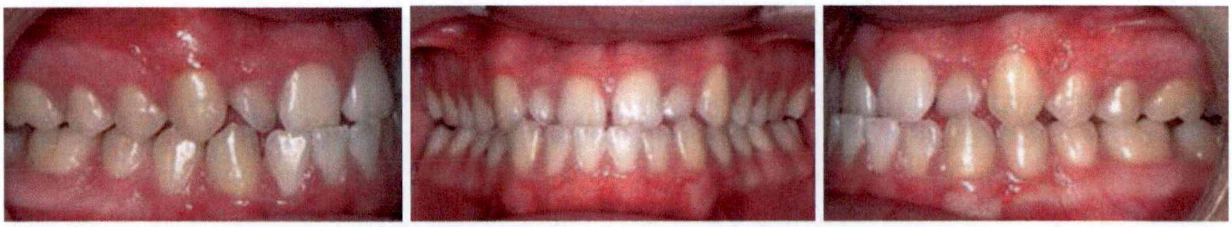

Fig. 4 A class III malocclusion is clinically associated with reverse overjet due to deficient maxillary growth or excessive mandibular growth. Occlusal interferences are present in both the sagittal and transverse planes due to the anterior and posterior crossbites, respectively

anterior disc displacement and eventually TMD. However, studies using magnetic resonance imaging (MRI) to analyze the condyle-disc-fossa relationship after the application of controlled forces with a chin cup have concluded that the appliance does not increase the risk for TMD [31, 32].

A hyperdivergent growth pattern of the mandible is associated with increased lower facial height, steep mandibular plane angle, and a tendency for an anterior open bite. On the other hand, a hypodivergent growth pattern is clinically associated with a deep overbite (Fig. 5). Both of these malocclusions in the vertical plane have a direct impact on the TMJ and the surrounding musculature. A systematic review reported an association between anterior open bite and TMJ disc displacement subsequently leading to degenerative TMJ disorders [33]. As mandibular growth and condyle position are closely interrelated, this is to be expected. The authors did, however, caution that their conclusion was based on low-quality evidence from heterogenous studies.

3.4 Condylar Position and Dental Occlusion

The relationship between the positions of the condyles in the glenoid fossa and the teeth in the dental arches has long been debated in dental literature. Consequently, definitions of often-used terms such as centric relation (CR) and maximum intercuspation (MI) have been repeatedly modified. For instance, over the past five decades, the definition of CR (the position of the condyles independent of tooth contact) has evolved from describing the condylar position in the glenoid fossa as being the most posterior to posterior-superior to the currently accepted anterior-superior [34].

The importance of accurately defining, as well as clinically finding, CR in dentistry lies in the assumption that this condylar position refers to the ideal and reproducible relationship between the mandible and cranium [35]. This forms the basis of the gnathological view that in order to prevent TMD after any dental procedure such as orthodontic treatment, CR and MI must coincide [36]. Thus, proponents of this theory have used various CR bite registration procedures and occlusal deprogramming oral appliances to obtain centric relation records [37, 38]. However, evaluation of condylar position in the glenoid fossa using magnetic resonance imaging (MRI) showed that chair-side manipulation of the jaw into a centric relation position is not reliable and cannot be used to prevent TMDs [39].

Based on the contemporary scientific evidence, there is no rationale for mounting orthodontic patients' maxillary and mandibular casts on a dental articulator to determine and treat a malocclusion to an arbitrary CR [40]. Additionally, TMD signs and symptoms are not related to a particular position of the mandibular condyle in the glenoid fossa, whether it be posterior, superior, or anterior [41, 42]. Not surprisingly, authors of a recent review on the clinical implications of centric relation recommended that the term "CR" should not be used at all. To maintain TMJ health, each orthodontic patient should instead be treated to establish a unique TMJ position that is determined by maximum intercuspation of the teeth [43].

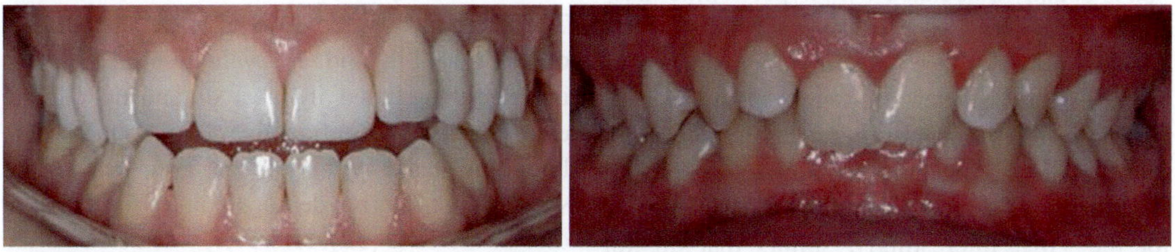

Fig. 5 Both anterior open bite and deep overbite malocclusions in the vertical plane can predispose to the development of TMD

3.5 Functional Occlusion

Among the various definitions of occlusion that have been put forth over the years, one that has been promoted as "functional occlusion" particularly by gnathologists is canine guide/protected occlusion. By definition, in a canine or mutually protected occlusion, the posterior teeth are not in contact during excursive movements of the mandible. This is achieved by the horizontal and vertical overlap between the maxillary and mandibular canines [34]. Proponents of this occlusal scheme believe that when the posterior teeth are not in contact during lateral mandibular movements, less forces are placed on the TMJ [44, 45]. This, in turn, is suggested to both alleviate preexisting TMD symptoms and prevent the initiation of new joint problems. However, there is no evidence in the scientific literature to support a relationship between any form of functional occlusion (including canine-protected occlusion) and the development of TMD symptoms [46]. As a result, there is no evidence-based rationale for aiming to establish a preordained occlusal scheme with the underlying notion that it will somehow have an effect on TMJ health.

3.6 Occlusal Appliance Therapy

Occlusal appliances that are fabricated to address TMD symptoms are more commonly referred to as "splints." Occlusal splints vary in design and relieve pressure on the TMJ by dis-occluding the posterior teeth and/or relaxing the muscles of mastication [47]. This can help in repositioning the joints and in redistributing the loads within the joint. Patients presenting with a deep overbite that is usually associated with hypertrophic masticatory muscles and excessive pressure on the TMJs could benefit from this treatment approach. Splint therapy is often followed by alteration of the occlusal relationships between the maxillary and mandibular teeth in an effort to establish occlusal contacts that are considered to be better for the TMJ. Interestingly, splints that do not have any occlusal coverage, and are thus a sham or placebo appliance/therapy, were found to be quite effective in relieving TMD symptoms [48]. Similarly, "mock" equilibration (adjustment of occlusal relationships) relieved TMD symptoms in more than half of the participants in a clinical study [49]. These highlight the importance of underlying psychosocial factors in the etiology and treatment of TMD.

3.7 Psychosocial Considerations

Patient expectations are important to recognize and address during any medical intervention, including the treatment of TMDs. This relies heavily on an accurate diagnosis and consideration of all possible etiological factors. Irreversible dental treatment such as occlusal equilibration should not be attempted in all patients, particularly when an etiological factor cannot be clearly established. In these situations, it is best to offer conservative treatment potions that are symptomatic and palliative, to address TMD symptoms [50]. Orthodontic treatment aimed at alleviating TMD symptoms is included in the category of irreversible treatment options, as are orthognathic surgical interventions. In situations where the muscles of mastication are responsible for some or all of the TMD symptoms, these irreversible treatments are unlikely to offer long-lasting relief to patients. Diagnostic imaging modalities such as MRI should be used prior to considering any invasive intracapsular procedures [51]. The bottom line is that a clinician must first provide TMD patients relief from pain and distress prior to considering any invasive procedures.

4 Diagnosis: TMJ Sounds

TMJ "sounds" are considered to be an indicator of joint health, and an evaluation of these is invariably included in most diagnostic clinical examinations. Traditionally, joint sounds have been correlated with TMD as both a sign and symptom of internal derangement of the articular disc of the TMJ [52]. However, research over the years has showed that commonly heard clicking and popping sounds are not limited to joints with dysfunction and thus cannot be used to diagnose joint pathology [53, 54]. A detailed classification of TMJ sounds takes into account the nature (click or crepitus), quality (hard or soft), location (relative to mandibular movement), and timing (opening or closing of the jaws) of sounds [55]. Based on this classification, a soft, subtle sound is a routine finding in most joints and can be attributed to various causes such as sudden movement of the TMJ ligaments or surface irregularities of the articulating surfaces. Clicking and popping sounds should only be considered as indicators of TMD when these are associated with other factors such as joint pain, muscle tenderness, and decreased range of mandibular movement [56, 57]. Considered by itself, TMJ clicking commonly occurs in over one-third of the population and does not routinely progress to a serious condition [58, 59].

5 The OPPERA Study

5.1 Rationale

The continuing stress on evidence-based treatment approaches in medicine and dentistry was the driving force behind a unique clinical study titled "Orofacial Pain: Prospective Evaluation and Risk Assessment" (OPPERA) study [60]. This longitudinal, multi-site, prospective study on TMDs was continuously funded for over 12 years by the National Institute of Dental and Craniofacial Research (NIDCR), a branch of the U.S. National Institutes of Health (NIH). The aim of the study was to identify the signs and symptoms as well as the potential risk factors (genetic and environmental) that predispose individuals to the development of painful TMJ disorders. The transition from acute to chronic states, and TMD associations with other systemic chronic conditions, were also investigated. Following the publication of some of the study results in two special issues of the *Journal of Pain* in 2011 [60] and 2013 [61], multiple additional scientific articles have reported various aspects of the vast findings from the study. Collectively, all this information has improved our understanding of TMD and has established that these disorders should be categorized as biopsychosocial and not just as dental conditions localized to the jaws.

5.2 Materials and Methods

OPPERA was originally designed to recruit 3200 individuals without TMD. Study participants were scheduled to be followed up for 5 years in an attempt to identify 200 new TMD cases from this cohort [62]. For the case-control arm of the study, 200 individuals with chronic, symptomatic TMD were recruited. The researchers then analyzed the predictors of TMD in each group.

5.3 Results

Many contributing factors were identified that play a role in the development of TMD. Among these, psychological distress and pain amplification are the two prominent variables that predispose to the condition(s). Individuals with these personality traits appear to be more susceptible to the onset and continuation of TMD [60]. Additional contributions to this process from the environment include both physical (such as trauma and infection) and social (such as daily stress) factors. Interactions between varying magnitudes of distress and pain amplification give rise to painful TMD that can be subclinical, transient, or persistent [60].

The key findings from OPPERA are the following:

- TMD has a high prevalence as 4% of the study participants developed the condition annually.
- TMD prevalence is not uniform across all age groups as those between 35 and 44 years of age have a higher prevalence compared to the 18- and 24-year-old age group.
- There is a strong female predilection with women four times as likely as men to develop TMD.

- Considering racial differences, TMD is more prevalent in non-Hispanic whites compared to African Americans and Hispanics.
- TMD patients have decreased jaw function, reduced mouth opening, and increased muscle sensitivity. Other physical symptoms include headache, chest pain, lethargy, and difficulty sleeping.
- There are multiple chronic overlapping pain conditions (COPCs) that are associated with TMD. Based on the number and severity of these pain conditions, patients can be divided into the following three groups:
  - Group 1: Patients in the "Adaptive" group are the least symptomatic and have few COPCs. They report less pain than the other groups, have little psychological distress and do not have significant muscle pain sensitivity. There are more men compared to women in this group, and their pain is mostly localized to the TMJ and surrounding muscles.
  - Group 2: Patients in the "Pain Sensitive" group present with enhanced sensitivity to muscle pain compared to the previous group. Both psychological stress and COPCs are increased as well, and there are more women compared to men in this group.
  - Group 3: Patients in the "Global Symptoms" group experience the most severe pain and dysfunction. More women than men are affected, and, as expected, psychological stress, COPCs, and muscle tenderness are the most severe in these patients. Cardiovascular complications, jaw injuries, and an increased likelihood of smoking are other routine findings in this group.

Besides the abovementioned phenotypic risk factors that contribute to an increased incidence of TMD, genotypic factors are also receiving attention. In the OPPERA study, 358 genes that regulate pain were identified [61]. Varying degrees of genetic associations between these genes are likely to give rise to intermediate phenotypes. For instance, the catechol-O-methyltransferase (COMT) gene was found to be associated with TMD onset, while six single nucleotide polymorphisms (SNPs) were identified as risk factors for chronic TMD [63]. Thus, in the quest for the identification of the underlying biological pathways that contribute to TMD, new risk factors for the condition(s) could be identified as well.

6 Clear Aligners and TMD

Orthodontic "treatment" was long considered to refer primarily to the correction of malocclusion using fixed orthodontic appliances. However, over the past few years, clear aligners have become increasingly popular in orthodontics to treat a variety of malocclusions [64]. Nowadays, adult patients are likely to opt for and specifically request clear aligners at an orthodontic practice as these are more esthetic than fixed orthodontic appliances. When using clear aligners, the plastic that covers the occlusal surfaces of the teeth can have an effect on related oral structures and function as well. For instance, patients with sleep bruxism and clenching have been postulated to benefit from occlusal coverage that protects the tooth surfaces against dental wear [65]. A recent clinical study, however, concluded that clear plastic orthodontic retainers are not very beneficial in individuals with sleep bruxism [66]. Increased masticatory muscle activity was observed during sleeping in individuals wearing clear orthodontic retainers.

A clinical study was conducted to evaluate the effect of treatment with clear aligners on oral parafunctional behaviors and electromyographic (EMG) activities of masticatory muscles [67]. After wearing clear aligners for a minimum of 6 months, increased EMG activity of the masticatory muscles was observed. Similarly, a randomized controlled trial analyzed the effect of clear aligners on sleep bruxism in orthodontic patients [68]. Study participants were followed up for 6 months with a portable EMG device. Similar to the previous study, increased EMG activity was observed. As early as 1 month into treatment with clear aligners, study subjects reported increased muscle tenderness. Most of these effects appear to be transient, but the long-term impact of these on the TMJ and the surrounding oral musculature will likely be influenced by the overall duration of clear aligner wear.

Although a clear consensus cannot be reached in this area due to a lack of high-quality clinical studies, the current evidence indicates that clear aligners increase masticatory muscle activity. Thus, the use of aligners in orthodontic patients with a history of masticatory muscle pain should be approached with caution. Also, as there is insufficient evidence of any advantage in sleep bruxism patients [68], clear aligners should not be prescribed to this group as a possible treatment modality. The bottom line, based on the current scientific evidence, is that orthodontic treatment can neither cause nor treat TMD [69].

7 Conclusion

The term "temporomandibular disorder(s)" is a very broad categorization of problems affecting the TMJs. The diverse clinical presentation is due to the multifactorial etiology that often involves both hard and soft tissue components of the joints. Advances in research over the past few years have shifted the focus from classifying TMDs as purely dental conditions (and treating them with dental appliances) to considering the underlying medical and biophysical contributory factors as well. Orthodontists must be cognizant of the ongoing research in this area and take the current evidence into account when treatment planning patients with either preexisting TMDs or at risk for developing TMDs. These patients will undoubtedly benefit the most from the collaborated and concerted efforts of medical professionals including orthodontists.

Suggested Readings

1. Pollack B. Cases of note: Michigan jury awards $850,000 in ortho case: a tempest in a teapot. J Mich Dent Assoc. 1988;70(11–12):540–2.
2. Costen JB. A syndrome of ear and sinus symptoms dependent upon disturbed function of the temporomandibular joint. Ann Otol Rhinol Laryngol. 1934;43(1):1–15.
3. Block LS. Diagnosis and treatment of disturbances of the temporomandibular joint especially in relation to vertical dimension. J Am Dent Assoc. 1947;34(4):253–60.
4. Thompson J. Temporomandibular disorders: diagnosis and treatment. Temporomandibular Joint. 1964:146–184.
5. Christensen J. Effect of occlusion-raising procedures on the chewing system. Dent Pract Dent Rec. 1970;20(7):233–8.
6. Sved A. Changing the occlusal level and a new method of retention. Am J Orthod Oral Surg. 1944;30(10):527–35.
7. McCollum BB. Factors that make the mouth and teeth a vital organ. J Am Dent Assoc (1922). 1927;14(7):1261–71.
8. Ahlgren J. Pattern of chewing and malocclusion of teeth. A clinical study. Acta Odontol Scand. 1967;25(1):3–14.
9. Sheppard IM, Sheppard SM. Range of condylar movement during mandibular opening. J Prosthet Dent. 1965;15(2):263–71.
10. Stallard H. Functions of the occlusal surfaces of the teeth. J Am Dent Assoc (1922). 1926;13(10):1392–412.
11. Greene CS, Menchel HF. The use of oral appliances in the management of temporomandibular disorders. Oral Maxillofac Surg Clin North Am. 2018;30(3):265–77.
12. Roth RH. Temporomandibular pain-dysfunction and occlusal relationships. Angle Orthod. 1973;43(2):136–53.
13. Roth RH. The maintenance system and occlusal dynamics. Dent Clin N Am. 1976;20(4):761–88.
14. Roth RH. Functional occlusion for the orthodontist. J Clin Orthod. 1981;15(1):32.
15. Proffit WR, Fields Jr HW, Sarver DM. Contemporary orthodontics. Elsevier Health Sciences; 2006.
16. Thilander B, Bjerklin K. Posterior crossbite and temporomandibular disorders (TMDs): need for orthodontic treatment? Eur J Orthod. 2012;34(6):667–73.
17. Farella M, Michelotti A, Iodice G, Milani S, Martina R. Unilateral posterior crossbite is not associated with TMJ clicking in young adolescents. J Dent Res. 2007;86(2):137–41.
18. Iodice G, Danzi G, Cimino R, Paduano S, Michelotti A. Association between posterior crossbite, masticatory muscle pain, and disc displacement: a systematic review. Eur J Orthod. 2013;35(6):737–44.
19. Sonnesen L, Bakke M. Bite force in pre-orthodontic children with unilateral crossbite. Eur J Orthod. 2001;23(6):741–9.
20. Michelotti A, Iodice G, Piergentili M, Farella M, Martina R. Incidence of temporomandibular joint clicking in adolescents with and without unilateral posterior cross-bite: a 10-year follow-up study. J Oral Rehabil. 2016;43(1):16–22.
21. Olliver SJ, Broadbent JM, Thomson WM, Farella M. Occlusal features and TMJ clicking: a 30-year

evaluation from a cohort study. J Dent Res. 2020;99(11):1245–51.
22. Michelotti A, Rongo R, Valentino R, et al. Evaluation of masticatory muscle activity in patients with unilateral posterior crossbite before and after rapid maxillary expansion. Eur J Orthod. 2019;41(1):46–53.
23. Farronato G, Giannini L, Galbiati G, Sesso G, Maspero C. Orthodontic-surgical treatment: neuromuscular evaluation in skeletal class II and class III patients. Prog Orthod. 2012;13(3):226–36.
24. Manfredini D, Lombardo L, Siciliani G. Temporomandibular disorders and dental occlusion. A systematic review of association studies: end of an era? J Oral Rehabil. 2017;44(11):908–23.
25. Beattie JR, Paquette DE, Johnston LE Jr. The functional impact of extraction and nonextraction treatments: a long-term comparison in patients with "borderline," equally susceptible class II malocclusions. Am J Orthod Dentofacial Orthop. 1994;105(5):444–9.
26. Gianelly AA. Orthodontics, condylar position, and TMJ status. Am J Orthod Dentofacial Orthop. 1989;95(6):521–3.
27. Gianelly AA, Anderson CK, Boffa J. Longitudinal evaluation of condylar position in extraction and nonextraction treatment. Am J Orthod Dentofacial Orthop. 1991;100(5):416–20.
28. Hirsch C. No increased risk of temporomandibular disorders and bruxism in children and adolescents during orthodontic therapy. J Orofac Orthop. 2009;70(1):39–50.
29. Kim M-R, Graber TM, Viana MA. Orthodontics and temporomandibular disorder: a meta-analysis. Am J Orthod Dentofacial Orthop. 2002;121(5):438–46.
30. Luecke PE 3rd, Johnston LE Jr. The effect of maxillary first premolar extraction and incisor retraction on mandibular position: testing the central dogma of "functional orthodontics". Am J Orthod Dentofacial Orthop. 1992;101(1):4–12.
31. Arat ZM, Akçam MO, Gökalp H. Long-term effects of chin-cap therapy on the temporomandibular joints. Eur J Orthod. 2003;25(5):471–5.
32. Gokalp H, Arat M, Erden I. The changes in temporomandibular joint disc position and configuration in early orthognathic treatment: a magnetic resonance imaging evaluation. Eur J Orthod. 2000;22(3):217–24.
33. Manfredini D, Segu M, Arveda N, et al. Temporomandibular joint disorders in patients with different facial morphology. A systematic review of the literature. J Oral Maxillofac Surg. 2016;74(1):29–46.
34. The glossary of prosthodontic terms: ninth edition. J Prosthet Dent. 2017;117(5S):e1-e105.
35. Rinchuse DJ, Kandasamy S. Centric relation: a historical and contemporary orthodontic perspective. J Am Dent Assoc. 2006;137(4):494–501.
36. Klar NA, Kulbersh R, Freeland T, Kaczynski R. Maximum intercuspation-centric relation disharmony in 200 consecutively finished cases in a gnathologically oriented practice. Semin Orthod. 2003;9(2):109–16.
37. Cordray FE. Three-dimensional analysis of models articulated in the seated condylar position from a deprogrammed asymptomatic population: a prospective study. Part 1. Am J Orthod Dentofacial Orthop. 2006;129(5):619–30.
38. Karl PJ, Foley TF. The use of a deprogramming appliance to obtain centric relation records. Angle Orthod. 1999;69(2):117–24; discussion 24–5.
39. Kandasamy S, Boeddinghaus R, Kruger E. Condylar position assessed by magnetic resonance imaging after various bite position registrations. Am J Orthod Dentofacial Orthop. 2013;144(4):512–7.
40. Kandasamy S, Greene CS, Obrez A. An evidence-based evaluation of the concept of centric relation in the 21st century. Quintessence Int. 2018;49(9):755–60.
41. McNeill C, Mohl ND, Rugh JD, Tanaka TT. Temporomandibular disorders: diagnosis, management, education, and research. J Am Dent Assoc. 1990;120(3):253, 255, 257 passim.
42. Mohl ND, Dixon DC. Current status of diagnostic procedures for temporomandibular disorders. J Am Dent Assoc. 1994;125(1):56–64.
43. Zonnenberg AJJ, Turp JC, Greene CS. Centric relation critically revisited-what are the clinical implications? J Oral Rehabil. 2021;48(9):1050–5.
44. Cordray FE. Centric relation treatment and articulator mountings in orthodontics. Angle Orthod. 1996;66(2):153–8.
45. Roth RH, Rolfs DA. Functional occlusion for the orthodontist. Part II. J Clin Orthod. 1981;15(2):100–23.
46. Rinchuse DJ, Kandasamy S, Sciote J. A contemporary and evidence-based view of canine protected occlusion. Am J Orthod Dentofacial Orthop. 2007;132(1):90–102.
47. Clark GT. Classification, causation and treatment of masticatory myogenous pain and dysfunction. Oral Maxillofac Surg Clin North Am. 2008;20(2):145–57, v.
48. Greene CS, Laskin DM. Splint therapy for the myofascial pain-dysfunction (MPD) syndrome: a comparative study. J Am Dent Assoc. 1972;84(3):624–8.
49. Goodman P, Greene CS, Laskin DM. Response of patients with myofascial pain-dysfunction syndrome to mock equilibration. J Am Dent Assoc. 1976;92(4):755–8.
50. Greene CS. The etiology of temporomandibular disorders: implications for treatment. J Orofac Pain. 2001;15(2):93–105; discussion 6–16.
51. Larheim TA. Role of magnetic resonance imaging in the clinical diagnosis of the temporomandibular joint. Cells Tissues Organs. 2005;180(1):6–21.
52. Gay T, Bertolami CN, Donoff RB, Keith DA, Kelly JP. The acoustical characteristics of the normal and abnormal temporomandibular joint. J Oral Maxillofac Surg. 1987;45(5):397–407.

53. Ogutcen-Toller M. Sound analysis of temporomandibular joint internal derangements with phonographic recordings. J Prosthet Dent. 2003;89(3):311–8.
54. Tallents RH, Hatala M, Katzberg RW, Westesson PL. Temporomandibular joint sounds in asymptomatic volunteers. J Prosthet Dent. 1993;69(3):298–304.
55. Watt DM. Temporomandibular joint sounds. J Dent. 1980;8(2):119–27.
56. Greene CS, Laskin DM. Long-term status of TMJ clicking in patients with myofascial pain and dysfunction. J Am Dent Assoc. 1988;117(3):461–5.
57. Vincent SD, Lilly GE. Incidence and characterization of temporomandibular joint sounds in adults. J Am Dent Assoc. 1988;116(2):203–6.
58. de Leeuw R. Internal derangements of the temporomandibular joint. Oral Maxillofac Surg Clin North Am. 2008;20(2):159–68. v
59. Rinchuse DJ, Abraham J, Medwid L, Mortimer R. TMJ sounds: are they a common finding or are they indicative of pathosis/dysfunction? Am J Orthod Dentofacial Orthop. 1990;98(6):512–5.
60. Maixner W, Diatchenko L, Dubner R, et al. Orofacial pain prospective evaluation and risk assessment study—the OPPERA study. J Pain 2011;12(11 Suppl):T4–11.e1–2.
61. Slade GD, Fillingim RB, Sanders AE, et al. Summary of findings from the OPPERA prospective cohort study of incidence of first-onset temporomandibular disorder: implications and future directions. J Pain. 2013;14(12 Suppl):T116–24.
62. Slade GD, Bair E, By K, et al. Study methods, recruitment, sociodemographic findings, and demographic representativeness in the OPPERA study. J Pain. 2011;12(11 Suppl):T12–26.
63. Slade GD, Ohrbach R, Greenspan JD, et al. Painful temporomandibular disorder: decade of discovery from OPPERA studies. J Dent Res. 2016;95(10):1084–92.
64. Lagravere MO, Flores-Mir C. The treatment effects of Invisalign orthodontic aligners: a systematic review. J Am Dent Assoc. 2005;136(12):1724–9.
65. Macedo CR, Silva AB, Machado MA, Saconato H, Prado GF. Occlusal splints for treating sleep bruxism (tooth grinding). Cochrane Database Syst Rev. 2007;2007(4):CD005514.
66. Manfredini D, Lombardo L, Vigiani L, Arreghini A, Siciliani G. Effects of invisible orthodontic retainers on masticatory muscles activity during sleep: a controlled trial. Prog Orthod. 2018;19(1):24.
67. Liu P, Wu G, Liu J, Jiao D, Guo J. Assessment of oral parafunctional behaviors and electromyographic activities of the masticatory muscles in young female patients with orthodontic invisalign treatment. Int J Clin Exp Med. 2017;10(11):15323–8.
68. Castroflorio T, Bargellini A, Lucchese A, et al. Effects of clear aligners on sleep bruxism: randomized controlled trial. J Biol Regul Homeost Agents. 2018;32(2 Suppl 2):21–9.
69. Suvinen TI, Reade PC, Kemppainen P, Kononen M, Dworkin SF. Review of aetiological concepts of temporomandibular pain disorders: towards a biopsychosocial model for integration of physical disorder factors with psychological and psychosocial illness impact factors. Eur J Pain. 2005;9(6):613–33.

An Overview of Chronic Neuropathic Orofacial Pain

Revathi Shekar

1 Introduction

A May 2023 news release from the National Institutes of Health reported findings from a study that found that the incidence of chronic pain exceeded the incidence of other common chronic conditions like high blood pressure, diabetes, and depression among US adults. As the opioid epidemic continues to grow, understanding pain and recognizing chronic orofacial pain in the dental setting also warrant discussion, better understanding, as well as adapting evidence-based patient management strategies. This chapter provides a brief overview of chronic neuropathic orofacial pain conditions with the intent to help the oral healthcare provider look beyond the dentition when patients present with chronic pain.

2 Pain Is Protective

Pain is a subjective and complex experience involving emotional, physical, and cognitive aspects (Fig. 1). Pain is defined by the International Association for the Study of Pain (IASP) as "an unpleasant sensory and emotional experience associated with actual or potential tissue damage or described in terms of such damage."

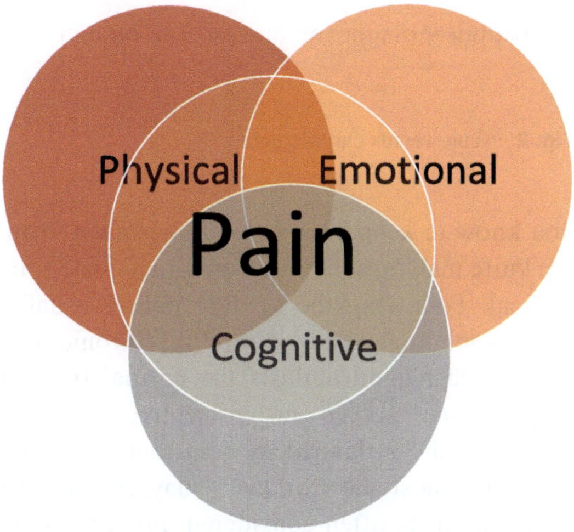

Fig. 1 Pain is a complex, multifaceted experience

Acute pain is caused by a specific injury or disease. It serves a useful purpose and is protective. Consider a situation where you are in the kitchen slicing vegetables with a knife and you accidentally cut your index finger. The injured finger becomes sensitive to light touch (allodynia) and hypersensitive to painful stimuli (hyperalgesia). The pain that ensues also helps

R. Shekar (✉)
Department of Diagnostic Sciences, University of Pittsburgh School of Dental Medicine, Pittsburgh, PA, USA

B. C. Stack Jr. et al. (eds.), *Craniofacial Pain*, https://doi.org/10.1007/978-3-031-57563-1_4

Acute Pain	Chronic Pain
• Is provoked by a specific disease or injury	• Pain outlasts the normal time of healing (when associated with disease/injury)
• Serves useful biologic purpose Injured area is: • Sensitive to light touch (**allodynia**) • Hypersensitive to painful stimuli (**hyperalgesia**)	• Serves no biologic purpose • Has no recognizable endpoint
• Is self-limited	• Chronic pain is considered a disease state
• Therapy- treat underlying cause	• Therapy - **multi-disciplinary approach**
• Ex. Pulpal pain from caries or trauma (routinely diagnosed and treated by dentists)	• Ex. neuralgia, neuropathic pain

Fig. 2 Acute versus chronic pain

you know to keep your index finger away from the knife making sure that there is adequate time to heal. Following the healing phase, usually, there is minimal, if any, disability. Chronic pain on the other hand outlasts the normal time of healing and serves no protective purpose. Chronic pain is defined as pain that is experienced on most days or every day in the past 3 months. It is often considered a disease state and not just a symptom. Figure 2 illustrates the differences between acute and chronic types of pain.

3 Dentoalveolar Pain (Toothache) Versus Chronic Orofacial Pain

Toothaches are commonly reported conditions. When patients seek care for this "typical" type of dental pain, the cause is usually pulpal/periapical infection that resolves following root canal therapy. Diagnosing dentoalveolar pain involves:

1. Eliciting a comprehensive history: the patient's chief complaint, medical history, a history of the nature, and location of pain symptoms
2. Performing a thorough clinical and radiographic assessment including the application of hot, cold, or electrical stimulus to the tooth, palpating the area, and percussion with an instrument

Although this sounds straightforward, there may be several confounding factors, including pain symptoms that fluctuate from one location to another and referred pain. Sometimes, non-odontogenic orofacial pain can masquerade as dentoalveolar. Therefore, the dentist must be aware of the possibility that the site of the patient's pain may be different (and distant) from the source and that a central cause for the patient's chronic, persistent pain symptoms can exist. Patients with these types of pain symptoms in the orofacial region can pose a diagnostic challenge to the provider. The orofacial region represents one of the more common sites of chronic pain in the body. The diagnosis of *orofacial pain* is complicated by the *closeness* and innervation of the anatomical structures in these areas.

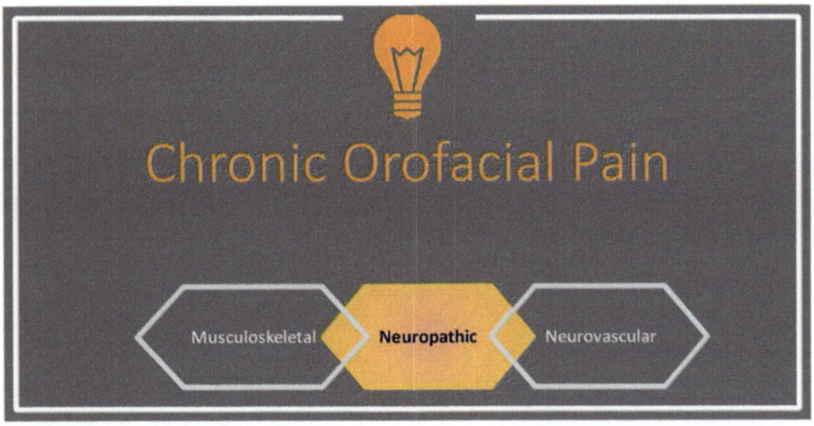

Fig. 3 The many faces of chronic orofacial pain

4 The Many Faces of Chronic Orofacial Pain

Chronic orofacial pain can originate from different regions in the face, head, and cervical regions, as well as from different etiologies (Fig. 3). Temporomandibular disorders involve the masticatory muscles and/or the temporomandibular joints. Neurovascular disorders like headaches can present as chronic orofacial pain, as seen in the case of facial migraines. Neuropathic pain conditions can arise from damage to the patient's peripheral nervous system. The peripheral nervous system is a network of neural pathways that carry signals to and from the central nervous system and the rest of the body. Neuropathy occurs when nerves are damaged, and as a result, they degenerate and fail to send and receive signals to function normally. This nerve damage could occur secondary to dental procedures, infection, a tumor, or a dysfunction of the nervous system.

5 Chronic Neuropathic Orofacial Pain

Neuropathic pain is defined as pain arising due to nerve damage or dysfunction of the somatosensory nervous system. The most important factor in arriving at an accurate diagnosis of neuropathic pain is a thorough patient history. Determining the location of pain is vital to making the correct diagnosis. Within the orofacial complex, there are several diagnoses for neuropathic pain, ranging across trigeminal neuralgia, painful post-traumatic trigeminal neuropathy, postherpetic neuralgia, burning mouth syndrome, and other neuropathies related to systemic diseases like diabetes and cancer. The diversity of the patient's pain complaints in this region often begs for collaboration and multidisciplinary management to best serve the patient. This chapter focuses on trigeminal neuralgia, glossopharyngeal neuralgia, persistent idiopathic dentoalveolar pain, painful post-traumatic trigeminal neuropathy, and burning mouth syndrome. For ease of understanding, we can classify these conditions as shown in Fig. 4.

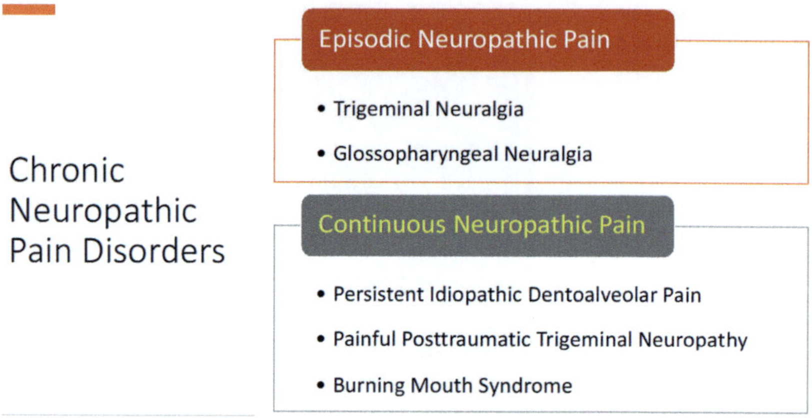

Fig. 4 Classification of chronic neuropathic pain disorders

6 Episodic Neuropathic Pain

6.1 Trigeminal Neuralgia

Trigeminal neuralgia is an episodic type of chronic neuropathic pain condition characterized by sudden, paroxysmal, short-lasting, lancinating/stabbing electric shock-like pain involving one or more branches of the trigeminal nerve. Diagnosis is made by history and identifying its very characteristic presenting features. First-line therapy relies on pharmacotherapy with carbamazepine. Figure 5 is a snapshot of the epidemiology and diagnostics of trigeminal neuralgia.

The trigeminal nerve is the fifth (CN V) cranial nerve and is also the largest cranial nerve. There are two trigeminal nerves—one on either side of the face. The nerve has three branches, the ophthalmic (V1), maxillary (V2), and mandibular (V3) nerves. These branches convene at the trigeminal ganglia, in Meckel's cave, in the middle cranial fossa. The primary function of the trigeminal nerve is to provide sensory innervation to the face, to detect touch, pain, temperature, and pressure sensations. The ophthalmic and maxillary branches are purely sensory, while the mandibular branch has both motor and sensory fibers, with the motor portion innervating the muscles of mastication.

6.1.1 Clinical Presentation of Trigeminal Neuralgia

Trigeminal neuralgia is a dysfunction of the fifth cranial nerve presenting as paroxysmal, excruciating pain in trigeminal dermatomes (innervated by the three branches of CN V), and accompanying spasm of the ipsilateral facial muscles. The symptoms are often unilateral in location. The pain symptoms begin and end abruptly, lasting anywhere between a fraction of a second to several minutes. They are triggered in the trigger areas in the dermatomes of the affected nerve branches. The triggers include the face, chewing, brushing, shaving, or even just the light touch of the breeze against the skin of the face. The maxillary and mandibular branches are more commonly affected. Patients can go into spontaneous remissions for weeks to years.

6.1.2 Diagnostic Criteria for Trigeminal Neuralgia (ICHD-3: International Classification of Headache Disorders, 3rd ed.)

1. Recurrent paroxysms of unilateral facial pain in the distribution(s) of one or more divisions of the trigeminal nerve, with no radiation beyond
2. Pain has the following characteristics:
   - Lasting from a fraction of a second to 2 min

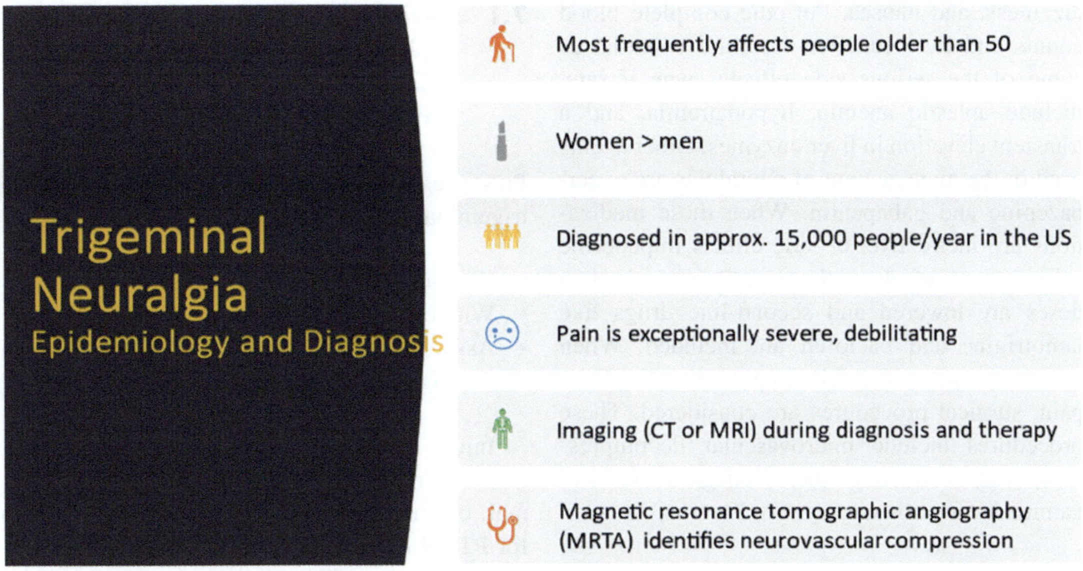

Fig. 5 A snapshot of the epidemiology and diagnostics of trigeminal neuralgia

- Severe intensity
- Electric shock-like, shooting, stabling, or sharp in quality
- Precipitated by innocuous stimuli within the affected trigeminal distribution

6.1.3 Types of Trigeminal Neuralgia

- **Classical trigeminal neuralgia** is caused by a compression of the trigeminal nerve by a blood vessel. Over time, this causes degeneration of the nerve's myelin sheath.
- **Secondary trigeminal neuralgia** arises as a complication of multiple sclerosis, a tumor in the area, or an arteriovenous malformation or by physical damage to the trigeminal nerve from a stroke, surgery, or facial trauma.
- **In a recently recognized form of trigeminal neuralgia**, there are the typical paroxysmal attacks, but against a background of dull, constant pain.

6.2 Glossopharyngeal Neuralgia

The glossopharyngeal nerve is the ninth paired cranial nerve (CN IX). The nerve has sensory, motor, and parasympathetic functions. It originates in the medulla oblongata of the brain and terminates in the pharynx where it divides into branches that it sends to the posterior one-third of the tongue, throat, tonsil, external ear canal, and carotid body.

Glossopharyngeal neuralgia is a rare condition characterized by paroxysmal, unilateral, severe pain in the tongue, throat, ear, and tonsils. Symptoms are usually described as sharp, stabbing, shooting, or lancinating and last from a few seconds to a few minutes. It has a milder natural history and course than trigeminal neuralgia, and most patients go into remission. The trigger areas encompass the tonsillar region and posterior pharynx. The triggers include swallowing, talking, coughing, yawning, touching the ear, or clearing the throat.

6.3 Management of Neuralgias

Antiepileptic medications are the drugs of choice. Carbamazepine (Tegretol) is used as first-line therapy. The common side effects include lightheadedness, confusion, blurred vision, sedation, dizziness, and nausea. Periodic complete blood counts and liver function tests are essential as some of the serious side effects, even if rare, include aplastic anemia, hyponatremia, and a transient elevation in liver enzymes. Other agents used in the management of neuralgias are oxcarbazepine and gabapentin. When these medications are ineffective, or side effects impede the achievement of drug therapeutic ranges, then doses are lowered and second-line drugs like lamotrigine and baclofen are included. When medical management fails to provide relief from pain, surgical procedures are considered. These procedures include microvascular decompression, radiofrequency thermocoagulation, and gamma knife radiosurgery.

7 Painful Post-traumatic Trigeminal Neuropathic Pain (PTTN)

Previously used terms: anesthesia dolorosa; painful post-traumatic trigeminal neuropathy

PTTN occurs following injury to the sensory division of the trigeminal nerve. It presents as unilateral or bilateral facial or oral pain that is persistent and/or recurring for more than 3 months and accompanied by other symptoms and signs of trigeminal nerve dysfunction. Patients present with allodynia, hyperpathia, and/or hyperalgesia. Allodynia is a painful response to a normally non-painful stimulus, hyperpathia is a complex painful response to repetitive non-painful stimuli, and hyperalgesia is a hypersensitive response to painful stimuli due to a lowered pain threshold.

Injuries to the trigeminal nerve can occur following:

- Root canal therapy
- Local anesthetic injections—physical trauma by the needle or due to chemical insult from the anesthetic solution
- Dental implant surgery
- Orthognathic surgery
- Fractures of the facial skeleton

7.1 Diagnostic Criteria for PTTN (2020 International Classification of Orofacial Pain, 4.1.2.3)

Presence of persisting or recurring pain within trigeminal nerve distribution

- For more than 3 months' duration
- With onset within 6 months of injury
- Associated with somatosensory symptoms and signs or both

Injury to trigeminal nerve's peripheral branches may be secondary to mechanical, thermal, or chemical insult. The diagnostic workup for PTTN includes performing chair-side neurosensory testing. This may be accomplished by using instruments and items that are easily available in the dentist's office—a cotton swab or filaments from cotton pellets to test changes in light touch (allodynia); using the dental probe to test for hypersensitivity to a noxious stimulus; and warm and cool instruments for thermal sensation. Each of these tests will have to be performed bilaterally, making note of the findings and recording them as normal, increased, or reduced on each of the sides. It is recommended that the clinician map and keep a record of regions of abnormal sensations.

7.2 Clinical Features of PTTN

- **Pain Location:** usually unilateral around injury/at distal dermatome of injured nerve. Initially precisely located, it may become diffuse and spread across dermatomes over time
- **Pain Intensity**: moderate to severe (visual analog scale, 5–9)
- **Pain Quality:** usually burning, but also stabbing during exacerbation
- **Positive or Negative Local Neurological Signs**: clinically demonstrable sensory dysfunction (allodynia, hyperalgesia, or paresthesia)

7.3 Risk Factors for PTTN

- **Preoperative phase** (specific to the patient): psychosocial factors, genetic/pain modulatory mechanisms, comorbidities like sleep disorders
- **Intraoperative phase:** surgical or procedural technique, associated nerve/tissue injury, and analgesic regimens
- **Postoperative phase:** patient's coping ability, postoperative pain intensity

7.4 Preventing PTTN

Some strategies that can be employed to prevent PTTN include providing preemptive analgesia to reduce discomfort and heightened pain perception, selecting an alternative surgical approach that can minimize tissue damage and nerve injury, providing adequate local or regional anesthesia, and adequate postoperative analgesics to ensure minimal to no perioperative pain.

7.5 Management of PTTN

Patient education is crucial to the successful management of PTTN. Informing the patient of the condition and the likely etiology and clear communication of the prognosis and various management strategies available help the patient understand that less than a 100% pain relief is an expected outcome.

Pharmacotherapy includes using tricyclic antidepressants like amitriptyline, serotonin norepinephrine reuptake inhibitors like duloxetine, or anticonvulsants like gabapentin as first-line therapy. Topical medications delivered using neurosensory stents for intraoral PTTN have been reported.

PTTN is a chronic, persistent neuropathic pain condition requiring long-term management. There are reports of its association with an increased risk for development of depression. As such, employing multiple modalities for its management including cognitive behavioral therapy (CBT), acupuncture, physical therapy, and psychosocial interventions has been recommended.

8 Continuous Neuropathic Orofacial Pain

8.1 Persistent Idiopathic Dentoalveolar Pain

Previously used terms: atypical odontalgia, persistent idiopathic facial pain

Persistent idiopathic dentoalveolar pain is a continuous type of chronic orofacial pain localized to a dentoalveolar area that is frequently misdiagnosed, leading to incorrect and unnecessary dental treatments aimed at reliving the patient's "dental" pain. This type of persistent, chronic pain is not attributable to any other disorder, and that is why the term "idiopathic" is used which refers to a condition or disorder that "arises spontaneously or from an obscure or unknown cause." Diagnosis is made after history, exam, and radiographic assessment fail to identify a cause for the pain. The likely pathologic mechanism is thought to be short-circuiting or a dysfunction of nerves that carry pain sensations from the teeth and jaws.

The 2020 International Classification of Orofacial Pain (ICOP 6.3) defines persistent idiopathic dentoalveolar pain (PIDP) as a "persistent unilateral intraoral dentoalveolar pain, rarely occurring at multiple sites, with variable features but recurring daily for more than 2 hours per day for more than 3 months, in the absence of any preceding causative agent."

8.2 Diagnostic Criteria

A. Intraoral dentoalveolar pain fulfilling criteria B and C (below).
B. Recurring daily for more than 2 h/day and for more than 3 months.
C. Pain has both of the following characteristics:

1. Localized to a dentoalveolar site (tooth or alveolar bone)
2. Deep, dull, pressure-like quality

D. Clinical and radiographic examinations are normal, and local causes have been excluded.
E. Not better accounted for by another ICOP or International Classification of Headache Disorders-3 (ICHD-3) diagnosis.

However, persistent idiopathic dentoalveolar pain is a diagnosis of exclusion based on an observational study that found that patients with persistent idiopathic dentoalveolar pain shared a few common features including the following:

- Most patients reported no nocturnal awakening due to the pain.
- The sulcus surrounding the affected tooth/teeth being painful to light touch in a significant proportion of patients.
- Females being more commonly affected than males.
- Pain being described as throbbing, burning, and pulsating.

8.3 Management of Persistent Idiopathic Dentoalveolar Pain

The first step in the management of PIDP is to reassure the patient that their pain is real. Often, the patient has already visited several providers who have either not offered them a diagnosis or been dismissive of their concerns. It is also important to educate the patient that the pain is not of dental origin and, therefore, they are not going to benefit from any dental and/or surgical intervention.

The first-line pharmacologic therapy is a tricyclic antidepressant such as amitriptyline. Serotonin-norepinephrine reuptake inhibitors such as duloxetine can also be employed. Alternative systemic medications include anticonvulsants/membrane stabilizers like gabapentin and pregabalin.

Psychosocial therapy techniques like cognitive behavioral therapy (CBT) are aimed at improving the patient's management of their pain and reducing the resultant impact on their quality of life. Clinicians should recognize that patients with persistent idiopathic dentoalveolar pain are long-term chronic pain patients and require continued support with a multidisciplinary team involving orofacial pain specialists and neurologists along with psychiatric and psychological evaluations to identify comorbidities like depression and anxiety.

8.4 Continuous Neuropathic Orofacial Pain

8.4.1 Burning Mouth Syndrome

Burning mouth syndrome is a chronic neuropathic pain condition affecting the oral mucosa in the absence of any clinically evident pathology. In most cases, symptoms are localized to the anterior two-thirds of the tongue, but other oral mucosa may be involved including the hard palate, labial and buccal mucosa, gingiva, and floor of the mouth. Patients often describe their symptoms as a painful burning sensation over these sites. Burning mouth syndrome can also present as tingling, itching, pricking, or numbness in these areas. The pain is often intractable, though often linked to a stressful or traumatic event like the loss of a family member, a divorce, or even a dental procedure. The International Headache Society defines burning mouth syndrome as "an intraoral burning or dysesthesia sensation, recurring daily for more than 2 hours per day over more than 3 months, without clinically evident causative lesions."

The clinician is required to perform comprehensive diagnostic and laboratory tests, examining psychological, local, and systemic factors such as parafunctional habits, dysgeusia, salivary changes, nutritional deficiencies, diabetes, and hormonal deficiencies or imbalances. A complete blood count and panel workup, with tests for blood glucose, iron, ferritin, vitamin B12, vitamin D, and thyroid hormone/panel, should be performed and investigated. Burning mouth syndrome is a diagnosis of exclusion where a diagnosis is arrived at after all other possible causes for the burning symptoms have been eliminated based on a comprehensive history, physical evaluation, imaging (when indicated), and specific laboratory tests.

8.5 Management

Burning mouth syndrome is a challenging condition for the clinician to manage as well as an ordeal for the patient. Having empathy for your patient and reassuring them that a diagnosis has been achieved and that it is not a malignancy or cancer, which is often what the patient is concerned about, are helpful.

A crucial step in the management of burning mouth syndrome is to have a frank conversation with the patient, setting expectations and realistic treatment goals. Inform them that treatments are symptomatic and not curative, and although complete remission is the goal, it may not always be achieved. Also, with any therapy or combination of therapies, it may take several weeks to months before maximum benefits are achieved. There is no known cure for burning mouth syndrome, but some symptomatic relief may be achieved using a variety of medications.

Clonazepam (Klonopin) is a benzodiazepine agent with a long duration of action. Oral disintegrating clonazepam tablets are used at 0.5–3.0 mg daily, starting with 0.5 mg. One tablet is cut in half and dissolved in a glass of water. The solution is rinsed/swished in the mouth and then expectorated, starting initially once daily at night before bedtime. This regimen may be repeated three times daily depending on side effects and tolerance. Clonazepam has the potential to cause dependence and should not be prescribed to patients with a substance dependence problem. Alternative medications that can be used are amitriptyline (nortriptyline) and gabapentin. Drowsiness is a side effect of these medications, especially in the first couple of weeks. Patients should be instructed to take the medication once daily at bedtime, initially, and not drink alcohol or drive.

Capsaicin is another medication that may be used to manage burning mouth syndrome. It is an alkaloid present in chili peppers and pepper sauces and is the active ingredient in Zostrix. Capsaicin rinses can be formulated at home by dissolving 5–6 drops of Tabasco (R) sauce in 1 teaspoon of water and rinsing or swishing in the mouth, four times a day. The initial feeling is one of burning, but within a few minutes, some patients report that the overall burning is much reduced. However, capsaicin is not easily palatable for many patients due to the burning pain associated with its application leading to low adherence.

Alpha-lipoic acid, also known as lipoic acid, is a potent antioxidant with neuroprotective properties that has been used in the management of burning mouth syndrome. Although it is synthesized naturally, the quantities are insufficient for metabolic needs. Dietary supplements in doses of 200–600 mg are available and are typically well tolerated with little or no adverse effects.

Non-pharmacologic approaches to management may be used alone or in combination with medications. Stress management/reduction, meditation, yoga, exercise, and psychotherapy are all helpful in the management of burning mouth syndrome. Patient reassurance and education are critical factors in the optimal management of burning mouth syndrome. Treatment should be multimodal and multidisciplinary to manage all aspects of this condition, with conservative options being attempted first to minimize adverse drug reactions.

9 Summary

Although the focus of this text is the temporomandibular joint, its dysfunction, and its associated symptoms, it is critical for the treating dentist or physician to appreciate that craniofacial pain is a complex matter requiring a deep understanding of head and neck anatomy as well as an understanding of the complete differential diagnosis. Limits placed upon the potential elements of a differential diagnosis will result in a delay or failure to achieve the correct diagnosis and associated patient distress and suffering.

Suggested Readings

1. https://www.nih.gov/news-events/news-releases/nih-study-finds-high-rates-persistent-chronic-pain-among-us-adults. Accessed 21 Oct 2023.
2. Nahin RL, Feinberg T, Kapos FP, Terman GW. Estimated rates of incident and persistent chronic pain among US adults, 2019-2020. JAMA Netw Open. 2023;6:e2313563.
3. Okeson JP. Bell's orofacial pains. The clinical management of orofacial pain. 6th ed. Carol Stream: Quintessence Publishing; 2005.
4. Okeson JP. The classification of orofacial pains. Oral Maxillofac Surg Clin North Am. 2008;20(2):133–44.
5. International Classification of Orofacial Pain, 1st ed (ICOP). Cephalalgia. 2020;40(2):129–221. https://doi.org/10.1177/0333102419893823.
6. Baad-Hansen L, Benoliel R. Neuropathic orofacial pain: facts and fiction. Cephalalgia. 2017;37(7):670–9.
7. Sanner F, Sonntag D, Hambrock N, Zehnder M. Patients with persistent idiopathic dentoalveolar pain in dental practice. Int Endod J. 2022;55(3):231–9. https://doi.org/10.1111/iej.
8. Baad-Hansen L, Pigg M, Ivanovic SE, Faris H, List T, Drangsholt M, et al. Chairside intraoral qualitative somatosensory testing: reliability and comparison between patients with atypical odontalgia and healthy controls. J Orofac Pain. 2013;27:165–70.
9. Baad-Hansen L, Pigg M, Yang G, List T, Svensson P, Drangsholt M. Reliability of intra-oral quantitative sensory testing (QST) in patients with atypical odontalgia and healthy controls—a multicentre study. J Oral Rehabil. 2015;42:127–35.
10. Neal TW, Zuniga JR. Post-traumatic trigeminal neuropathic pain: factors affecting surgical treatment outcomes. Front Oral Health. 2022;3:904785. https://doi.org/10.3389/froh.2022.904785.
11. Tan HL, Renton T. Burning mouth syndrome: an update. Cephalalgia Rep. 2020;3:1–18. https://doi.org/10.1177/2515816320970143.
12. Freilich JE, Kuten-Shorrer M, Treister NS, et al. Burning mouth syndrome: a diagnostic challenge. Oral Surg Oral Med Oral Pathol Oral Radiol. 2020;129:120–4.
13. Miller CS, Farag AM, Chmieliauskaite M, et al. Is burning mouth a syndrome or a disorder? A commentary. Oral Surg Oral Med Oral Pathol Oral Radiol. 2019;127:361–3.
14. Headache Classification Committee of the International Headache Society (IHS). The international classification of headache disorders, 3rd edition. Cephalalgia. 2018;38:1–211.
15. International Association for the Study of Pain (IASP). Classification of chronic pain, 2nd edition (revised). 2011. https://www.iasp-pain.org. Assessed 19 Apr 2020.
16. The Orofacial Pain Classification Committee. International classification of orofacial pain, 1st edition (ICOP). Cephalalgia. 2020; 40: 129–221.
17. Klasser GD, Grushka M, Su N. Burning mouth syndrome. Oral Maxillofac Surg Clin North Am. 2016;28:381–96.
18. Nasri-Heir C, Khan J, Benoliel R, et al. Altered pain modulation in patients with persistent postendodontic pain. Pain. 2015;156:2032–41.
19. OFHPSIG, IASP, INfORM, AAOP, IHS. International Classification of Orofacial Pain. 2019. https://www.ihs-headache.org/binary_data/3468_the-international-orofacial-pain-classification-committee-icop-1-betafor-review.pdf.
20. Nixdorf D, Moana-Filho E. Persistent dento-alveolar pain disorder (PDAP): working towards a better understanding. Rev Pain. 2011;5:18–27.
21. Singh PM, Dehran M, Mohan VK, Trikha A, Kaur M. Analgesic efficacy and safety of medical therapy alone vs combined medical therapy and extraoral glossopharyngeal nerve block in glossopharyngeal neuralgia. Pain Med. 2013;14(1):93–102. https://doi.org/10.1111/pme.12001.
22. Woolf CJ. Central sensitization: implications for the diagnosis and treatment of pain. Pain. 2011;152(3, Suppl):S2–S15.
23. Khan M, Nishi SE, Hassan SN, Islam MA, Gan SH. Trigeminal neuralgia, glossopharyngeal neuralgia, and myofascial pain dysfunction syndrome: an update. Pain Res Manag. 2017;2017:7438326. https://doi.org/10.1155/2017/7438326.
24. Melis M, Lobo SL, Ceneviz C, et al. Atypical odontalgia: a review of the literature. Headache. 2003;43:1060–74.
25. International Classification of Orofacial Pain, 1st edition (ICOP). Cephalalgia. 2020;40(2):129–221.
26. Crooks DA, Miles JB. Trigeminal neuralgia due to vascular compression in multiple sclerosis—Post-mortem findings. Br J Neurosurg. 1996;10(1):85–8. https://doi.org/10.1080/02688699650040575.
27. Woolf CJ, Mannion RJ. Neuropathic pain: aetiology, symptoms, mechanisms, and management. Lancet. 1999;353:1959–64.
28. Toda K. Etiology of trigeminal neuralgia. Oral Sci Int. 2007;4(1):10–8. https://doi.org/10.1016/S1348-8643(07)80007-3.
29. Love S, Coakham HB. Trigeminal neuralgia: pathology and pathogenesis. Brain. 2001;124(12):2347–60. https://doi.org/10.1093/brain/124.12.2347.
30. Zakrzewska JM, Linskey ME. Trigeminal neuralgia. Am Fam Physician. 2016;94(2):133–5.
31. Hamlyn PJ, King TT. Neurovascular compression in trigeminal neuralgia: a clinical and anatomical study. J Neurosurg. 1992;76(6):948–54. https://doi.org/10.3171/jns.1992.76.6.0948.

Imaging of the Common Conditions of the Temporomandibular Joint

Husniye Demirturk and Anitha Potluri

1 Introduction

The temporomandibular joint (TMJ) stands out as a distinctive anatomical structure, being the sole diarthrodial synovial joint within the human body. It remains under constant load, even during periods of inactivity, necessitating robust biomechanical integrity to withstand the substantial mechanical stresses it encounters during its functioning.

The TMJ consists of extracapsular elements, including nerves, vessels, ligaments, and a capsule, which will not be discussed in this chapter because they are not easily visualized on TMJ imaging. The intracapsular components (Figs. 1 and 2) can be categorized into two groups: osseous elements and soft tissue components. The osseous components encompass (1) the glenoid (mandibular) fossa and articular eminence and (2) the mandibular condyle. Cross-sectional hard tissue imaging techniques like cone beam CT (CBCT) or traditional CT are recommended to assess these osseous components effectively. CBCT is often preferred due to its lower radiation exposure. It offers the advantage of generating sub-millimetric custom cross sections from the same dataset which aids in the early detection of articular surface deterioration.

This chapter discusses the common conditions of TMJ and the radiographic methods employed to investigate potential deterioration in TMJ's biomechanical stability. This chapter will not cover trauma, cysts, and neoplasm of TMJ.

H. Demirturk · A. Potluri (✉)
Department of Diagnostic Sciences,
University of Pittsburgh School of Dental Medicine,
Pittsburgh, PA, USA
e-mail: hud25@pitt.edu

B. C. Stack Jr. et al. (eds.), *Craniofacial Pain*, https://doi.org/10.1007/978-3-031-57563-1_5

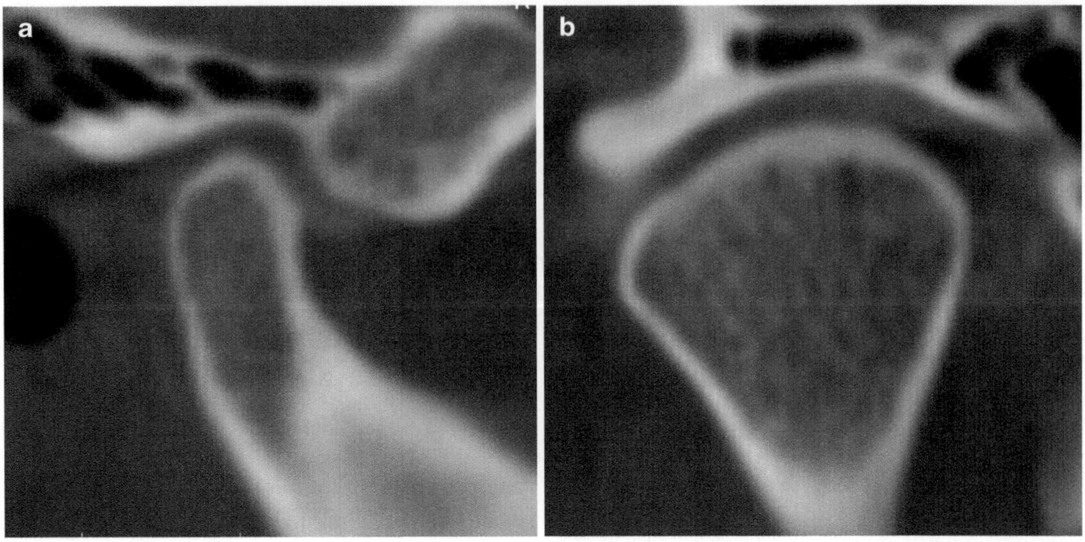

Fig. 1 CBCT sagittal and coronal views demonstrate the TMJ normal anatomy. In sagittal (**a**) and coronal (**b**) planes, the bony elements appear rounded and create an irregular joint structure. In adult condyles, the outer cortex of the condylar articulation is notably thin. The marrow spaces exhibit uniformity and lack any signs of sclerosis. In the sagittal view, the expected normal disc space should resemble the shape of a bow tie, representing the disc positioned between the joint surfaces. Meanwhile, in the coronal view, it should resemble the crescent shape of the posterior band of the disc

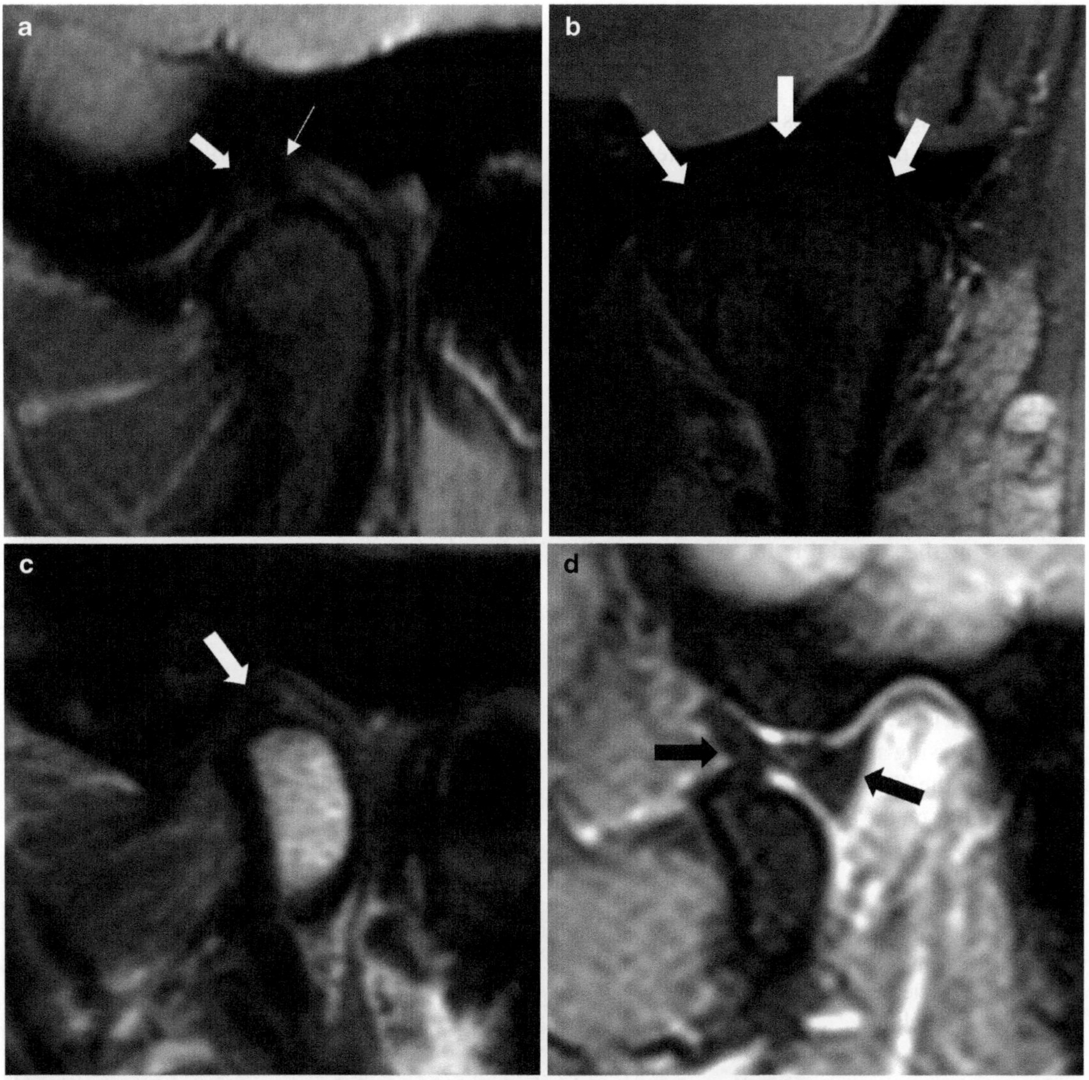

Fig. 2 MRI axially corrected sagittal and coronal views demonstrate the TMJ normal anatomy in open and closed positions. In a closed sagittal MRI (**a** and **c**), the posterior band of the bow tie-shaped disc is positioned at the 12 o'clock position on the condyle (arrow). The intermediate zone is between the incongruent articulations, while the anterior band rests on the lateral pterygoid muscle fibers. The posterior attachment (line arrow) is connected to the posterior band of the disc, and the marrow spaces exhibit low to intermediate signals on the PDWI (**a** and **b**) and T2WI (**d**) and high signals on T1WI (**c**). The cortical outlines are continuous and uniform (**a**). In a coronal closed MRI (**b**), the posterior band of the disc takes on a crescent shape (arrow) and is positioned evenly superior to the condyle. It tapers toward the poles and attaches to the neck of the condyle with the medial and lateral collateral ligament. In an open sagittal MRI (**d**), the condyle translates to the crest of the articular eminence, and the disc is positioned between the crest of the eminence and the condyle. (Courtesy K. Orhan, DDS)

2 Imaging Techniques and Protocols

Various imaging techniques exist for examining the TMJ. Some traditional plain-film techniques including transcranial, Towne, submentovertex, and lateral tomographic projections have been superseded by three-dimensional imaging methods that provide superior precision regarding tissue morphology and spatial relationships and will not be discussed in this chapter.

A. **Panoramic radiography**: A panoramic radiograph can provide basic information about the osseous components of the TMJ. However, it falls short in accurately assessing the spatial relationships of the TMJ because the teeth are in a protrusive position during image capture to align both jaws within the focal trough.
B. **Cone beam computed tomography (CBCT)**: CBCT offers a comprehensive view encompassing not only the osseous components of the TMJ but also the impact of TMJ conditions on the entire craniofacial complex. Evaluation of asymmetry (whether one side is enlarged or decreased in size and length), changes in growth, alterations in occlusion (bite), neck posture, and risk factors associated with sleep-disordered breathing are analyzed (Fig. 3).

Imaging protocol: To assess all of the abovementioned aspects, a field of view of at least 16 cm or larger is necessary to visualize these structures and their interplay within a single volume. During imaging, the teeth should be in maximum intercuspation, and the head posture should closely mimic the natural head posture. Common standard reformations aid in the evaluation of TMJ and craniofacial complex:

- Custom cross-sectional images of the TMJs
- Sagittal and coronal oblique sections of the TMJs
- TMJ axial view
- Panoramic reformation
- 3D frontal and lateral reformations
- Analyses of airway morphology and volume

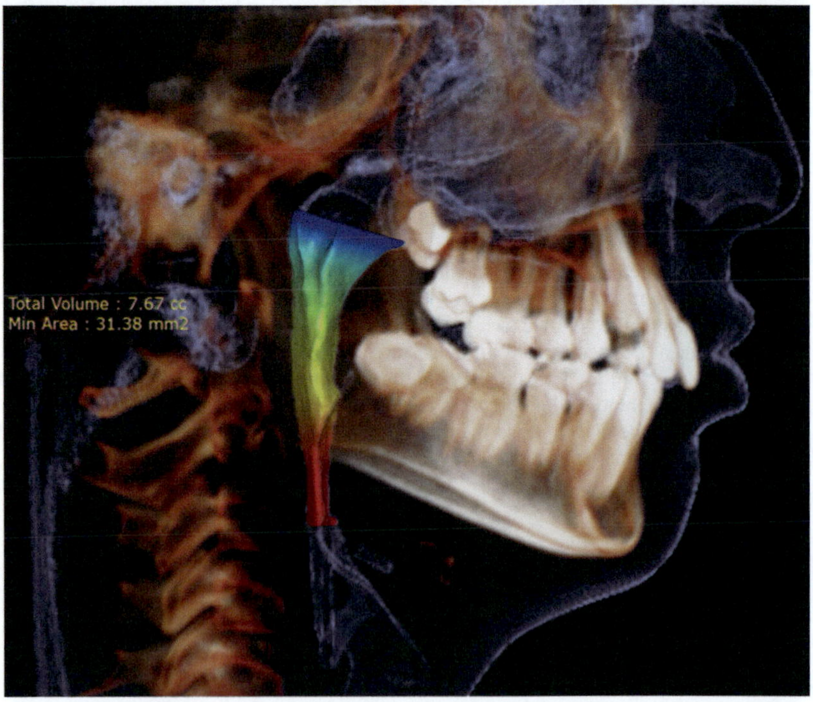

Fig. 3 CBCT airway analysis, highlighting the anatomical structures and dimensions relevant to the assessment of the upper airway

C. **Multidetector computed tomography (MDCT)**: MDCT images can fulfill the same objective as CBCT; however, MDCT involves higher radiation exposure. Therefore, whenever CBCT is available, it should be the preferred choice as it provides the same information with lower radiation exposure for the patient. MDCT has similar imaging protocols to CBCT.
D. **Magnetic resonance imaging (MRI)**: MRI provides valuable information and is considered the gold standard about the state and positioning of the soft tissue components within the temporomandibular joint (see also chapter "The Neurological Aspects of the Trigeminal Cranial Complex and Its Role in the TMJ Dysfunction and Multiple Movement Disorders").

Articular disc: The normal articular disc is clearly visible in fast spin echo sequences, appearing as a hypointense (low signal intensity) fibrocartilaginous biconcave structure positioned between the temporal bone and the mandibular condyle. When viewed in sagittal oblique images, the disc resembles a bow tie, where a thinner central intermediate zone connects the anterior and posterior triangular bands. Normally, in a closed-mouth position, the posterior band of the disc is typically situated at approximately the 11–12 o'clock position in relation to the condyle (Fig. 2). However, when the mouth opens, both the condyle and the disc translate forward beneath the articular eminence. This results in the central portion of the disc aligning over the apex of the condyle. The section of the disc positioned between the articular surfaces should constitute the junction between the anterior band and the intermediate zone. Simultaneously, the condyle should be situated inferior to the level of the articular eminence (Fig. 2). In the coronal view, the posterior band of the disc should appear like a crescent positioned on top of the condyle, tapering gently toward the poles of the condyle (Fig. 2).

Indications: Assessing the disc and its attachments, other soft tissues, joint effusion, soft tissue neoplasia, or neoplastic-like lesions. The morphology of osseous components and bone marrow integrity can be evaluated. However, subtle osseous alterations indicative of early active degenerative change or joint disease are better seen with CBCT.

Common imaging protocols: T1 or proton density (PD) and T2 and/or short tau inversion recovery (STIR) in both closed-mouth (maximal intercuspal) and open-mouth positions. Cross-sectional images should be acquired, including axially corrected sagittal oblique and coronal oblique sections along the long axes of the condyles and at right angles to them.

The closed-mouth position with the teeth in maximum intercuspation shows the condition and position of the disc and other soft tissues, aiding in determining disc displacement. The open-mouth position shows whether a displaced disc has been recaptured by the condyle during the opening of the jaw.

3 Imaging of Common TMJ Pathological Conditions

3.1 Developmental Disturbances of TMJ

TMJs are not fully developed at birth, making them susceptible to developmental disturbances before and after birth. Kaneyama and colleagues have classified developmental disturbances as follows:

- Hypoplasia or aplasia of the condyle
  - Congenital or primary hypoplasia or aplasia
  - Acquired or secondary hypoplasia or aplasia
- Condylar hyperplasia
- Bifid condyle

1. **Condylar hypoplasia or aplasia**

   Condylar aplasia refers to the absence or nondevelopment of the mandibular condyle, while condylar hypoplasia indicates insufficient growth or underdevelopment of the condyle. Both aplasia and hypoplasia can manifest as congenital or acquired conditions and may affect one side or both sides (Fig. 4).

Various congenital conditions associated with hypoplasia or aplasia include the Pierre Robin sequence, hemifacial macrosomia, Treacher Collins syndrome, oculo-auriculo-vertebral syndrome, and Hurler syndrome. In congenital cases, bilateral TMJs are often affected; however, the predominant clinical presentation may be seen as unilateral. On the other hand, acquired or secondary hypoplasia or aplasia can occur due to various factors, such as local factors that disrupt condyle development, including trauma, infections affecting the mandible or middle ear, and therapeutic radiation.

Imaging:

- Affects the condyle along with underdevelopment of the same-side ramus and mandibular body.
- Condyle is small but retains its normal shape and morphology.
- Small mandibular fossa.
- The posterior border of the ramus and the condylar neck may display a posterior inclination.
- Unilateral cases are more common than bilateral.
- Mandibular asymmetry and TMJ dysfunction.
- Extent of resulting asymmetry varies based on the age at which condylar growth is affected.
- Chin frequently deviates toward the affected side, and on opening, mandible deviates toward the affected side.

2. **Condylar hyperplasia**

Condylar hyperplasia is characterized by the unilateral enlargement of the condyle (Fig. 5). While the exact cause remains unclear, some theories suggest that mild, chronic inflammation may play a role, triggering a condition akin to proliferative osteomyelitis, and may stimulate condylar growth or surrounding structures. The unilateral nature strongly indicates a localized phenomenon. Obwegeser and Makek have classified condylar hyperplasia as follows:

- **Type A**: Hemimandibular hyperplasia, resulting in vertical plane asymmetry. This type is characterized by unilateral vertical growth with minimal chin deviation.
- **Type B**: Hemimandibular elongation, leading to transverse plane asymmetry. This type causes chin deviation toward the opposite side without vertical asymmetry.
- **Type C**: Combination of types A and B, showing hyperplastic characteristics either unilaterally or bilaterally.
- **Imaging:**
- Large condylar process with normal subchondral bone and cortical outline.
- Condylar process is notably larger in comparison to the dimensions of the corresponding fossa.
- Unilateral enlargement of condylar process, ascending ramus, and mandibular body on the same side.
- Osseous midline of the mandible may deviate toward the opposite side.
- Instead of being concave, ramus posterior border and mandible inferior border often exhibit a convex shape.

Fig. 4 3D volume renderings from anterior (**a**) and lateral (**b**) view, sagittal (**c** and **d**) and coronal (**e** and **f**) CBCT images show mandibular asymmetry associated with right condylar hypoplasia. 3D volume renderings illustrate mild mandibular asymmetry, where the right side is smaller than the left due to right condylar hypoplasia. Right condyle (**c** and **e**) is small compared to the left (**d** and **f**) but has a normal morphology. When aligning the two sides of the skull base, orbits, and zygomas on the lateral view, the lower border of the right mandible appears higher relative to the left (**b**, arrow). Any alteration in the dimensions of a condyle, regardless of its underlying origin—whether developmental, degenerative, or inflammatory—will lead to mandibular asymmetry

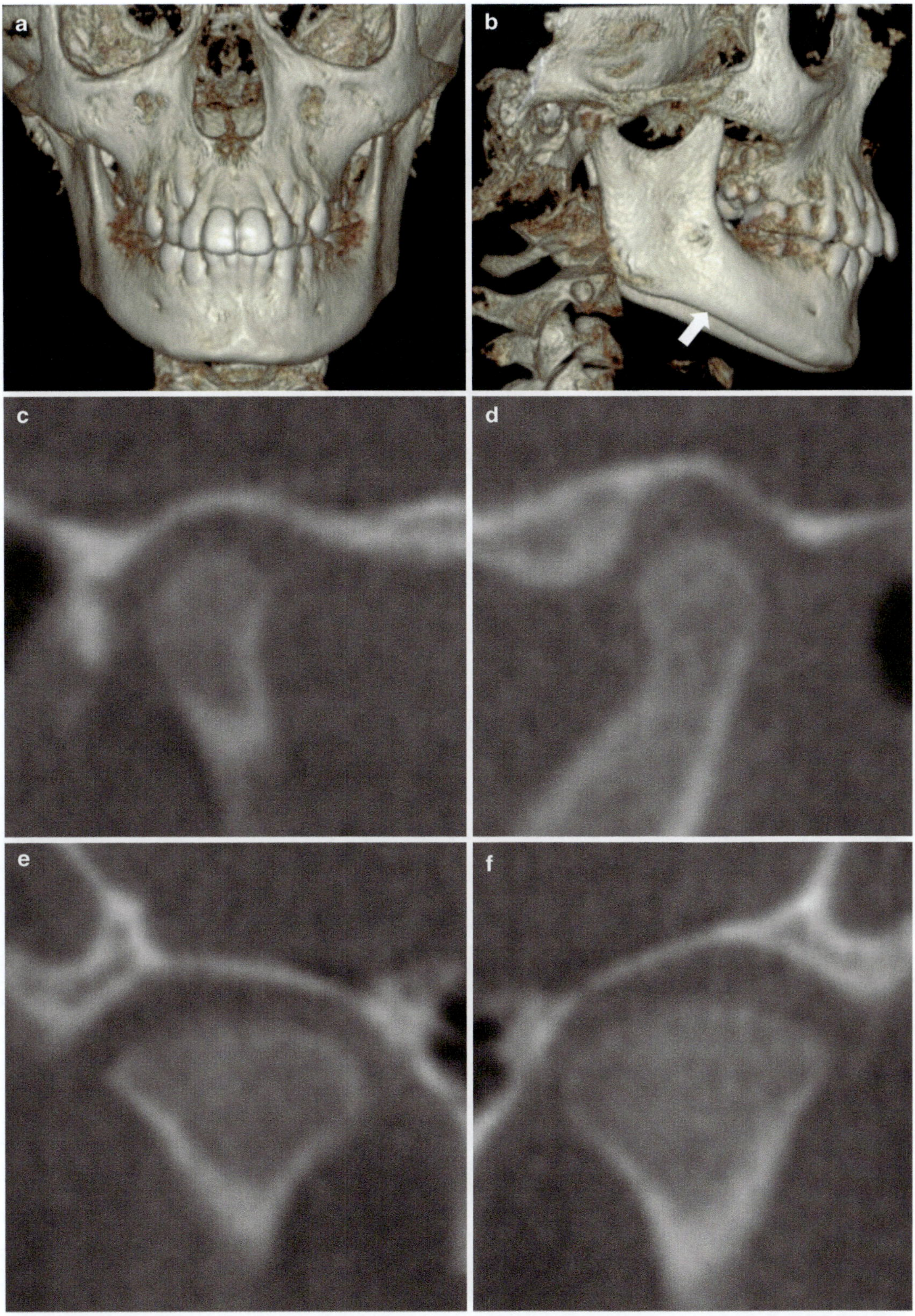
a
b
c
d
e
f

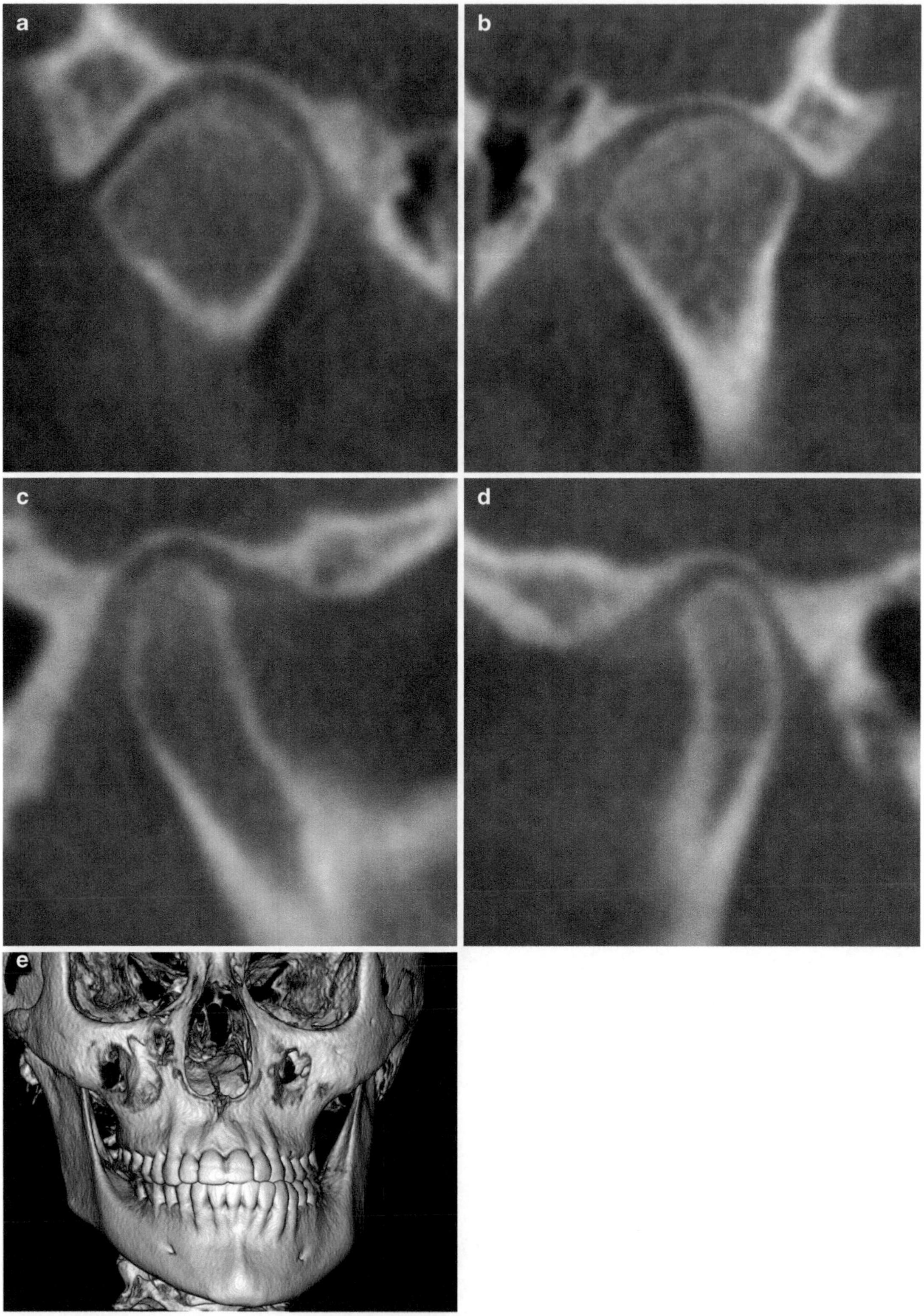

Fig. 5 Coronal (**a** and **b**), sagittal (**c** and **d**), and 3D volume rendering (**e**) CBCT images show right condylar hyperplasia accompanied by hemimandibular elongation resulting in transverse plane asymmetry, leading to chin deviation toward the contralateral side. Right condylar process is large (**a** and **c**) compared to the normal left side (**b** and **d**) with normal cortical borders and subchondral bone

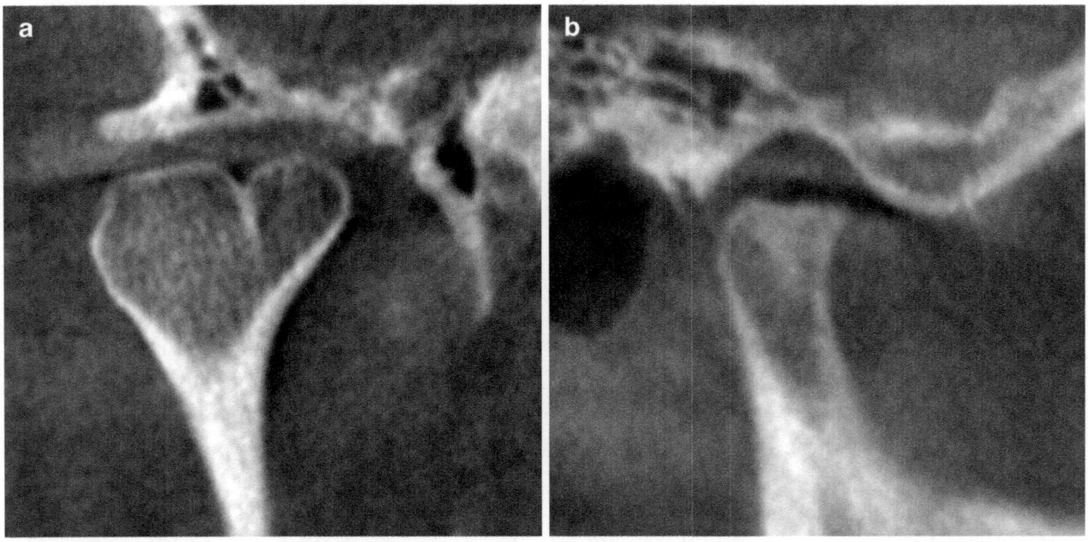

Fig. 6 CBCT images illustrate a bifid condyle in a mediolateral orientation. The coronal image (**a**) depicts a heart-shaped condyle, while the sagittal image (**b**) reveals flattening and minor depression in the center of the superior aspect of the right condyle

3. **Bifid condyle**

Bifid condyle is characterized by the presence of a groove or depression of varying depth on the mandibular condyle, resulting in partial division of the condyle (Fig. 6). Condition is usually observed unilaterally, although there have been reports of bilateral bifid condyles. Trifid condyles have also been documented, but they are a rare phenomenon compared to bifidity. Bifidity's cause is still debated, with theories ranging from possible embryonic origins tied to limited blood supply to the condylar head, trauma, or microtrauma from sources like birth-related injuries or condylar head fractures to factors such as genetic or systemic conditions, infections, and radiotherapy.

Imaging:

- Depression or notch on the superior condylar surface or a complete duplication with continuous cortex.
- Orientation of the condyles can be either in the mediolateral or in the anteroposterior plane. In the mediolateral case, they resemble a heart shape in coronal images, while in the anteroposterior case, they appear as two condyles, one located anterior to the other in sagittal reformat images.
- Mandibular fossa can undergo remodeling to adapt to the changed condylar morphology.
- Traumatic causes may lead to bony ankylosis.
- Condyle appears lobulated in panoramic radiograph.

3.2 TMJ Internal Derangements

Internal derangements, characterized by alterations in the disc's morphology or position within the TMJ, can be triggered by factors such as trauma, malocclusion, ligament laxity, or other conditions that exert pressure on the disc causing it to shift from its normal location. Once the disc is displaced, it initiates a breakdown in the usual joint function. The following discussion will outline the progression from internal derangement to degenerative joint disease, along with the different forms of these derangements and the various stages of degenerative joint disease.

Disc displacement is considered to have four clinical stages:

- Stage I (disc displacement with reduction): The articular disc is displaced when the mouth is closed but returns to its normal position when the mouth is opened; the central narrow zone of the disc is in contact with the condylar head and articular eminence when the mouth is opened.
- Stage II (disc displacement with reduction with intermittent locking): The disc is displaced when the mouth is closed and intermittently locked in position when the mouth is opened.
- Stage III (disc displacement without reduction): The disc is displaced when the mouth is closed and does not return to its normal position when the mouth is opened. This condition is sometimes referred to as a "closed lock."
- Stage IV (disc displacement without reduction): In the final stage, the disc is permanently displaced and does not return to its normal position, with perforation of the disc or posterior (band) attachment tissues.

Degree of Disc Displacement: Disc displacement can manifest as either partial or complete. In cases of partial displacement, the disc undergoes morphological changes, adopting either a biplanar appearance (characterized by the flattening of the posterior band) or a biconvex shape (associated with thickening of the posterior band, typically observed when the condyle is positioned posteriorly). Conversely, a completely displaced disc that has been acutely displaced retains its biconcave appearance (Figs. 7 and 8). However, over time, it may gradually lose its original shape and anteroposterior length, eventually leading to atrophy (Fig. 9).

Direction of Disc Displacement: Disc displacement can be presented in multiple directions. The most common form is anterior disc displacement (Figs. 7, 8, 9, and 10). Other forms include anterior rotational displacement where the disc slides off of just one pole while maintaining a normal relationship with the remaining portions of the condyle (Fig. 11), sideways displacement in either a purely lateral or medial direction (Fig. 12), or posterior displacement which should be distinguished from the thickening of the intermediate posterior attachment, also referred to as "pseudodisc formation" (Fig. 9).

Disc Displacement with Reduction (DDWR): DDWR is among the most prevalent intra-articular disorders. DDWR can be found in approximately 33% of asymptomatic individuals. In individuals with DDWR, the disc is displaced relative to the condyle when the mouth is closed. However, when the mouth is opened, the disc returns to the intermediate position between the condyle and the articular tubercle. The disc returns to its displaced state once again upon closing the mouth (Figs. 10 and 13).

Following the reduction of the disc during condylar translation, there is typically no restriction in the range of motion. However, mandibular movements may not exhibit the same level of smoothness as in a normal condition due to the momentary sliding of the condyle on and off the disc. Nevertheless, once the mouth reaches the fully open position, the ultimate alignment of the condyle and the disc in a joint with DDWR is nearly identical to that in a joint without displacement. Clinically, DDWR is associated with TMJ noise. The movement of the disc onto and off of its proper position can produce clicking, snapping, and/or popping sounds, collectively known as opening and closing "clicks."

Disc Displacement Without Reduction (DDWOR): In the closed-mouth position, the disc is displaced relative to the condyle, and the disc does not return to its normal position with mouth opening. The displaced disc mechanically hinders the condyle's translation, resulting in restricted jaw opening and a jaw deviation toward the affected side.

Signs encompass a maximum assisted mouth opening of less than 40 mm, mandibular deflection to the ipsilateral side during opening and protrusion, and limited movement toward the contralateral side. Symptoms may involve sharp, sudden, and intense pain localized around the ear area and a sudden reduction in mandibular movement due to the "closed lock." As time passes and

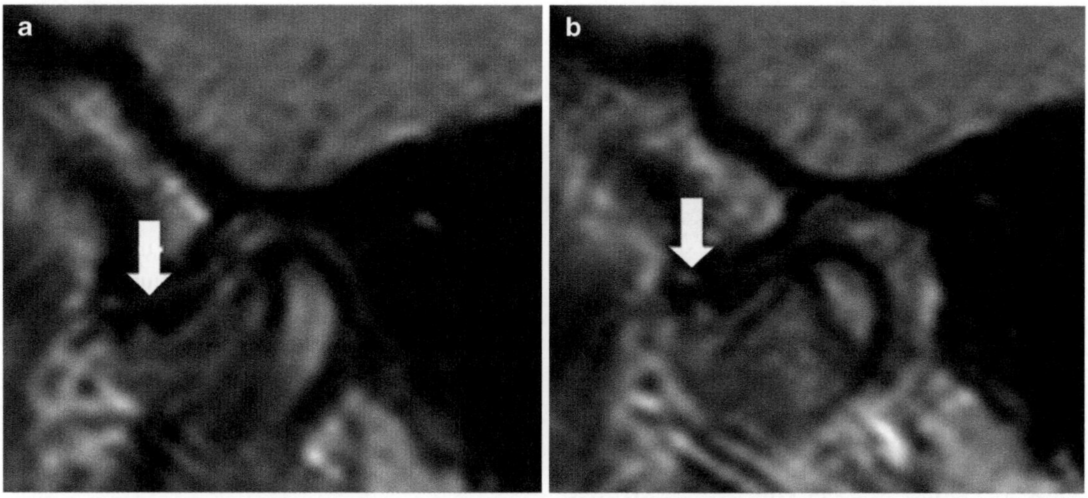

Fig. 7 Sagittal T1WI closed-mouth image (**a**) shows anterior disc displacement, with the disc (white arrow) positioned inferior to the crest of the articular eminence and the condyle situated posteriorly within the mandibular fossa. Assessment of the condylar position should consider its relationship with the fossa and the disc, not just the disc's relation to the condyle. In the sagittal T1WI open-mouth image (**b**), the disc (white arrow) exhibits a slight anterior movement yet remains inferior to the crest of the eminence, while the condyle remains positioned posterior to the crest of the eminence, indicating anterior disc displacement without reduction and limited mouth opening. The disc relatively retains its biconcave shape and anteroposterior dimension, suggesting an acutely displaced disc. (Courtesy P. Celenk, DDS)

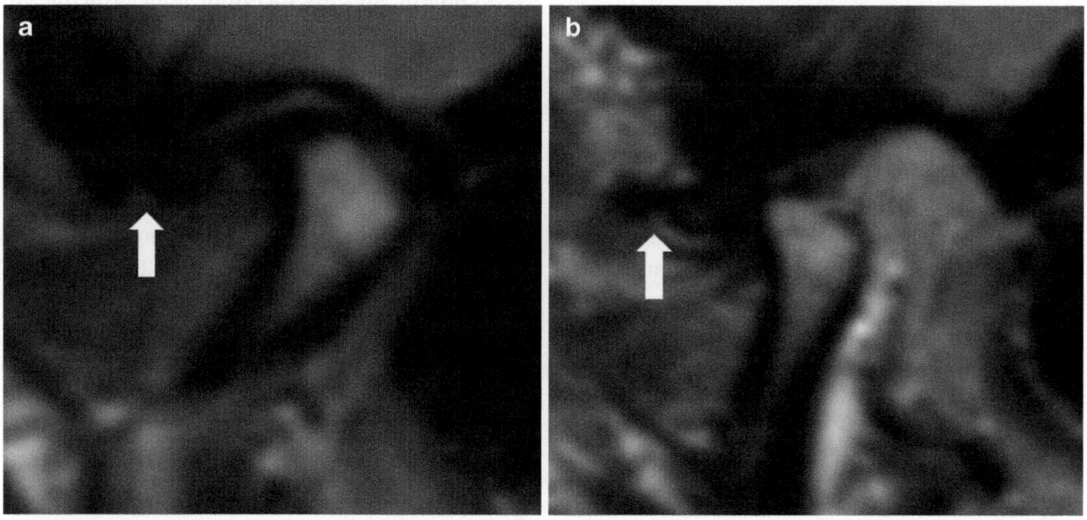

Fig. 8 (**a**) and (**b**) show anterior disc displacement without reduction on sagittal closed (**a**) and open (**b**) PD MR images. In the closed position, the condyle is positioned posteriorly in the mandibular fossa, and the disc (arrow) is slightly posterior to the crest of the articular eminence. In the open position, the condyle translates posterior to the crest of the articular eminence, and the disc (arrow) is anterior to the condyle and anteroinferior to the crest of the articular eminence. The disc maintains its biconcave appearance and anteroposterior dimension suggestive of an acutely displaced disc

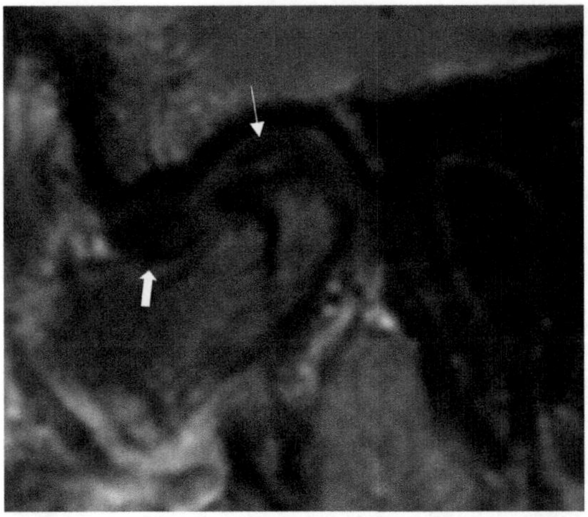

Fig. 9 The sagittal closed T1 MR image reveals osteophyte, sclerosis, and vertical height loss of the condyle, and flattening of the eminence consistent with degenerative joint disease, as well as a chronically anteriorly displaced disc (arrow) that has altered shape. A pseudodisc formation (thin arrow) can be seen posterior to the displaced disc and superior to the condyle. The thickening and fibrosis of the posterior attachment create a disclike appearance, which in some instances may be misinterpreted as a posteriorly displaced disc. (Courtesy ST Gokdeniz and K. Orhan, DDS)

tissues adapt, the range of motion is gradually regained, leading to a subsiding of symptoms (Figs. 7 and 8).

3.2.1 Bone Marrow Edema and Joint Effusion

During growth, the composition of bone marrow in the mandible undergoes a transformation, initially being predominantly hematopoietic marrow and gradually transitioning to mostly fatty marrow. On imaging sequences like T1WI and fluid-sensitive images such as T2WI with fat saturation or STIR, the signal intensity of the temporal and mandibular bones reflects the changing proportions of hematopoietic and fatty marrow. In infants, bone marrow signal intensity appears low on T1-weighted images (similar to muscle) and intermediate on fluid-sensitive sequences (appearing brighter than muscle but darker than fluid). As individuals age and the proportion of fatty marrow increases, the signal intensity eventually becomes the same as subcutaneous fatty tissue across all imaging sequences.

In acute trauma cases, the bone marrow can become edematous, resulting in a high signal intensity in the subchondral bone on T2WI. This signal is typically intermediate to low on T1WI or PDWI.

Joint Fluid

Similar to other synovial joints, the TMJ also contains a small quantity of joint fluid. This fluid is derived from plasma through a process known as dialysis and is secreted by the synovial membrane. Normal, physiological amount of joint fluid may not be apparent on T1WI. However, it becomes easily detectable on T2WI, where it appears as an area with high signal intensity, similar to other fluids (i.e., showing an isointense signal compared to cerebrospinal fluid). Small dots or lines of high signal intensity within the joint recesses, not exceeding 1 mm in width, can be considered a physiological amount of joint fluid. These should not be misinterpreted as joint effusion, which typically involves a larger fluid accumulation and can indicate an underlying medical condition.

Synovitis and the resulting joint effusion are best seen on T2WI, presenting as regions of increased signal intensity (hyperintensity) (Fig. 14). This fluid accumulation can happen within a single compartment or affect both, creating an "arthrographic effect" that accentuates the disc shape (Fig. 14).

If there is effusion in just one joint compartment, it can reveal a perforation in the disc or its attachments when the fluid leaks into the other compartment. Additionally, this fluid can demonstrate movement within a compartment during jaw opening, aiding in visualizing the detachment of the temporal posterior attachment (TPA) from the glenoid fossa. In cases of acute micro- or macro-trauma, the bone marrow can exhibit edematous changes, leading to a high signal intensity in the subchondral bone on T2-weighted images, while appearing intermediate to low signal intensity on T1- or PD-weighted images.

3.2.2 Subluxation

The most frequent TMJ subluxation or dislocation in a non-fractured mandible involves bilat-

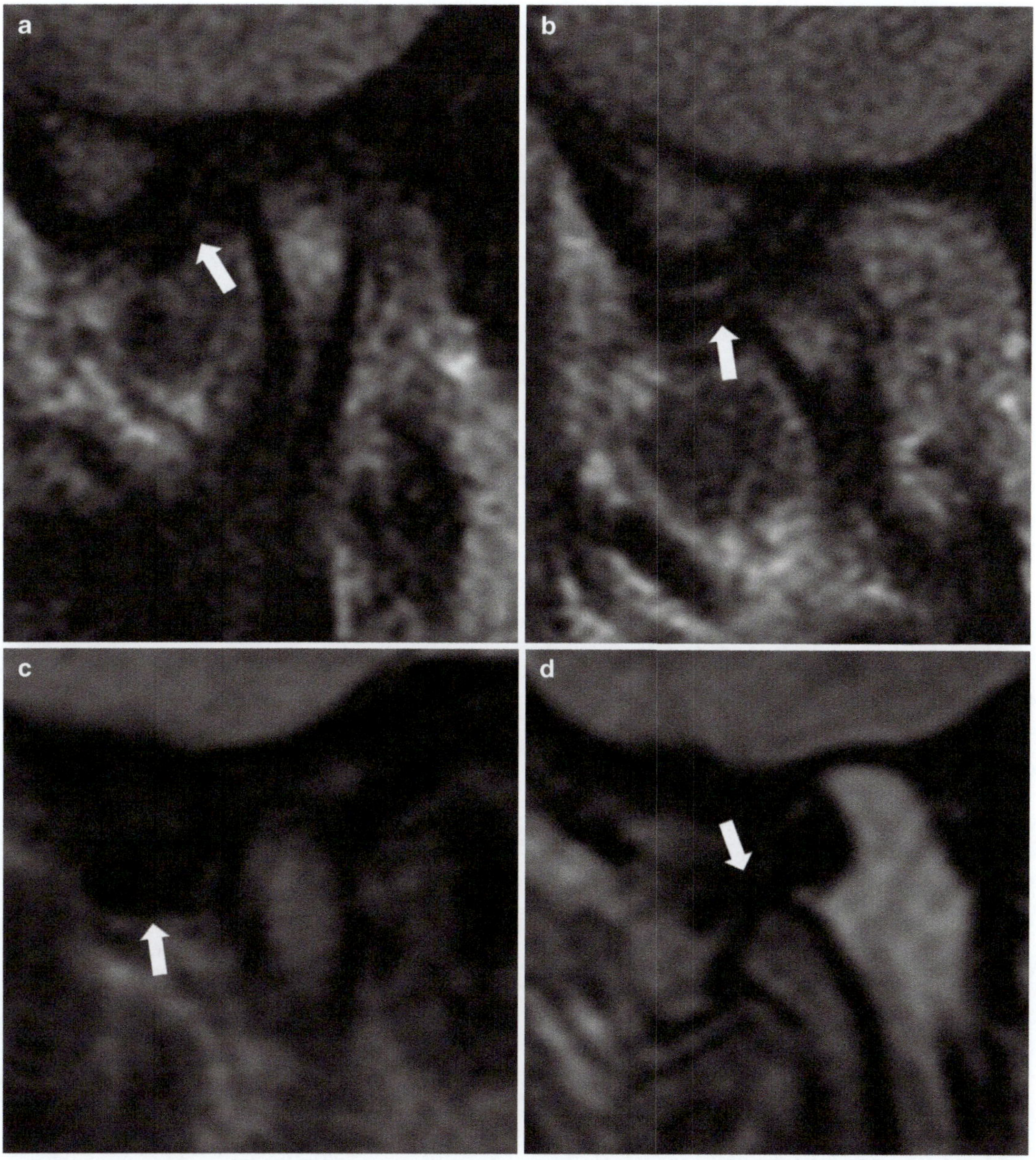

Fig. 10 Sagittal PD MR images show anterior disc displacement with reduction: In the closed view (**a**), the posterior band of the disc is located at the 9 o'clock position relative to the condyle. In the open view (**b**), the condyle translates to a position slightly posterior to the crest of the eminence, and posterior band of the disc is located between anterosuperior aspect of the condyle and posterior slope of the articular eminence consistent with partial reduction and slightly limited opening. (**c**) Sagittal view shows anteriorly displaced disc in the closed position. Upon opening (**d**), the condyle translates to a position just inferior and posterior to the articular eminence's crest suggestive of mild decrease in the range of motion, while the disc, situated between the joint surfaces, corresponds to the junction between the anterior band and the intermediate zone. In open-mouth position, the point of intersection between intermediate zone and anterior band should be positioned between the articular surfaces

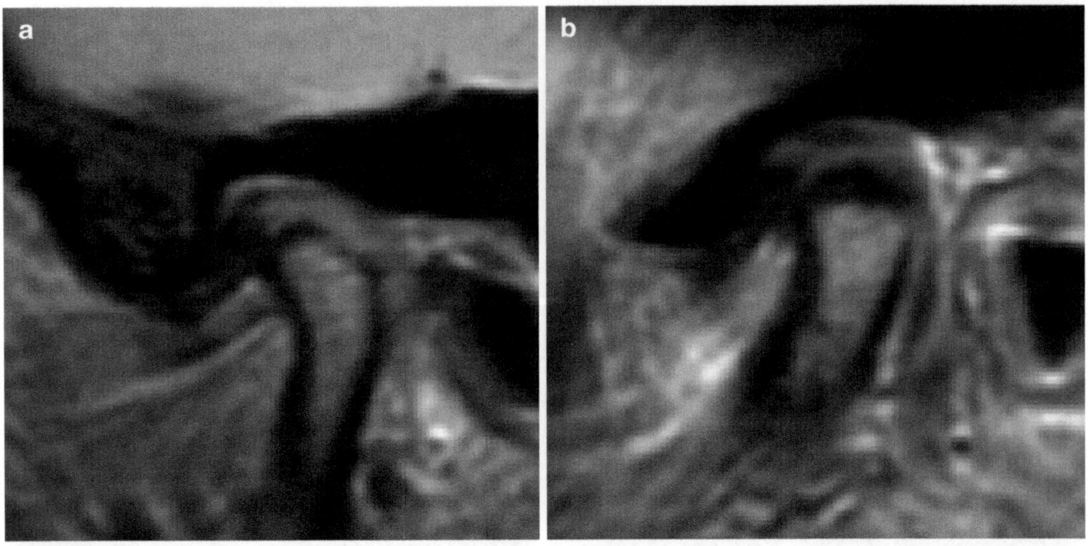

Fig. 11 PDWI sagittal images show anterior rotational disc displacement. (**a**) The central area of the TMJ displays a relatively normal disc-condyle relationship (11 o'clock position). (**b**) Meanwhile, in the lateral region of the TMJ, the posterior band of the disc is anterior to the condyle

eral dislocation of the mandibular heads anteriorly to the articular tubercles without spontaneous reduction.

The condyle is situated in an anterior and superior position relative to the crest of the eminence. Within this context, the part of the disc located between the bony elements is referred to as the anterior band, and it often sits between the posterior aspect of the condyle and the anterior slope of the eminence (Figs. 13 and 15). This hypermobility can be observed in patients with Ehlers-Danlos syndrome and joint laxity. In addition to neurological and neuromuscular conditions, the absence of posterior support due to advanced tooth loss is considered a predisposing factor for TMJ dislocation.

Typically, individuals in the age range of 25–45 years are affected. The most common triggers are routine activities that involve wide mouth opening, such as yawning, laughing, or biting. During clinical examination, an empty TMJ socket can be observed. Additionally, long-term dislocation may manifest signs of malnutrition in some cases.

Patients with symptoms that could suggest other differential diagnoses should undergo imaging examinations, including panoramic radiography, CBCT, and MRI. These diagnostic procedures can help to rule out facial fractures and give information for further treatment plans.

3.2.3 Disc Adhesion

To achieve a full range of jaw movement, it is essential for the condyle to rotate, moving along the inferior part of the disc. Furthermore, the mandibular condyle/disc pair must glide smoothly along the posterior aspect, vertex, and lower portion of the articular eminence. This arrangement provides wide mouth opening, lateral movement, protrusion, and retrusion.

Disc adhesion refers to the bands of connective tissue that connect the disc with the intracapsular structures. The fibrous connection of the disc can happen either in the superior compartment (which is more common and restricts motion to a greater extent) or in the inferior compartment. Jaw may deviate to the affected side during mouth opening. In cases of superior compartment adhesions, when the jaw opens, the condyle moves, but the position of the disc remains unchanged in comparison to its closed position (Fig. 16).

Adhesion of the disc to the articular fossa can eventually prevent the gliding of the disc, result-

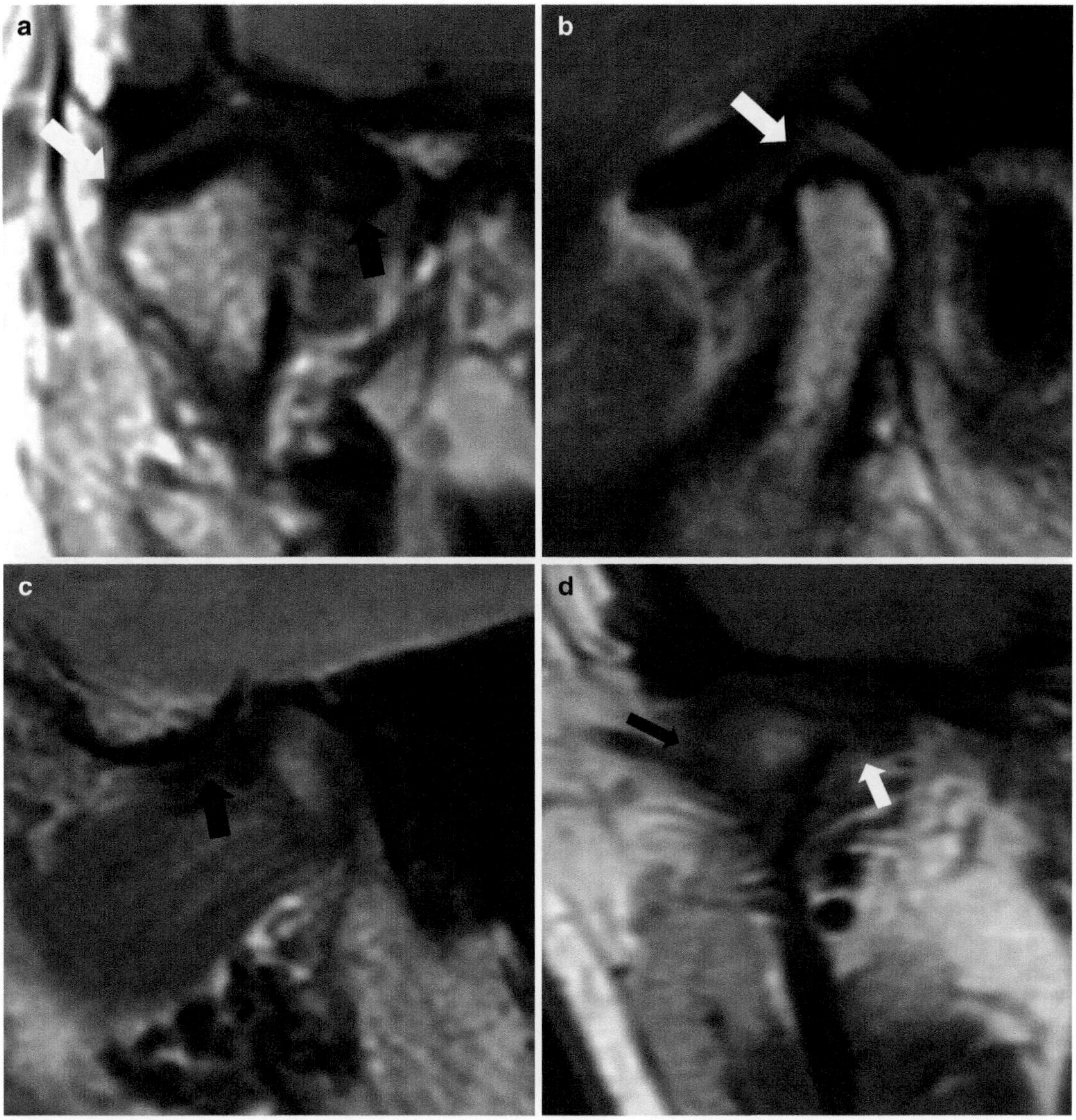

Fig. 12 PDWI coronal and sagittal images show sideways disc displacement: (**a**) Coronal image reveals a low-signal medial portion of the disc (black arrow), which is folded over the medial pole while the lateral superior portion is lacking the disc (white arrow). (**b**) Sagittal image depicts the absence of a posterior band of the disc superior to the condyle in the lateral portion of the TMJ (white arrow). (**c**) Sagittal image reveals a low-signal disc that is folded over the lateral pole in the lateral aspect of the TMJ (black arrow). (**d**) T1WI coronal view in a different patient illustrates anteromedial disc displacement. Medial portion of the disc folded over the medial pole (white arrow) while the lateral pole lacking the disc (black arrow). (Courtesy T Gokdeniz and K Orhan, DDS)

ing in a significant restriction of mouth opening. This attachment could mark the initial phase of a progression that may develop into anterior displacement with adhesion or even progress to osteoarthritis.

3.2.4 Functional Remodeling of the Temporomandibular Joint

Functional remodeling of the TMJ denotes the adaptive adjustments in the joint due to changes

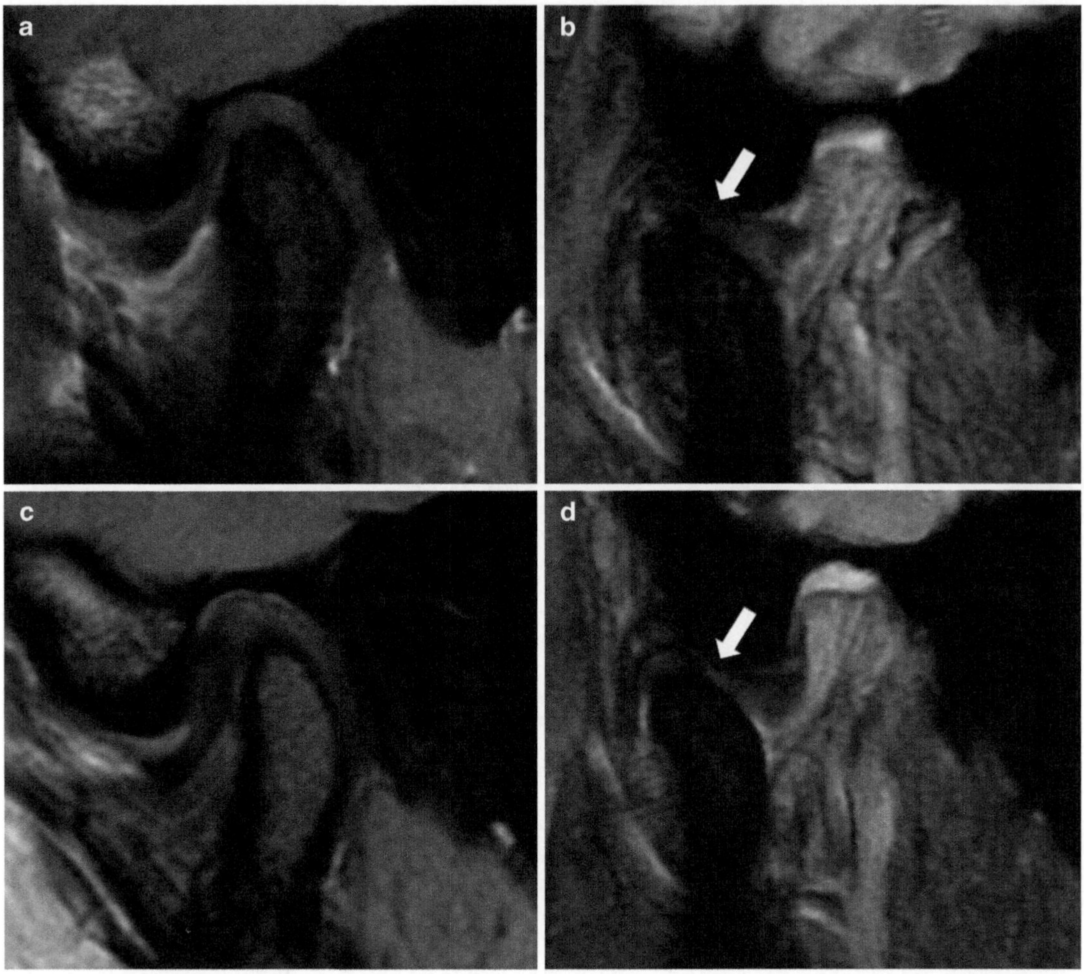

Fig. 13 T1WI (**a**) and PDWI (**b–d**) sagittal images show bilateral hypermobility and anterior disc displacement with reduction. In the closed-mouth position, the right condyle is centered (**a**), while the left condyle is posteriorly positioned (**c**) within the fossa, and the disc is anteriorly displaced on both sides. In the open-mouth position (**b** and **d**), both condyles translate to a point anterior and superior to the crest of the eminence. The intermediate zone of the disc is positioned between the posterior aspect of the condyle and the anterior slope of the eminence (arrows)

in functional requirements or conditions (Fig. 17). This dynamic phenomenon encompasses the modification of different components within the TMJ, such as the joint surfaces, articular discs, and related ligaments.

Functional remodeling can be prompted by various factors, such as muscle activity, patterns of jaw movement, and occlusion (bite) alterations. For instance, when there is an irregular jaw movement or abnormal bite, the TMJ may adaptively change to accommodate these functional requirements. These adaptations may involve modifying the position and form of the joint surfaces, remodeling the articular disc, and adjusting the alignment and tension of the related ligaments.

Functional remodeling is a multifaceted process that can differ based on individual factors like genetic makeup, age, and overall health. Functional remodeling is a normal occurrence

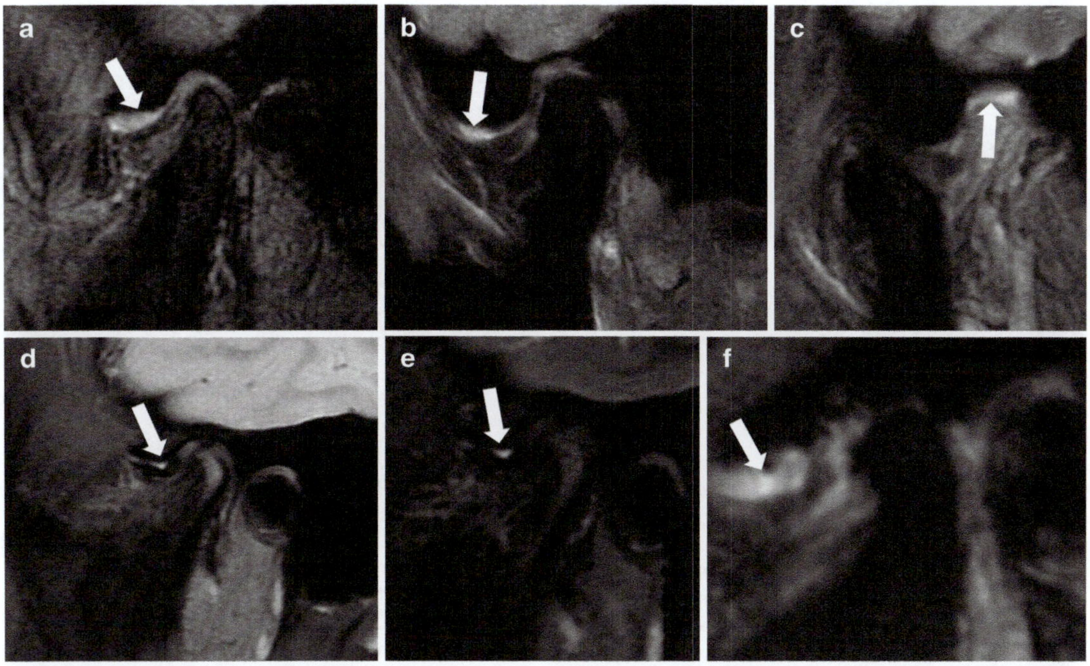

Fig. 14 Sagittal cross-section images show joint effusion. T2WI image (**a**) in closed position reveals mild to moderate joint effusion in the anterior recess of the superior compartment. MERGE image (**b**) in closed position shows the presence of synovial fluid within the anterior recess of the superior compartment, delineating the contours of the disc and its posterior attachment. In the MERGE image (**c**) of the same patient upon mouth opening, the fluid migrates to the posterior recess of the superior compartment. PD FS (**d**) and T2 STIR (**e**) images of a patient in open position illustrate mild joint effusion in the anterior recess of the superior compartment and limited condylar movement. MERGE image (**f**) of a different patient in closed position shows moderate joint effusion in the anterior recess of the superior compartment

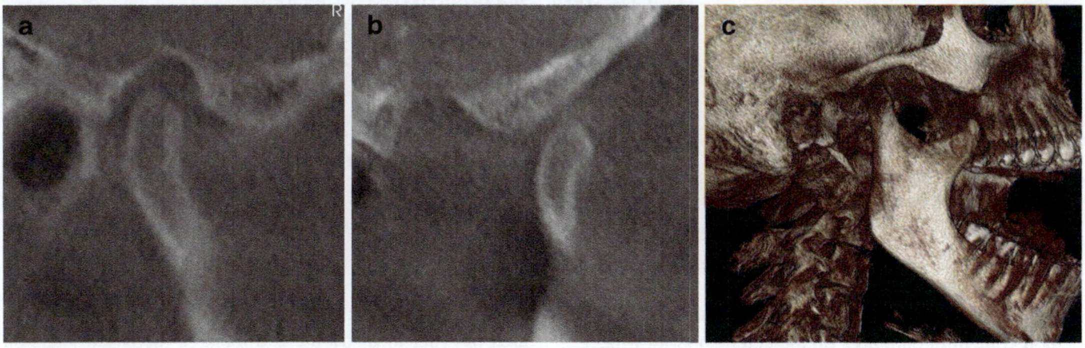

Fig. 15 CBCT sagittal cross-sectional images (**a** and **b**) and 3D volume rendering (**c**) show hypermobility. In the closed-mouth position (**a**), the condyle is located posteriorly within the fossa, while in the open-mouth position (**b**), the condyle translates to a point anterior and superior to the crest of the eminence (**b** and **c**)

that responds to functional needs and does not necessarily signify any pathology or dysfunction.

3.2.5 Degenerative Joint Disease

The terms degenerative joint disease (DJD), osteoarthritis, and osteoarthrosis are frequently

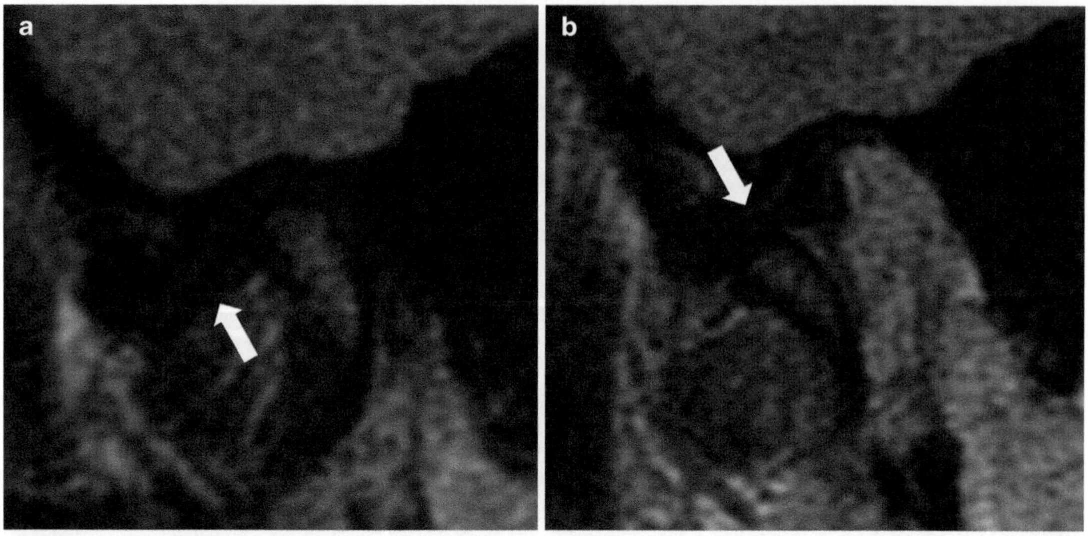

Fig. 16 PDWI sagittal views show hypomobility in the left TMJ. (**a**) In the closed position, the condyle is posteriorly positioned in the fossa, and the disc is anterior to the condyle (arrow). (**b**) In the open position, the position of the disc remains relatively unchanged relative to the fossa (arrow), while the condyle translates to the intermediate zone of the disc. These observations suggest adhesion in the superior compartment of the TMJ

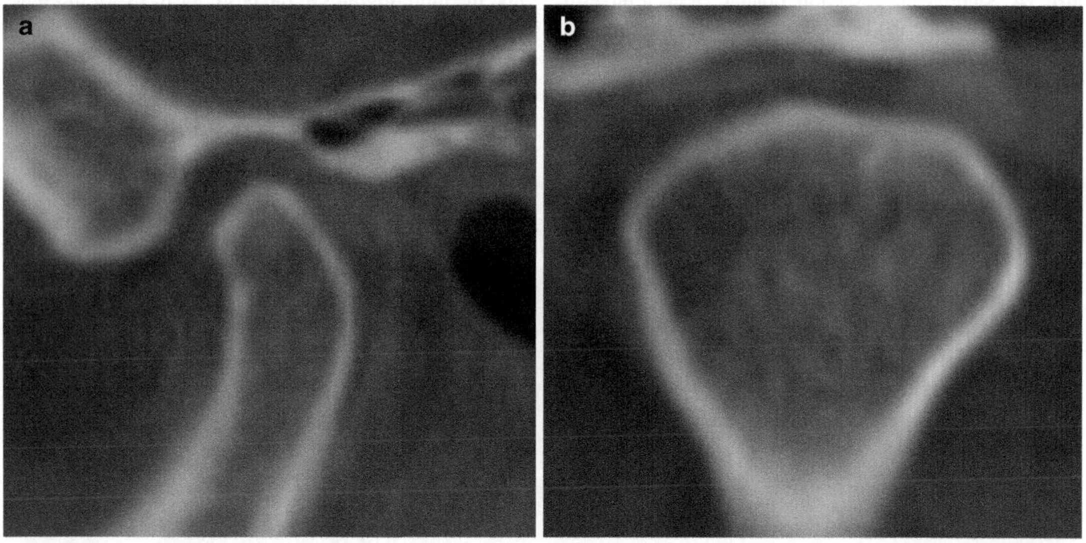

Fig. 17 CBCT axially corrected sagittal and coronal views demonstrate mild flattening on the anterosuperior aspect of the left condyle consistent with functional remodeling. This process represents the bone's effort to enlarge its surface area in order to distribute and manage increased loads on the joint surface. Sagittal (**a**) and coronal (**b**) views

used interchangeably. DJD is a noninflammatory degenerative condition that can develop in the TMJ. DJD occurs when the functional demands on the articular tissues exceed their remodeling capacity, leading to the destruction of these tissues. It can affect either a single joint or both joints bilaterally, and the progression of this condition may also vary between the two joints, leading to alterations in the shape and functionality of the mandible.

In the context of TMJs, primary DJD is considered idiopathic. Secondary DJD is generally assumed to occur after the displacement of the disc when there is bony contact between the condyle and the articular fossa. However, there have been reports suggesting that DJD can develop before disc displacement occurs.

DJD is typically diagnosed radiographically, as clinical signs and symptoms often have limited validity. Three key radiographic features indicative of a diagnosis of DJD include osteophytes, surface erosion, and subcortical pseudocysts. These features are illustrated in Figs. 9, 18, 19, 20, 21, and 22 and are described as follows:

- Osteophyte is characterized by marginal hypertrophy with sclerotic borders and angular, exophytic, osseous formation from the surface.

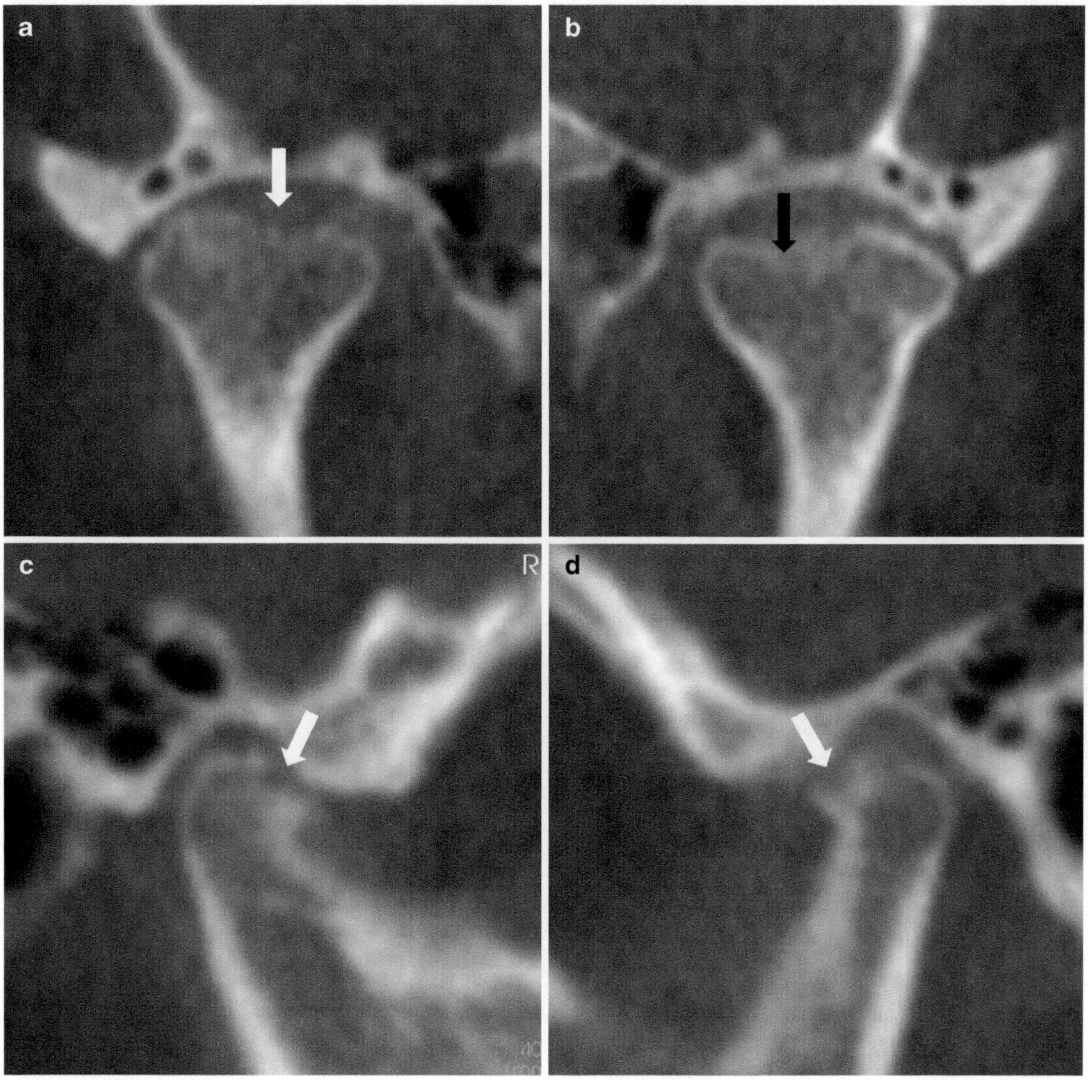

Fig. 18 Coronal (**a** and **b**) and sagittal (**c** and **d**) cross sections of right (**a** and **c**) and left (**b** and **d**) TMJs with active degenerative joint disease. Erosion and decortication are seen on anterosuperior articular surface of both condyles (white arrow), with visible hint of recortication and fuzzy appearance on the left (black arrow), indicative of healing process

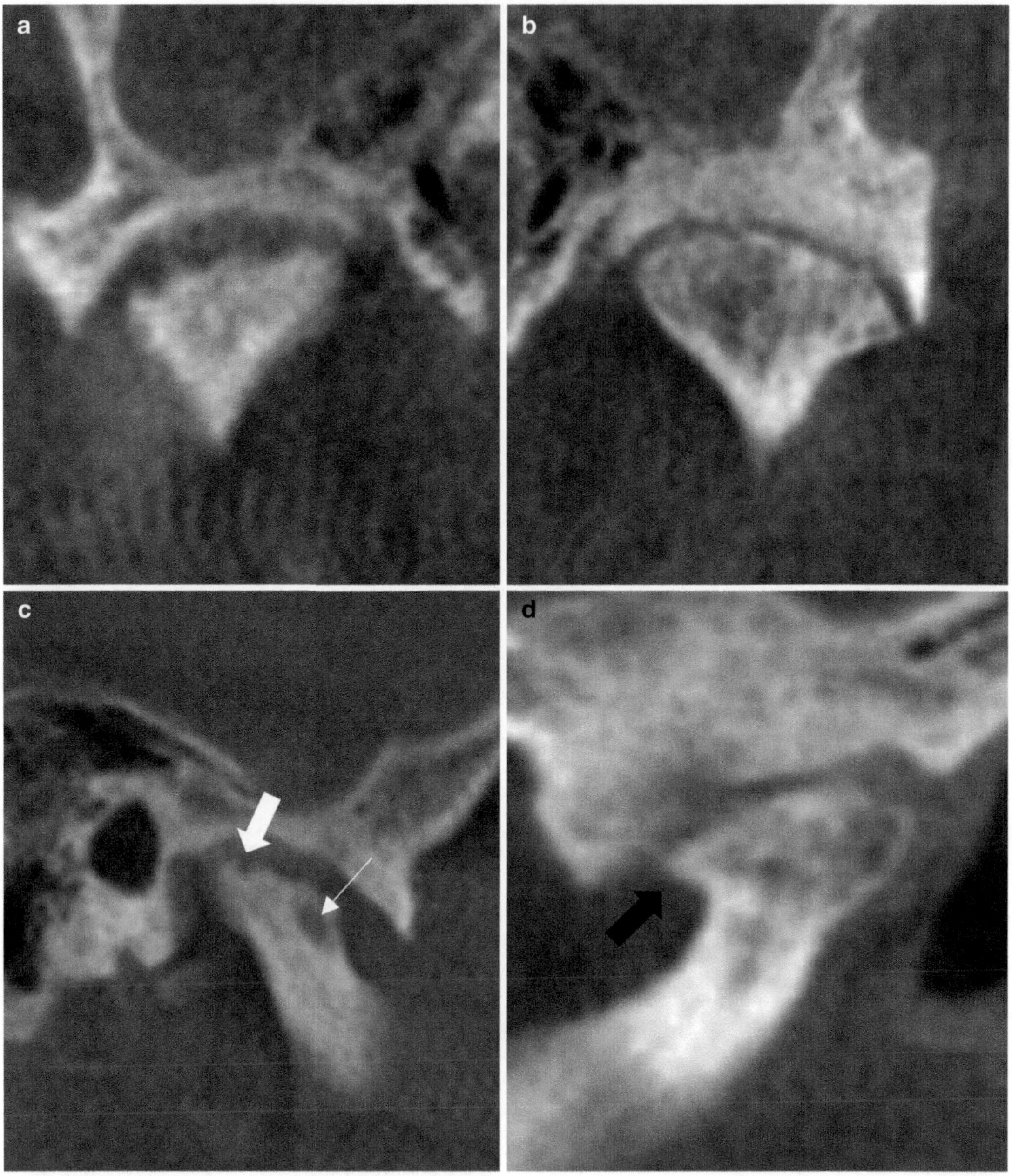

Fig. 19 Coronal (**a** and **b**) and sagittal (**c** and **d**) cross sections of right (**a** and **c**) and left (**b** and **d**) TMJs with severe degenerative joint disease. Bilateral condyles, articular eminences, and mandibular fossae show significant volume loss, severe flattening, and sclerosis. Notably, there is subchondral cyst on the right condyle (thin white arrow) close to proximal surface, thickening of the left mandibular fossa roof, vertical height loss in both condyles, and shallower mandibular fossae. Erosion and decortication on the superior articular surface of right condyle (white arrow) are consistent with active phase of the disease. Recortication and osteophyte on the anterior aspect of the left condyle (black arrow) showing that the disease has reached the stable stage

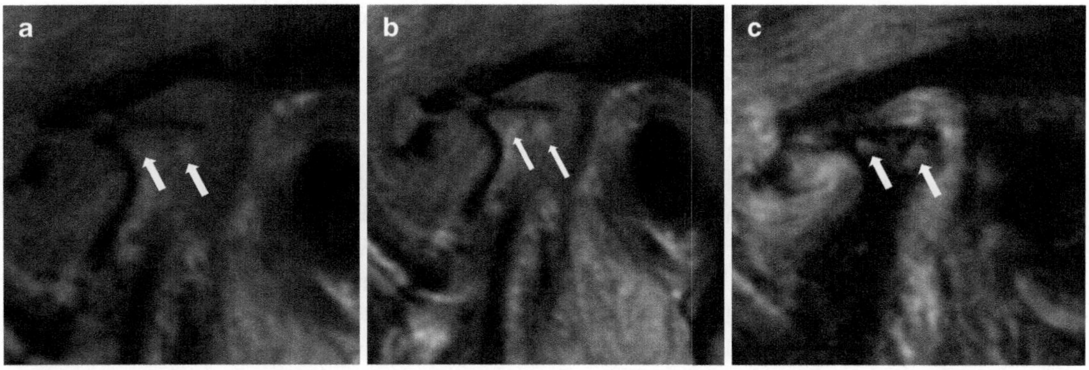

Fig. 20 Visualization of a subchondral bone cyst (arrows) using various MRI protocols on the same condyle; signal variations can be seen across different imaging sequences: (**a**) T1WI (**b**) PDWI, (**c**) MERGE. (Courtesy T. Gokdeniz, DDS and K. Orhan, DDS)

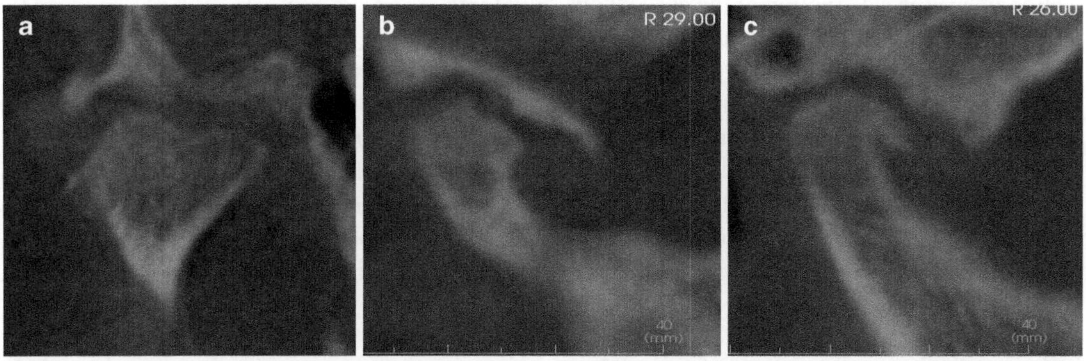

Fig. 21 Coronal (**a**) and sagittal (**b** and **c**) cross sections of the right TMJ show degenerative joint disease with significant vertical height and volume loss in the condyle and possible irregular cortical break on the mandibular fossa roof (**a** and **b**). Note large osteophyte in the anterior aspect of the condyle (**c**). The disease has not yet reached the stable phase

- Surface erosion refers to the loss of continuity in the articular cortex, which can occur in the condyle, fossa, or both.
- Subcortical pseudocyst (subchondral bone cyst, Ely cyst) is a cavity beneath the articular surface that deviates from normal marrow pattern. It is not a true cyst but rather represents the loss of trabecular bone structure in that area.

The above radiographic features play a critical role in diagnosing DJD.

Additional radiographic findings associated with potential osseous remodeling include articular surface flattening and subcortical sclerosis. These can be challenging to definitively diagnose as DJD because they may arise due to various factors, including aging, functional remodeling of the joints, or precursors to DJD. Over time, flattening and sclerosis can progress to DJD; as such, it would represent regressive remodeling or remain stable, reflecting adaptive remodeling (Fig. 17).

- Surface flattening refers to losing the rounded contour of the condyle or the articular eminence. It is important to note that this feature can be observed in normal, healthy joints and be a variation of the normal anatomy.
- Subcortical sclerosis is described as an increase in the thickness of the cortical plate in areas that bear the load in relation to adjacent non-load-bearing areas. This is often associated with increased loading of the joint or can occur with normal loading when there is disc displacement.

The initial phase of DJD begins on the superior surface of the mandibular condyle. It may be observed in axially corrected sagittal cross-section images as a disruption of the cortical outline and loss of trabecular structure beneath the surface (Figs. 18, 19, and 21). This stage is referred to as "active DJD." As the erosions go through a healing process and recorticate, the condyle undergoes a reduction in size, resulting in a loss of both vertical height and volume (Figs. 19 and 22). The process of recortication, whether partial or complete, on the articular surface is regarded as a component of the healing stage (Fig. 18).

When recortication is fully accomplished, DJD is considered in a "stable" phase (Figs. 19 and 22). Additional radiographic indicators of stable DJD include osteophytes, generally on the anterior aspect of the condyle, and loose articular bodies known as "joint mice," which can be considered synovial chondromatosis secondary to DJD (Fig. 23). It is important to note that if excessive forces are reintroduced, the entire process may reactivate, potentially leading to further erosion and loss of condylar volume. Reapplication of excessive forces can potentially reactivate the entire process, leading to new erosion and further loss of condylar volume.

3.2.6 Inflammatory Disorders

Rheumatoid Arthritis

Rheumatoid arthritis (RA) is a chronic inflammatory autoimmune condition with an unknown etiology. It is characterized by joint tenderness, swelling, and progressive destruction of synovial

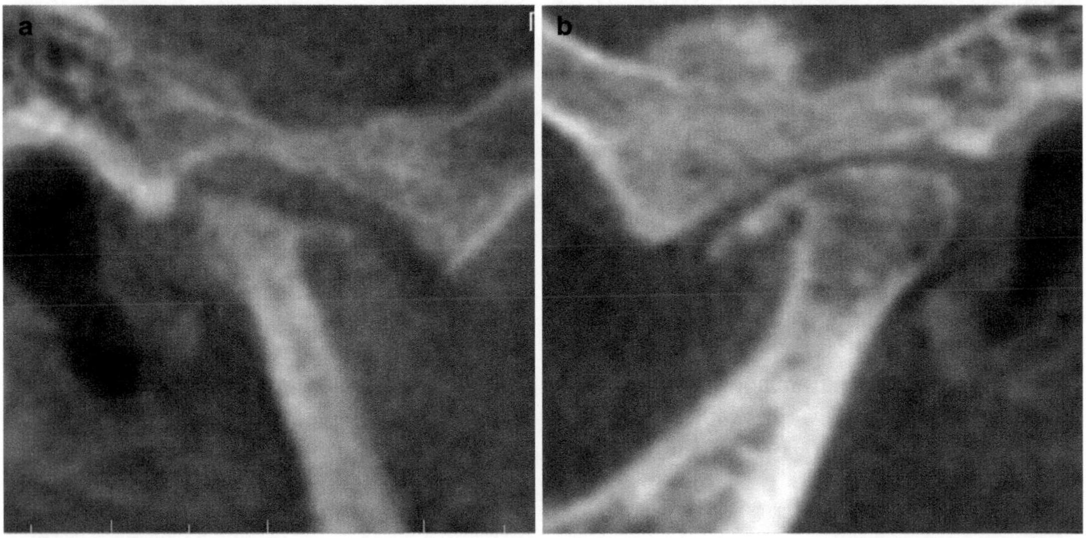

Fig. 22 The sagittal cross-sectional CBCT images (**a** and **b**) illustrate characteristic features of TMJ degenerative joint disease, including severe condylar flattening, vertical height loss, subchondral sclerosis, and presence of a large osteophyte. Recortication, more prominent on the left, is suggestive of a stable phase. The mandibular fossa and articular eminences are shallow and exhibit sclerosis, and flattening indicating the advanced nature of the disease

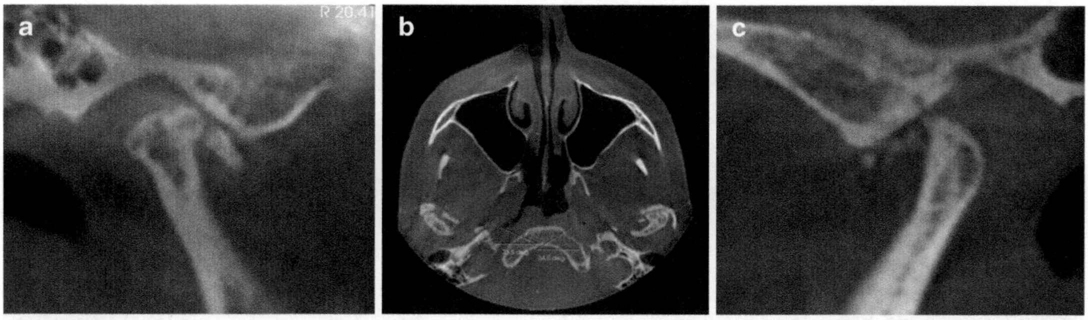

Fig. 23 CBCT sagittal (**a** and **c**) and axial (**b**) cross sections illustrate loose articular bodies (arrows) secondary to degenerative joint disease, also referred to as "secondary synovial chondromatosis" or "joint mice." While the osseous components of the TMJ exhibit degenerative joint disease changes, there is no mass effect typically associated with primary synovial chondromatosis

joints. This can result in severe disability and an increased risk of premature mortality. RA can result in synovitis, which, in turn, can lead to the formation of synovial granulation tissue, commonly referred to as pannus.

Joint involvement in RA typically follows a polyarticular distribution and often presents with symmetrically bilateral. Patients commonly experience chronic episodes of flare-ups and periods of remission. TMJ involvement in RA is rare despite the widespread polyarticular nature of the disease.

Juvenile idiopathic arthritis (JIA), also known as juvenile RA or Still's disease, is an autoimmune pediatric rheumatic condition. In JIA patients, TMJ involvement can be remarkably high, with rates reported as high as 87%, and TMJ can be the sole joint affected by JIA. Patients may be asymptomatic or show restricted jaw movement, mandibular asymmetry, and a class II malocclusion due to irreversible condylar resorption.

Imaging

The most frequent finding of RA is the erosion of the condylar head on a panoramic radiograph and flattening of the articular eminence, subchondral cyst, erosion, and reduced joint space on CT. On MRI, the most common findings are the abnormal (increased) signal intensity of the condylar bone marrow, high signal intensity in the joint space due to the fluid (synovitis), erosion of the condylar cortex, and resorption that may extend to more than half of the condylar head. The pannus usually exhibits an intermediate signal intensity on both T1- and T2WI. In JIA, CBCT can show bilateral flat and significantly misshapen condyles, often accompanied by a widened glenoid fossa, elongated and superiorly positioned coronoid processes, and clockwise rotation of the mandible, which can be attributed to the shortened condyles (Fig. 24).

In RA, there are some key differences compared to DJD:

- Disc position: In RA, the disc can remain in a normal position even in the presence of significant osseous changes. In contrast, in DJD, disc displacement is more common.
- Osteophyte formation: Osteophyte (bone spur) formation is not common in RA but is more frequent in DJD.
- Effusion: RA patients tend to have a higher frequency of joint effusion (accumulation of fluid in the joint) than patients with DJD.
- Condylar shape: The characteristic appearance of a condyle affected by RA resembles a "sharpened pencil." In DJD, the erosions on the condyle tend to display a pattern of focal erosions and subsequent loss of volume.

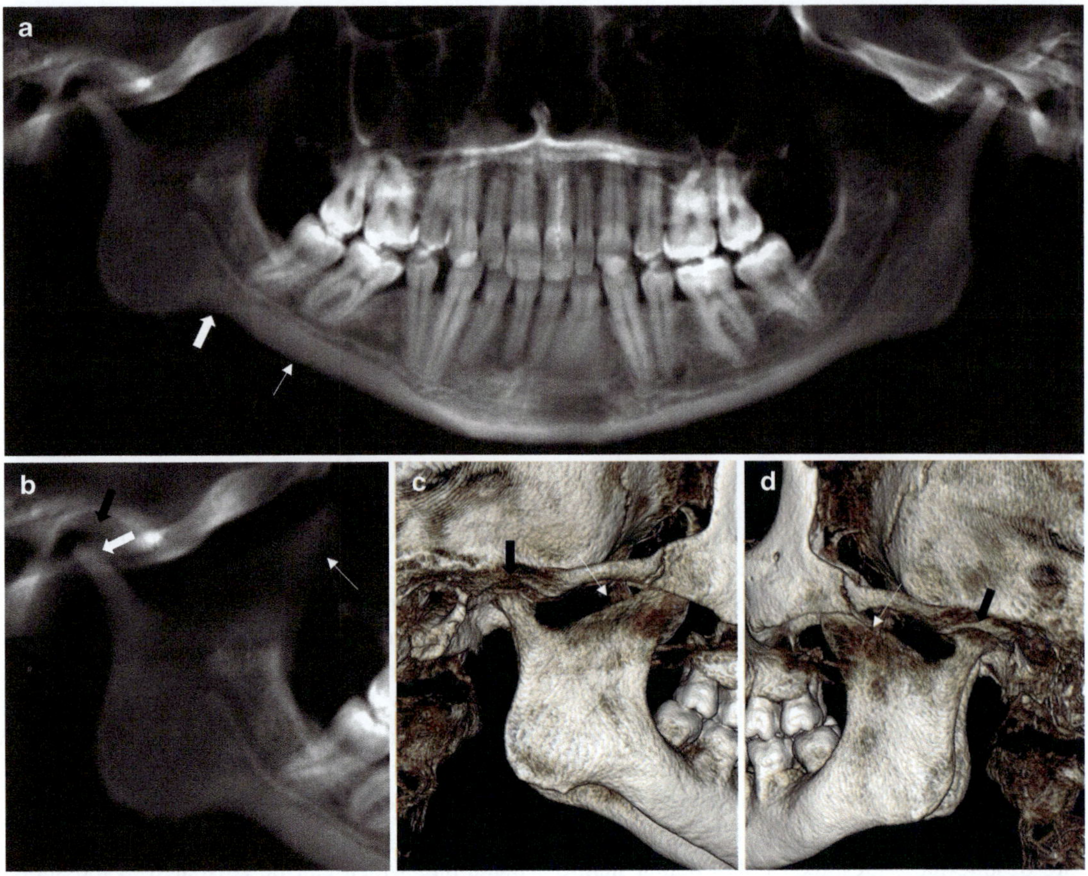

Fig. 24 CBCT reconstructions reveal marked changes in the bilateral TMJs in a young patient suspicious for juvenile rheumatoid arthritis and juvenile degenerative joint disease (idiopathic condylar resorption): panoramic reconstruction (**a**) demonstrates prominent antegonial notch (arrow), steep mandibular plane (thin arrow), and notably short mandibular rami. In a sagittal oblique view of the right mandible (**b**) and volume renderings of the right (**c**) and left (**d**) mandible, notable features include a condylar stump (white arrow), underdeveloped mandibular fossa, and eminence (black arrows) suggesting that this condition likely started earlier in life, prior to their full development and long coronoid process (thin arrows) compared to the condylar process

- Joint involvement: RA often affects TMJs bilaterally due to being a systemic autoimmune condition involving multiple joints throughout the body. DJD can affect either a single joint or both joints.

In certain instances, both conditions can coexist when there is a displacement of the disc and DJD develops simultaneously.

Synovial Chondromatosis

Synovial chondromatosis (SC) is a rare benign condition characterized by the proliferation of nodular cartilaginous or osteocartilaginous entities within the synovium of a joint. Over time, these entities ossify, detach, and are observed as loose bodies floating in the joint space.

Imaging

Panoramic radiographs can reveal signs of SC once the cartilage undergoes ossification. However, for a comprehensive diagnosis and treatment planning, CT and MRI are advised. MRI is particularly useful as it can display multiple nodular entities, whether cartilaginous or osseous in nature and joint effusion. On T1WI,

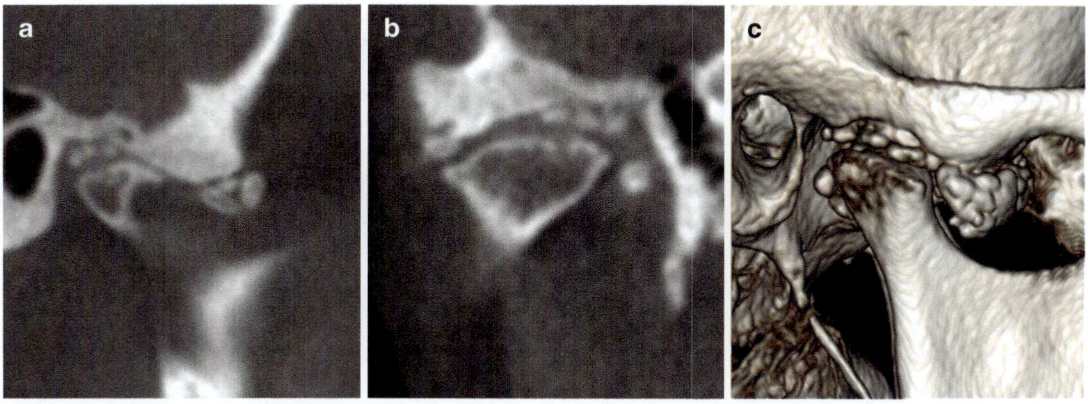

Fig. 25 Sagittal (**a**), coronal (**b**), and 3D volume-rendering (**c**) CBCT images illustrating primary synovial chondromatosis in the right (TMJ), displaying multiple well-defined calcified structures with low-density centers, in the superior, medial, and anterior aspects of the condyle and inferior to the crest of articular eminence. (Courtesy, M. Noujeim DDS)

heterogeneous and hypointense loose bodies are observed in the superior joint space. On T2WI, hyperintense effusion ± expansion and a "ring-like" signal caused by hyperintense fluid surrounding a group of hypointense loose bodies are commonly seen. These findings are indicative of the condition. On CT or CBCT, irregular joint surface, limited motion, widened joint space, calcified loose bodies, sclerotic mandibular condyle, and glenoid fossa can be seen (Fig. 25).

4 Summary

Imaging is a fundamental element in the assessment of the patient with suspected TMJ dysfunction and/or craniofacial pain. There are many imaging options available to characterize TMJ dysfunction, whether caused by congenital abnormalities or internal derangements. **Proceeding directly to imaging should be avoided**. A thorough physical exam is crucial for the formulation of a proper differential diagnosis and ordering of appropriate radiology.

Suggested Readings

1. Koenig LJ, Tamimi D, Perschbacher SE, Demirturk H. editors. Diagnostic imaging: oral and maxillofacial, 3rd ed. Elsevier; 2023.
2. Alsulaimani FF, Alswajy WA. Orthodontic management of anterior disc displacement without reduction. J Orthod Sci. 2022;11:30. https://doi.org/10.4103/jos.jos_24_22. eCollection 2022.
3. Ding L, Chen R, Liu J, Wang Y, Chang Q, Ren L. The effect of functional mandibular advancement for adolescent patients with skeletal class II malocclusion on the TMJ: a systematic review and meta-analysis. BMC Oral Health. 2022;22(1):51. https://doi.org/10.1186/s12903-022-02075-8.
4. Tamimi D, Kocasarac HD, Mardini S. Imaging of the temporomandibular joint. Semin Roentgenol. 2019;54(3):282–301. https://doi.org/10.1053/j.ro.2019.03.007. Epub 2019 Mar 11.
5. Poluha RL, Canales GT, Costa YM, Grossmann E, Bonjardim LR, Conti PCR. Temporomandibular joint disc displacement with reduction: a review of mechanisms and clinical presentation. J Appl Oral Sci. 2019;27:e20180433. https://doi.org/10.1590/1678-7757-2018-0433.
6. Kellenberger CJ, Junhasavasdikul T, Tolend M, Doria AS. Temporomandibular joint atlas for detection and grading of juvenile idiopathic arthritis involvement by magnetic resonance imaging. Pediatr Radiol. 2018;48(3):411–26. https://doi.org/10.1007/s00247-017-4000-0. Epub 2017 Nov 13.
7. Prechel U, Ottl P, Ahlers OM, Neff A. The treatment of temporomandibular joint dislocation. Dtsch Arztebl Int. 2018;115(5):59–64. https://doi.org/10.3238/arztebl.2018.0059.
8. Ahmad M, Schiffman EL. Temporomandibular joint disorders and orofacial pain. Dent Clin N Am. 2016;60(1):105–24. https://doi.org/10.1016/j.cden.2015.08.004. Epub 2015 Oct 21.
9. Melo DP, Oliveira LCAF, Carvalho ACA, Oenning ACC, Gonzaga AKG, Campos PSF. Temporomandibular joint disc adhesion: evi-

dence from magnetic resonance images. RGO—Rev Gaúch Odontol. 2014;62(2):169–72.
10. Barkin S, Weinberg S. Internal derangements of the temporomandibular joint: the role of arthroscopic surgery and arthrocentesis. J Can Dent Assoc. 2000;66(4):199–203.
11. Obwegeser HL, Makek MS. Hemimandibular hyperplasia-hemimandibular elongation. J Maxillofac Surg. 1986;14(4):183–208.

Temporomandibular Joint: Review of the Anatomy, Pathology, and Magnetic Resonance Imaging Techniques

Francisco Abaete Chagas-Neto, José Luiz de Sá Neto, and Paulo Moraes Agnollitto

1 Introduction: Acquisition Techniques and Protocols

MR is considered the most effective imaging technique for examining intra-articular processes within the temporomandibular joint (TMJ). **Its superior ability to provide high contrast resolution of soft tissues makes it the current gold standard for diagnosing disc disorders in the TMJ** [1, 2].

The assessment of the temporomandibular joint (TMJ) in a clinical setting may lack specificity due to the similarities in symptoms observed in cases of internal derangement and myofascial pain dysfunction. When there is a suspicion of an abnormality in the internal structure of the joint, it is advisable to include magnetic resonance imaging 1.5 or 3T (MRI) as a standard part of the evaluation process. MRI offers excellent resolution and tissue contrast, enabling a comprehensive assessment of both the anatomical and biomechanical aspects of the joint by capturing images with the mouth in both open and closed positions [1].

All patients undergoing TMJ MRI examination are positioned in a supine position with their arms adducted (Fig. 1). They are advised to remove any metallic objects, such as hairpins, coins, or earrings, to ensure accurate imaging and prevent interference. Before the procedure begins, the process is carefully explained to the patients to provide reassurance. They are informed about the duration of the examination and the importance of remaining still during the imaging process. This helps to minimize motion artifacts and obtain clear images [1, 3].

To conduct a dynamic study, patients are instructed to slowly open and close their mouths. This allows for the evaluation of movement and function during the examination. By following these instructions, patients can actively participate in the imaging process and contribute to the comprehensive assessment of their TMJs [4, 5].

When assessing the temporomandibular joints (TMJs), it is crucial to examine them while the mouth is closed and the teeth are in maximum intercuspation, meaning they are aligned in their most natural biting position (Fig. 2). This position allows for reliable evaluation of the spatial relationships between the TMJ components, ensuring an accurate diagnosis. Additionally, images taken with the mouth in the open position provide information about the position of the condyle (the round protrusion on the mandible) and the disc [4–6].

F. A. Chagas-Neto (✉)
TS Health Center, Hospital Geral de Fortaleza - HGF/One Laudos, Unifametro and Fatesa, Fortaleza, CE, Brazil

J. L. de Sá Neto
Department of Radiology and Diagnostic Imaging, Pontifical Catholic University's Hospital (PUC-Campinas), Campinas, SP, Brazil

P. M. Agnollitto
Radiology Division, Department of Medical Imaging, Hematology and Clinical Oncology, University of São Paulo, Ribeirão Preto Medical School, Ribeirão Preto, SP, Brazil

B. C. Stack Jr. et al. (eds.), *Craniofacial Pain*, https://doi.org/10.1007/978-3-031-57563-1_6

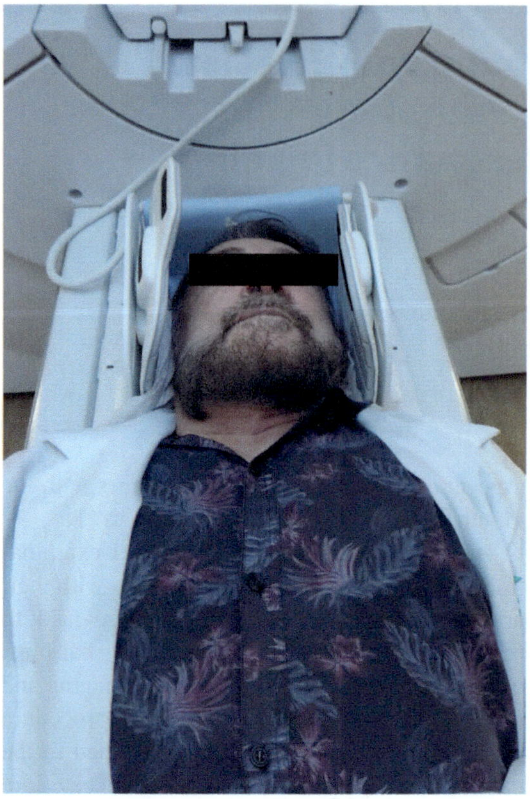

Fig. 1 Patient lying in supine position

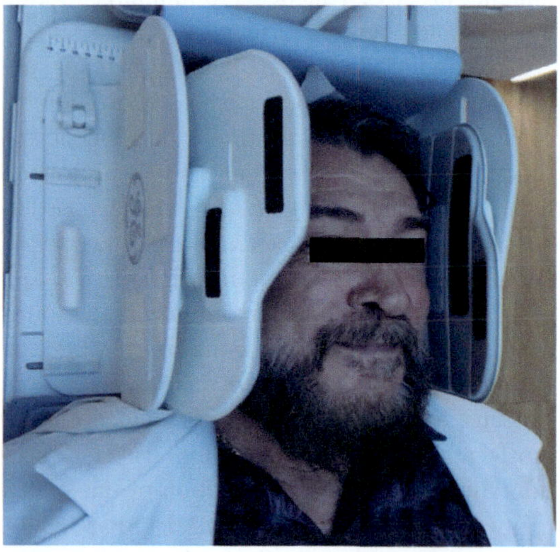

Fig. 2 Patient with closed mouth and aligned teeth in the natural biting position

For patients who are unable to maintain their mouths open and stable throughout the scanning process, a prefabricated mouth prop can be used

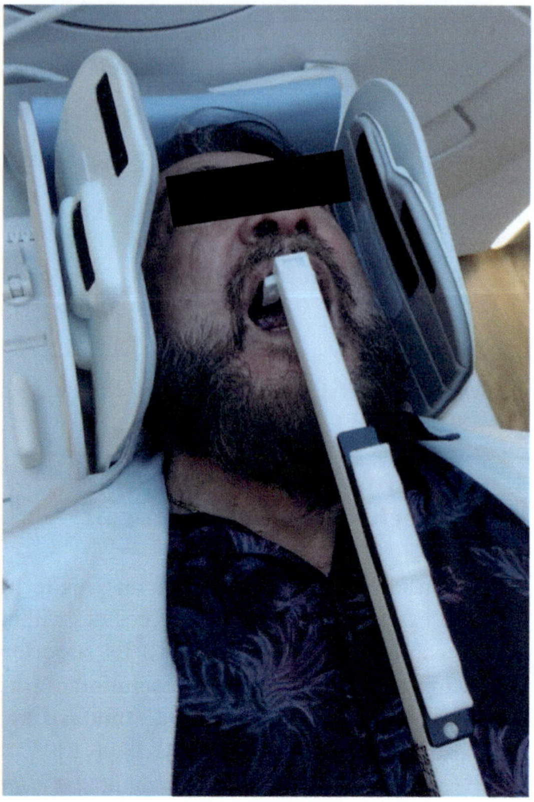

Fig. 3 Mouth prop device to evaluate the TMJ in the open mouth position

(Fig. 3). This device is designed to mimic and sustain the patient's maximum mouth opening, effectively stabilizing it during imaging. In some cases, a third scan may be requested with a splint inserted between the teeth. This splint, created by a dentist, alters the relationship between the condyle and the fossa (the concave depression in the temporal bone). It helps evaluate the impact of the splint on the position of the condyle and the surrounding soft tissues [5, 6].

Dual-surface coils are small bilateral coils used to provide excellent detail of the joint with a small field of view, high signal-to-noise ratio, and simultaneous bilateral acquisition (Fig. 4). Modern multichannel head coils and flexible coils with great parameters can also be used with satisfactory results (Fig. 5) [5].

The specific protocol for conducting an MR study of the temporomandibular joint (TMJ) can vary among different institutions. However, there are some key sequences that are com-

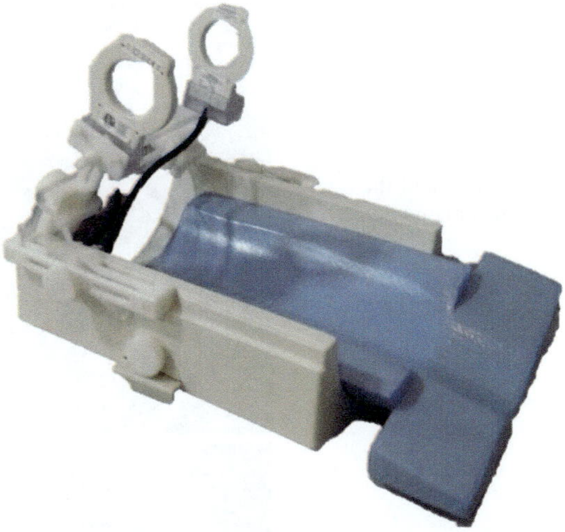

Fig. 4 TMJ's dual-surface coil

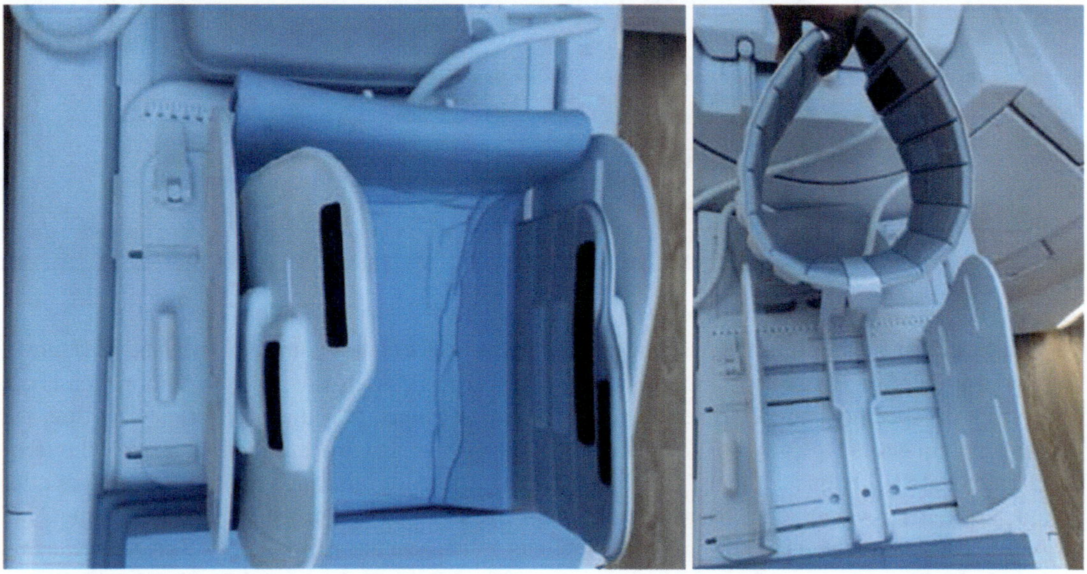

Fig. 5 Multichannel flexible coil

monly employed. Typically, the examination begins with an axial T1- or T2-weighted spin echo (SE) sequence, which uses a large field of view (FOV) to capture both temporomandibular joints. This sequence helps in planning the subsequent oblique sagittal and oblique coronal sequences (as shown in Fig. 6) and allows for comparison of the orientation of the mandibular condyles [7].

The next essential sequence is an oblique coronal T1-weighted sequence for each TMJ. This sequence is crucial for evaluating the morphology of the mandibular condyle and assessing the sagittal position of the disc relative to the condyle. Several oblique sagittal sequences are also fundamental. These sequences are used to evaluate the relative coronal position of the disc in relation to the condyle, which is often the most significant finding in TMJ assessment. Typically, a T1-weighted or proton density (PD)-weighted SE sequence is used, and some institutions opt to acquire both sequences to enhance the sensitivity and specificity of the examination. It is important to evaluate the relationship of the disc with the osseous structures both in the resting position and during the open-mouth position. Lastly, a

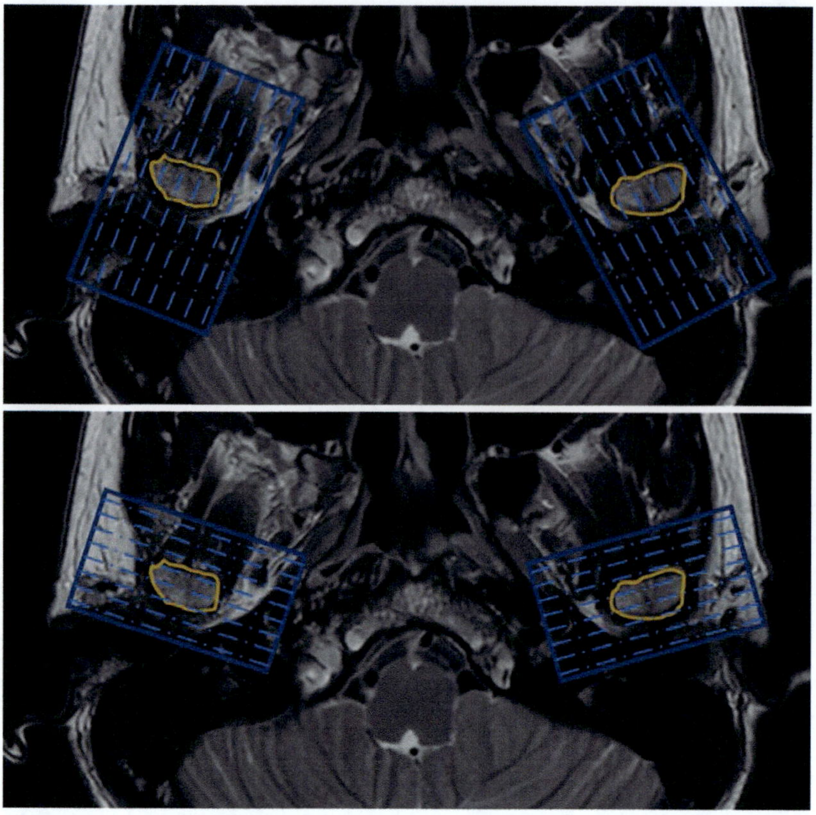

Fig. 6 Large FOV T2-weighted axial sequence. Planning of oblique coronal and oblique sagittal sequences according to the orientation of the mandibular condyle

T2-weighted fast spin echo (FSE) sequence is employed to identify and assess joint effusion.

Overall, the specific sequences used may vary, but the key sequences typically include axial T1- or T2-weighted SE, oblique coronal T1-weighted, oblique sagittal T1-weighted or PD-weighted SE (or both), and T2-weighted FSE for joint effusion evaluation [6, 8].

Dynamic information of the temporomandibular joint (TMJ) can be captured using MR imaging through a technique called progressive image acquisition. This involves acquiring static images using spin echo techniques at gradual intervals from the closed position to the open position. These images are then displayed sequentially in a back-and-forth closed cine loop, creating a dynamic visual representation of the TMJ movement [7, 8].

In addition to spin echo techniques, some researchers have explored the use of a balanced steady-state free procession (bSSFP) sequence for dynamic MR imaging of the TMJ. This sequence, typically performed at a magnetic field of 3T, offers advantages in terms of imaging speed and contrast. It allows for the assessment of dynamic TMJ movements and can provide valuable information about the joint function and any abnormalities. Both the progressive image acquisition with spin echo techniques and the utilization of bSSFP sequences offer ways to capture dynamic information during TMJ imaging, enabling a more comprehensive evaluation of the joint's movement and functionality [7, 8].

Intravenous contrast is ordinarily not needed and may be used in suspected inflammatory disorders (such as juvenile idiopathic arthritis) or in suspected malignancy. We provide at the end of the chapter some examples of protocols from different institutions [9].

While MR is a valuable imaging modality for evaluating temporomandibular joint (TMJ) disorders, it does have some limitations. MR is not capable of capturing biochemical alterations and early pathological changes in the TMJ disc and related muscles before structural damage becomes evident. Additionally, MR may be less sensitive in detecting bony components of the TMJ compared to cone beam CT. These limitations can result in a non-comprehensive evaluation, potentially leading to misdiagnosis and mistreatment of TMJ disorders. However, in recent decades, there have been advancements in MRI hardware and techniques, resulting in significant improvements in image quality and the ability to perform real-time dynamic imaging of TMJ disorders [10–12].

Furthermore, with the development of various MRI sequences and sophisticated post-processing algorithms, quantitative and functional evaluation of multiple biochemical properties of TMJ structures has become feasible. These advancements allow for a better understanding of the TMJ structures and a deeper comprehension of its disorders [8, 12].

Additionally, the novel technique of zero echo time (ZTE) has been introduced, which has achieved comparable diagnostic value for detecting osseous abnormalities in the TMJ within an MRI setting.

Overall, while MRI has its limitations, ongoing advancements in hardware, techniques, and post-processing algorithms have enhanced its capabilities, enabling improved image quality, real-time dynamic imaging, and quantitative assessment of TMJ structures. These developments contribute to a more comprehensive evaluation and better understanding of TMJ disorders and will ultimately help its early diagnosis, treatment planning, therapeutic efficacy evaluation, and even image-guided intervention. To validate the reliability of previous findings and delve deeper into the clinical significance of advanced MRI techniques in various temporomandibular disorder (TMD) scenarios, additional research involving a substantial number of patients is necessary. A summary of recent advanced MRI techniques in TMD is shown in Table 1 [4, 8, 12].

Table 1 Summary of recent advanced MRI techniques in TMD imaging

MR technique	Sequence	Basic principles	Advantages	Disadvantage	Applications in TMJ
DWI	FSE	Incorporates diffusion-sensitizing gradients into T2-weighted spin-echo (SE) sequences, typically utilizing echo planar imaging	– Measurement of diffusion properties	– Susceptibility artifacts	– Establishes a correlation between ADC values and the perception of pain in masticatory muscles
Real-time imaging	GRE, SE	Employs rapid sequences with high-efficiency k-space pathways (such as radial) and employ sophisticated reconstruction algorithms, occasionally incorporating parallel imaging techniques	– Optimal temporal resolution – Satisfactory image fidelity – Swift acquisition	– Restricted volumetric imaging capability – Complex reconstruction processes – Necessity for specialized computational hardware	– Captures the dynamic and natural motion of the TMJ under (patho) physiological conditions
DTI		Enhances the basic DWI by incorporating a minimum of six independent sensitizing gradients, followed by conducting an analysis of eigenvectors and eigenvalues	– Visualization of fiber orientations – Measurement of directional diffusion anisotropy	– Inadequate spatial resolution – Lack of a standardized protocol	– Visualizes collagen fibers within the TMJ disc and fiber bundles within masticatory muscles in vivo – Quantifies the alterations in DTI parameters before and after treatment

(continued)

Table 1 (continued)

MR technique	Sequence	Basic principles	Advantages	Disadvantage	Applications in TMJ
IVIM		Expands the mono-exponential DWI model to a biexponential model incorporating multiple b values	– Measurement of both diffusion and perfusion characteristics	– Geometric distortions	Establishes a connection between IVIM parameters and various TMD conditions
UTE	UTE sequence	Employs a brief radiofrequency (RF) pulse and initiate data acquisition promptly after the completion of excitation. The data collection takes place simultaneously with the activation of the readout gradient	– Collecting signals from tissues characterized by ultrashort T2 relaxation times	– Dependence on high gradient performance – Restricted availability of suitable software – Extended acquisition durations	– Visualize the TMJ disc, fibrocartilaginous surface, and condylar morphology – Evaluate osseous alterations associated with TMD – Measure the biochemical properties of the TMJ disc
T2 mapping	SE	Incorporates multiple TEs within a single TR and employ exponential decay curve fitting to ascertain T2 relaxation times using signals acquired at each TE	– Simple – Measurement and evaluation of biochemical characteristics	– Magic angle effect – Sensitivity to joint effusion	– Establishes a correlation between T2 values and the pain in masticatory muscles and alterations in condylar bone marrow – Facilitates ultrastructural analysis to examine the composition of the TMJ disc and retrodiscal tissue

TMD temporomandibular joint disorders, *TMJ* temporomandibular joints, *GRE* gradient echo, *SE* spin echo, *FSE* fast spin echo, *DWI* diffusion-weighted imaging, *ADC* apparent diffusion coefficient, *IVIM* intravoxel incoherent motion, *DTI* diffusion tensor imaging, *UTE* ultrashort echo time

2 MRI TMJ Anatomy and Biomechanics

Interpreting TMJ imaging requires an understanding of the normal anatomy of the joint. The TMJ is an unusual synovial joint in that the articular surfaces are covered with fibrocartilage rather than hyaline cartilage, located between the glenoid fossa of the temporal bone and the mandibular condyle. There are four main anatomical components of the temporomandibular joint. These components consist of the mandibular condyle, the mandibular fossa, the articular eminence of the temporal bone, and the articular disc (also known as the articular meniscus). The articular disc plays a crucial role in the function and dysfunction of the joint, as explained in the following sections. It is a biconcave fibrocartilaginous structure that can be divided into three distinct zones: an anterior thick band, a posterior thick band, and a thinner intermediate zone. By separating the articular synovial space into two separate compartments (superior and inferior) unless there is a disc rupture, the articular disc plays a critical role [13, 14].

Additionally, there are other significant anatomical structures within the temporomandibular joint. One such structure is the lateral pterygoid muscle, which is divided into two heads or bellies. While the attachments of these heads may vary, the inferior head typically inserts onto the anterior aspect of the mandibular condyle, while the superior head may attach exclusively to the anterior band of the articular disc or both the disc and the condyle. Both heads actively contribute to the mastication process and jaw movements. In cases of temporomandibular joint dysfunction, it is believed that the inferior head functions as a stabilizer of the joint and may undergo morphological changes due to hyperactivity, which should be assessed and reported in MRI scans [15–18].

Another important anatomical area is the bilaminar zone, also known as the retrodiscal tissue. This zone is located posteriorly to the posterior band of the articular disc and consists of two retrodiscal layers (superior and inferior) with neurovascular structures in between. These layers are continuous with the posterior band of the disc and act as ligaments that help maintain the proper placement of the disc. It is essential to actively evaluate this area in MRI scans because a rupture in these layers may be the cause or consequence of disc luxation and temporomandibular joint dysfunction.

In addition to these structures, the temporomandibular joint is further stabilized by various extra-articular structures, including the temporomandibular, sphenomandibular, and stylomandibular ligaments, as well as the medial pterygoid, masseter, temporal, and suprahyoid muscles. The mentioned anatomical structures of the temporomandibular joint are illustrated in Fig. 7 [13–15, 18].

On MRI scans, the condyle exhibits a high signal intensity on T1-weighted images due to the presence of marrow fat. Both the cortical bone and the disc display low signal intensity on both T1-weighted and T2-weighted images. This is attributed to their low proton density and short T2 relaxation times. However, there are instances where the central portion of the disc may exhibit

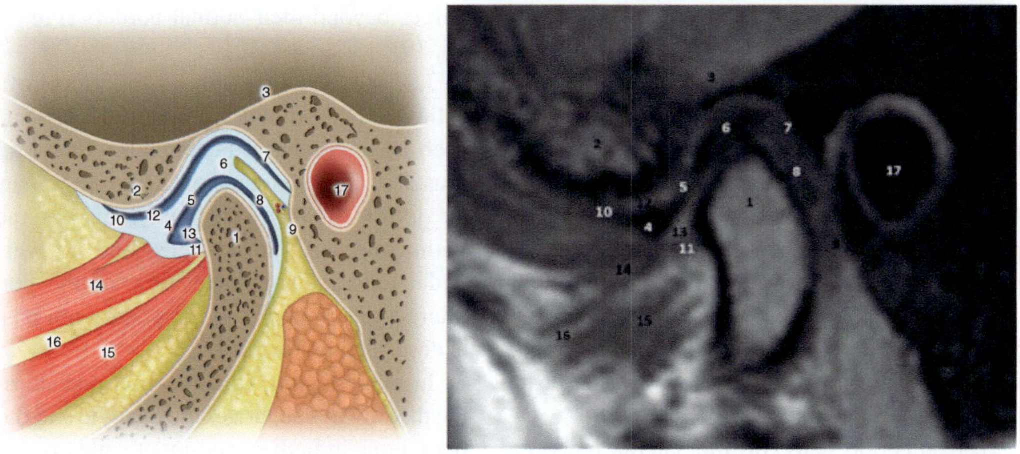

Fig. 7 Illustration and MRI of TMJ anatomy. (1) Mandibular condyle; (2) articular eminence of temporal bone; (3) mandibular fossa; (4) articular disc (anterior band); (5) articular disc (intermediate zone); (6) articular disc (posterior band); (7 and 8) bilaminar zone (superior and inferior retrodiscal layers); (9) bilaminar zone (neurovascular structures); (10 and 11) superior and inferior capsular insertions; (12 and 13) superior and inferior joint recesses; (14 and 15) superior and inferior heads of the lateral pterygoid muscle; (16) interpterygoid space; (17) external auditory canal

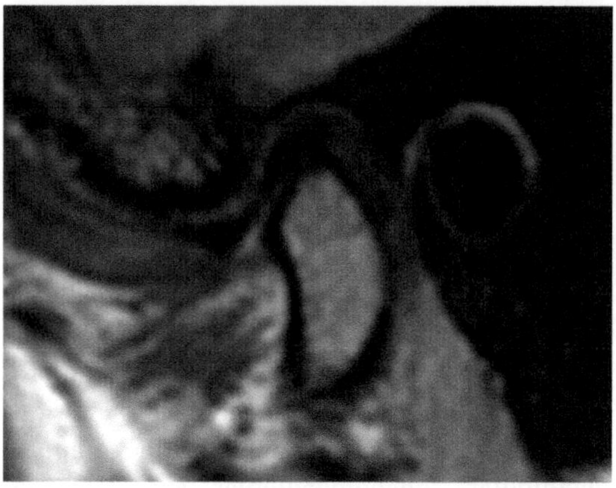

Fig. 8 MRI TMJ anatomy. Note the slightly hyperintense signal of the intermediate zone and the center of the posterior band

high signal intensity on T2-weighted and proton density images, resembling the hydration pattern seen in the central region of a vertebral disc. Apart from this, the disc appears homogeneous, hypointense, and biconcave in shape [15, 16].

The center of the posterior band of the disc may exhibit slight hyperintensity due to the presence of loose areolar tissue (Fig. 8). The posterior attachment of the disc appears to have higher signal intensity than muscle on proton density- and T1-weighted images, primarily due to the presence of fatty tissue. The bilaminar zone, seen as structures with intermediate signal intensity, is visible as well [14, 18].

In the closed-mouth position, the junction between the posterior band and the posterior attachment is typically located above the condylar head, close to the 12 o'clock position. The posterior band and retrodiscal tissue are best visualized in the open-mouth position. In this position, the intermediate zone of the disc lies between the condyle and the articular eminence, while the posterior band rests against the posterior surface of the condyle [19].

The superior belly of the lateral pterygoid muscle attaches to the anterior band of the disc, while the inferior belly of the lateral pterygoid attaches to the anterior surface of the condylar neck via a thin linear hypointense fibrous band (Fig. 7). This band is situated just below the position of the disc and can sometimes be mistaken

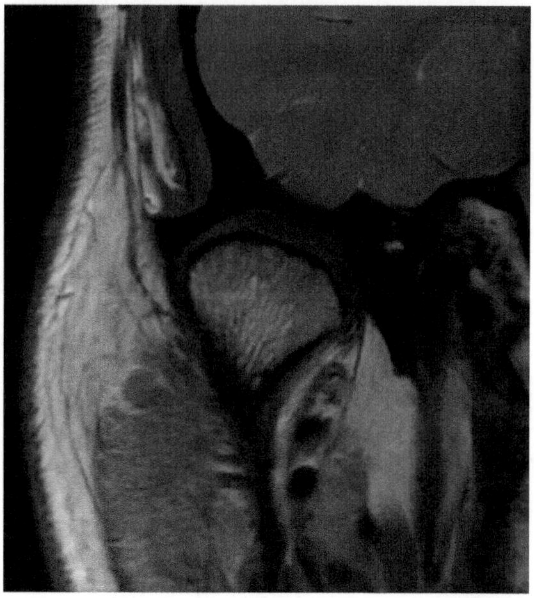

Fig. 9 MRI TMJ anatomy in the coronal plane. The disc is crescent shaped, and no abnormal bulges are seen beyond the borders of the lateral and medial capsules

for the disc, particularly when the disc is displaced medially or laterally. In the coronal plane, the disc appears crescent-shaped, with its medial and lateral borders attaching to the respective aspects of the condylar head and joint capsule. The lateral and medial capsules do not exhibit any outward bulges beyond their normal borders (Fig. 9) [14, 16, 19].

Jaw movement requires a high level of interaction and coordination among various structures such as the bilateral mandibular condyles, disc, muscles, and ligaments of the temporomandibular joints (TMJs). The functional interactions within the TMJ are complex and not yet fully understood. A simplistic view of the complex interactions in open- and closed-mouth positions is described below [20].

In a healthy joint, the thin intermediate zone of the disc always separates the condyle and the temporal bone in both closed-mouth and open-mouth positions to prevent articular damage. The disc is positioned between the condyle (inferiorly) and the glenoid fossa (superiorly), while the articular eminence is located anterior to the disc. Normally, the disc is aligned so that the anterior band is in front of the condyle, and the junction of the poste-

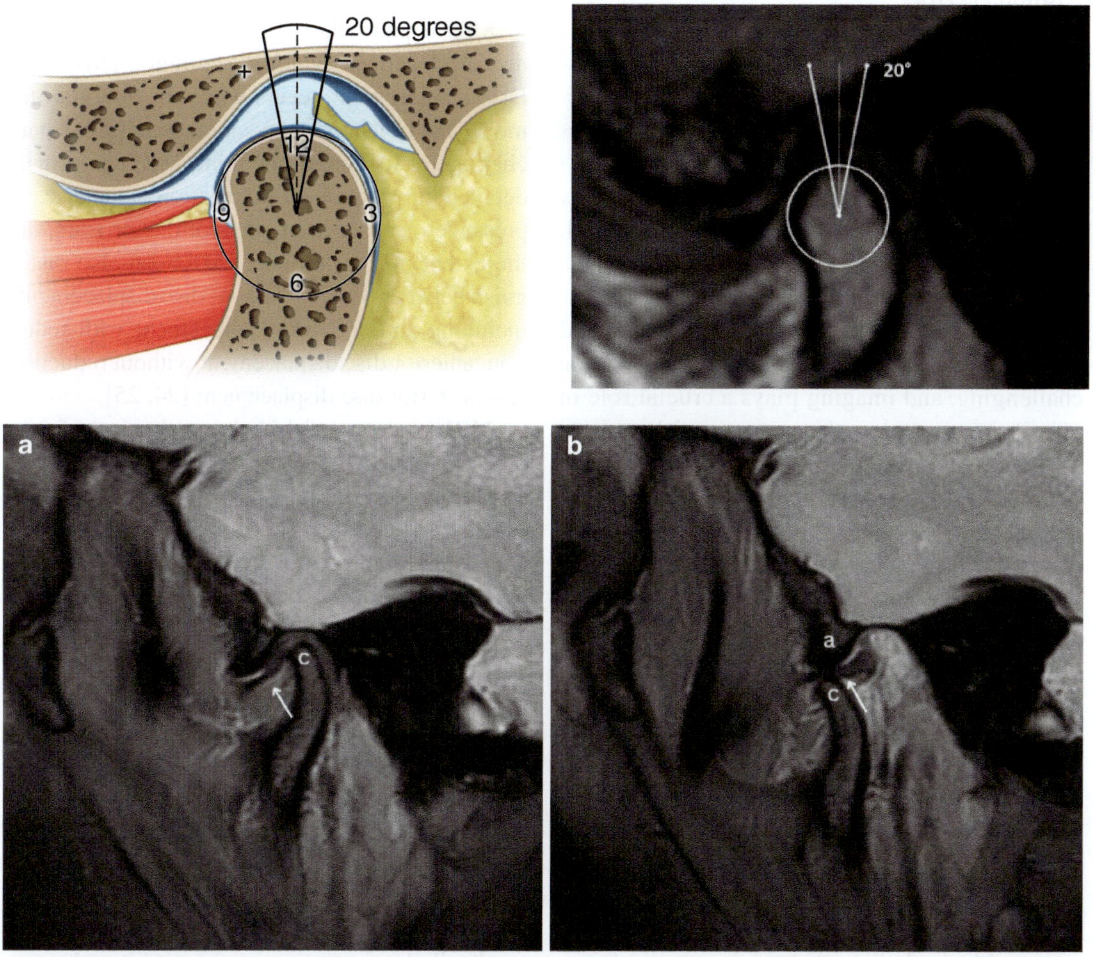

Fig. 10 (**a**) Normal position of the joint structures in closed-mouth position. The mandibular condyle is aligned with the mandibular fossa, and the posterior border of the disc is within 20° of a vertical line traced from the condyle to be within the 95th percentile of normal. Because the first definition may result in up to 30% false positives, Rammelsberg and colleagues suggested that a disc should be considered anteriorly displaced beyond 30° from the vertical. (**b**) Anterior displacement with reduction. (A) Sagittal proton density-weighted magnetic resonance imaging (MRI) in the closed-mouth position demonstrates anterior displacement of the disc (arrow) in front of the mandibular condyle (the letter, c). (B) Sagittal proton density-weighted MRI in the open-mouth position demonstrates reduction of the disc (arrow) between the articular eminence (a) and the mandibular condyle (c)

rior band and bilaminar zone lies just above the condylar head near the 12 o'clock position. It must be positioned with the limit of its posterior band aligned with a vertical line drawn from the center of circle with the condyle diameter, as shown in Fig. 10a. A variability of −10° to +10° is considered within normal limits [3, 13].

However, there is some controversy regarding the range of normal disc positions. In the normal population, there is significant variation in the relationship between the posterior band and bilaminar zone, leading to incorrect classification of anterior disc displacement. Rammelsberg et al. propose that disc positions up to +30° from the vertical should be considered normal. Other authors have suggested using the intermediate zone as the reference point, so that in a healthy joint, it is always interposed between the condyle and the temporal bone regardless of the joint position [1, 20].

3 Traumatic Lesions: Temporomandibular Joint

Temporomandibular joint (TMJ) is a complex joint that connects the mandible to the skull, responsible for the movements of the lower jaw. Traumatic injuries to the TMJ can cause significant morbidity and can lead to chronic pain and dysfunction. Diagnosis of TMJ injuries can be challenging, and imaging plays a crucial role in identifying the extent and severity of the injury. Various imaging modalities have been used to evaluate TMJ injuries, including conventional radiography, computed tomography (CT), and magnetic resonance imaging (MRI). Among these, MRI has gained popularity in recent times due to its ability to provide detailed information on soft tissue injuries. This essay aims to explore the role of MRI in the evaluation of traumatic injuries to the TMJ, including its advantages, limitations, and current advancements [10, 21].

Traumatic injuries to the TMJ can occur due to various reasons, including direct trauma, indirect trauma, or repetitive microtrauma. Direct trauma to the TMJ can occur due to a blow to the jaw or face, resulting in fractures of the mandible or the temporal bone. Indirect trauma can occur due to whiplash injuries, resulting in dislocation or subluxation of the joint. Repetitive microtrauma can occur due to chronic teeth grinding or clenching, resulting in joint degeneration and pain [19, 22, 23].

3.1 Role of MRI in TMJ Injury Evaluation

MRI is a noninvasive imaging modality that uses a strong magnetic field and radio waves to produce detailed images of soft tissues. MRI is useful in the evaluation of TMJ injuries as it can provide detailed information on the extent and severity of soft tissue injuries. MRI can also distinguish between acute and chronic injuries, which is essential in the management of TMJ injuries.

MRI is particularly useful in the evaluation of disc displacement, which is a common TMJ injury. Disc displacement occurs when the articular disc moves out of its normal position, resulting in pain, clicking, or locking of the joint. MRI can provide detailed information on the position of the disc, the presence or absence of perforations or tears, and the extent of joint effusion. MRI can also distinguish between various types of disc displacements, including anterior disc displacement with reduction, anterior disc displacement without reduction, and posterior disc displacement [24, 25].

MRI is also useful in the evaluation of joint degeneration, which is a common consequence of chronic TMJ injuries. Joint degeneration can result in osteoarthritis, which can cause significant pain and dysfunction. MRI can provide detailed information on the extent and severity of joint degeneration, including the presence or absence of bone erosions, joint effusion, and synovial hypertrophy [24, 25].

3.1.1 Advantages

1. Detailed soft tissue evaluation: MRI is particularly useful in the evaluation of soft tissue injuries, including ligamentous and muscular injuries, which are not visible on conventional radiographs or CT scans. MRI can provide detailed information on the extent and severity of soft tissue injuries, making it an excellent tool for the assessment of TMJ injuries.
2. Noninvasive: MRI is a noninvasive imaging modality that does not use ionizing radiation, making it a safe option for the evaluation of TMJ injuries, especially in children and young adults.
3. Multiplanar imaging: MRI can provide images in multiple planes, including axial, sagittal, and coronal, allowing for a comprehensive evaluation of the TMJ.
4. Differentiation between acute and chronic injuries: MRI can differentiate between acute and chronic injuries, which is essential in the management of TMJ injuries.
5. Improved patient comfort: MRI is a painless imaging modality that does not require the use

of contrast agents, making it a comfortable option for patients [5, 10, 11].

3.1.2 Limitations

1. Cost: MRI is an expensive imaging modality compared to conventional radiographs or CT scans, making it less accessible in some healthcare settings.
2. Time-consuming: MRI scans can take longer than conventional radiographs or CT scans, which can be a limiting factor in emergency situations.
3. Claustrophobia: Some patients may experience claustrophobia during MRI scans, which can limit the use of this imaging modality in some patients.
4. Metallic implants: Patients with metallic implants, such as dental implants or pacemakers, may not be eligible for MRI scans due to safety concerns [8, 10, 11].

3.2 Current Advancements in MRI for TMJ Injury Evaluation

Advancements in MRI technology have improved the accuracy and efficiency of TMJ injury evaluation. One such advancement is the use of high-resolution MRI, which provides detailed images of the TMJ structures, including the articular disc, ligaments, and muscles. High-resolution MRI is particularly useful in the evaluation of small or subtle injuries, which may be missed on conventional MRI scans. Another advancement is the use of functional MRI (fMRI), which can provide information on the functional status of the TMJ. fMRI can evaluate the TMJ during active mouth opening and closing, providing information on the movement patterns and muscle activation during these movements. This information can be useful in the assessment of TMJ dysfunction and in the planning of TMJ surgeries [26, 27].

3.2.1 TMJ Dislocation

TMJ dislocation occurs when the mandible (lower jawbone) becomes dislocated from the temporal bone (skull bone) that forms the joint. This can occur due to a variety of factors, including trauma, overuse, or underlying structural abnormalities. The symptoms of TMJ dislocation can range from mild discomfort to severe pain and functional impairment [18, 20, 21].

MRI can be a valuable tool for evaluating TMJ dislocation, as it provides detailed images of the joint and surrounding structures. These images can help healthcare professionals identify the underlying causes of the dislocation, as well as any structural abnormalities or damage to the joint that may be contributing to the problem [22, 23, 28].

3.2.2 Causes of TMJ Dislocation

TMJ dislocation can occur due to a variety of factors, including trauma, overuse, or underlying structural abnormalities.

Trauma: Trauma to the jaw or head can cause the mandibular condyle to become dislocated from the temporal bone. This can occur due to a blow to the face, a fall, or a car accident, among other things.

Overuse: Overuse of the TMJ can also lead to dislocation. This can occur due to excessive chewing or grinding of the teeth, or as a result of certain habits such as nail biting or clenching the jaw [18, 22, 23].

Structural abnormalities: Underlying structural abnormalities can also contribute to TMJ dislocation. These can include deformities of the mandibular condyle or temporal bone, as well as abnormalities of the articular disc or joint capsule [29].

Symptoms

The symptoms of TMJ dislocation can vary depending on the severity and underlying cause of the problem. Some common symptoms include [23, 27, 30]:

1. Pain or discomfort in the jaw joint or surrounding areas
2. Limited range of motion or difficulty opening and closing the mouth
3. Clicking, popping, or grating sounds when moving the jaw
4. Locking of the jaw in an open or closed position
5. Headaches

3.2.3 TMJ Fractures

Temporomandibular joint (TMJ) fractures are relatively uncommon but can be a significant source of pain and dysfunction. They can occur due to a variety of factors, including trauma, overuse, or underlying structural abnormalities. Magnetic resonance imaging (MRI) is a noninvasive diagnostic tool that can be used to evaluate TMJ fractures and aid in treatment planning [26].

Trauma: Trauma to the jaw or head can cause fractures to the mandibular condyle or other structures of the TMJ. This can occur due to a blow to the face, a fall, or a car accident, among other things.

Overuse: Overuse of the TMJ can also lead to fractures. This can occur due to excessive chewing or grinding of the teeth, or because of certain habits such as nail biting or clenching the jaw.

Structural abnormalities: Underlying structural abnormalities can also contribute to TMJ fractures. These can include deformities of the mandibular condyle or temporal bone, as well as abnormalities of the articular disc or joint capsule [27, 31].

Symptoms

The symptoms of TMJ fractures can vary depending on the severity and underlying cause of the problem. Some common symptoms include [27, 30]:

1. Pain or discomfort in the jaw joint or surrounding areas
2. Swelling or tenderness around the TMJ
3. Limited range of motion or difficulty opening and closing the mouth
4. Clicking, popping, or grating sounds when moving the jaw
5. Locking of the jaw in an open or closed position

3.2.4 MRI in the Evaluation of TMJ Fractures

MRI can be a valuable tool for evaluating TMJ fractures, as it provides detailed images of the joint and surrounding structures. These images can help healthcare professionals identify the location and extent of the fracture, as well as any associated soft tissue injuries. MRI can also help differentiate TMJ fractures from other causes of jaw pain and dysfunction, such as arthritis or muscle strain [26, 31].

4 Internal Derangements and Degeneration

Internal derangement (ID) refers to a joint malfunction that disrupts smooth joint function, caused by abnormal interaction of the articular disc, condyle, and articular eminence. Clinical features of ID include articular pain and noises. The most common cause of ID is disc displacement, but not all displaced discs are associated with derangement, and not all derangements are caused by disc displacement. Loose bodies, joint effusion, and adhesions in the joint can also cause derangement. Surprisingly, up to 34% of asymptomatic volunteers may have anterior disc displacement, and 23% of patients with derangement may have normal disc position [32–34].

Approximately 80% of patients referred for diagnostic imaging of the TMJ demonstrate some form of disc displacement in most large MRI series. MRI is the preferred imaging method for diagnosing ID, with a 95% accuracy rate for assessing the disc position and shape, and a 93% accuracy rate for assessing osseous changes [33–35].

4.1 Temporomandibular Joint Developmental Disorders

Temporomandibular joint (TMJ) developmental disorders are a group of conditions that affect the growth and function of the TMJ. The TMJ is the joint that connects the lower jaw to the skull and allows for movements such as chewing, speaking, and yawning. Magnetic resonance imaging (MRI) is a noninvasive imaging technique that uses a strong magnetic field and radio waves to produce detailed images of the soft tissues of the body. MRI has an important role in the diagnosis and management of TMJ developmental disorders [20, 26].

MRI can provide detailed images of the TMJ and its surrounding structures, including the bones, muscles, ligaments, and cartilage. This allows for the identification of abnormalities or changes in the TMJ that may be indicative of a developmental disorder. For example, MRI can reveal the presence of a disc displacement, which occurs when the disc that cushions the TMJ is displaced from its normal position. This condition is commonly associated with TMJ pain and dysfunction [28, 36].

MRI can also be used to assess the growth and development of the TMJ in children. This is particularly important in cases of developmental disorders such as condylar hyperplasia, which is a condition where there is an overgrowth of the mandibular condyle, the part of the jaw that articulates with the skull. MRI can provide information about the size and shape of the condyle, as well as any changes in the surrounding tissues [32, 33].

In addition, MRI can be used to monitor the progression of TMJ developmental disorders over time. This is important in cases where conservative treatments such as physical therapy and medications are being used. By tracking changes in the TMJ over time, clinicians can assess the effectiveness of treatment and make adjustments as necessary [36].

Overall, MRI plays a valuable role in the diagnosis and management of TMJ developmental disorders. Its ability to provide detailed images of the TMJ and its surrounding structures allows for the identification of abnormalities and changes that may be indicative of a developmental disorder. MRI can also be used to assess the growth and development of the TMJ in children and monitor the progression of TMJ developmental disorders over time. With its noninvasive nature and high level of detail, MRI is an important tool in the management of TMJ developmental disorders [12, 34].

4.2 Disc Displacement

Disc displacement is a common condition of the TMJ that can cause significant pain and dysfunction. It occurs when the articular disc that separates the condyle and the fossa of the TMJ moves out of position. The displacement can be anterior, medial, lateral, or posterior, and it can be associated with derangement of the joint [18, 27, 35].

Magnetic resonance imaging (MRI) is the preferred imaging modality for the diagnosis of disc displacement, as it provides excellent soft tissue contrast and can accurately depict the position, shape, and integrity of the articular disc and other joint structures. Several studies have demonstrated the high diagnostic accuracy of MRI in the evaluation of disc displacement, with reported sensitivity and specificity rates of up to 100% and 96%, respectively [27, 37].

The clinical significance of disc displacement is still a matter of debate, as not all displaced discs are symptomatic, and the association between disc displacement and joint pain is not always clear. Some studies have suggested that disc displacement alone may not be sufficient to cause pain and that other factors, such as joint loading and inflammation, may play a role in the development of symptoms [29, 35].

Disc displacement can be categorized into two subtypes: anterior displacement with reduction (Fig. 10b) or anterior displacement with no reduction (Fig. 11), depending on whether a normal relationship between the condyle and the disc is restored during mouth opening [38].

The extent of disc displacement can be classified as complete or partial. Complete displacement occurs when the entire mediolateral dimension of the disc is displaced, while partial displacement refers to the displacement of either the medial or the lateral portion of the disc. Partial disc displacement, commonly observed in anterior displacement with reduction, often involves the anterior displacement of the lateral part of the disc, while the medial part remains in its normal position, referred to as rotational disc displacement. The precise mechanism underlying disc displacement remains unclear; however, trauma resulting in injury to the posterior disc attachment is considered the most probable cause. Unenhanced MRI is the preferred imaging modality for assessing ID of the TMJ [20, 28].

In the early stages of ID, the disc initially maintains its normal shape, but over time, it undergoes deformations characterized by thickening of the posterior band and thinning of the anterior band.

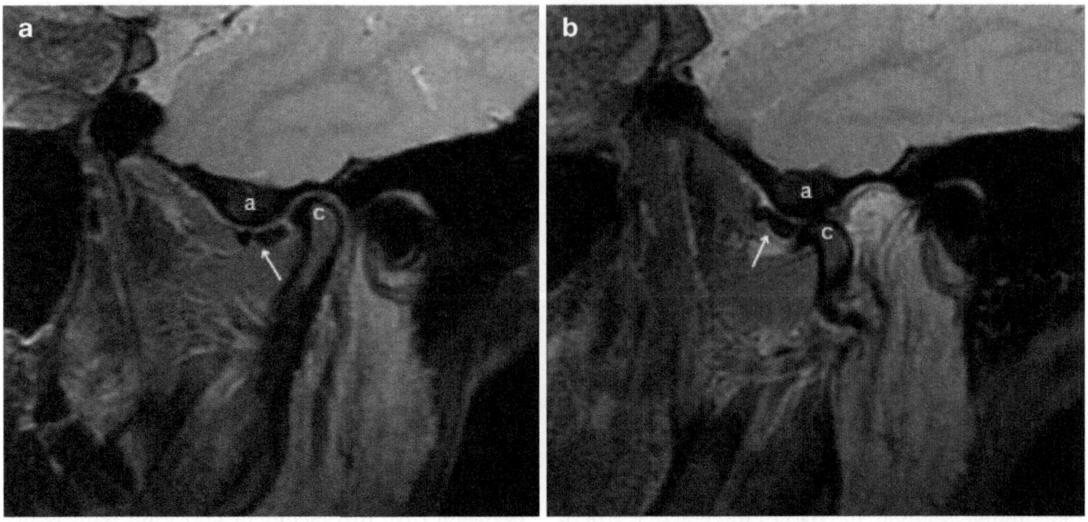

Fig. 11 Anterior displacement with no reduction. (**a**) Sagittal proton density-weighted magnetic resonance imaging (MRI) in the closed-mouth position demonstrates anterior displacement of the disc (arrow) related to the articular eminence (a) and anterior to the mandibular condyle (c). (**b**) Sagittal proton density-weighted MRI in the open-mouth position demonstrates no reduction of the disc (arrow) between the articular eminence (a) and the mandibular condyle (c)

This results in the disc assuming a biconvex, teardrop-shaped, or rounded appearance. As long as the disc remains positioned on top of the condyle during mouth opening, it maintains a normal biconcave shape. Consequently, the presence of an irregular and rounded disc typically indicates disc disease. Additional MRI findings suggestive of disc disease include disc flattening, a decrease in the normal intermediate to high signal intensity of the disc, and the presence of tears or perforations in the chronic stage [38, 39].

Posterior disc displacement is an uncommon occurrence (Fig. 12), representing only a small percentage of all disc displacements, ranging from 0.01 to 0.001%. The primary clinical manifestation is the sudden onset of a locked jaw in the open position. The use of MRI is valuable in diagnosing this condition as it reveals the displacement of the posterior band beyond the 1 o'clock position on the clock face. It is essential to review the patient's clinical information before interpreting the images to avoid mistaking a previous posterior disc plication for an acquired posterior disc displacement [38, 39].

Rotational displacements encompass anterolateral and anteromedial disc displacements, whereas sideways displacements include pure lateral and medial displacements. Isolated lateral displacement is a rare occurrence. Once again, these rotational and sideways displacements can be classified as complete or partial and can occur with or without disc reduction. Among these patterns, anterolateral displacement is the most commonly observed [24, 39].

4.3 Pseudo-Disc

Pseudo-disc (Fig. 13) is a term used to describe the presence of a band-like structure with low signal intensity, replacing the typically bright signal of the posterior disc attachment. It is observed in certain patients who have anteriorly displaced discs and is believed to be an adaptive reaction to the displacement, resulting from connective tissue thickening and hyalinization within the posterior disc attachment [37, 40].

4.4 Stuck Disc

The condition known as the "stuck disc" refers to a pathological state where the disc remains immobile in relation to the glenoid fossa and the articular eminence. This condition can be

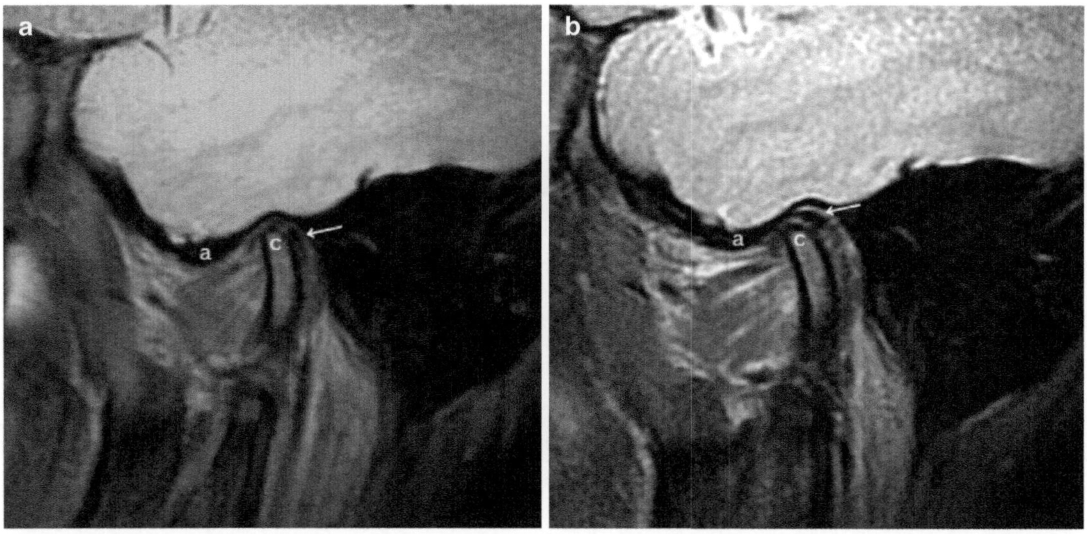

Fig. 12 Posterior displacement with no reduction. (**a**) Sagittal proton density-weighted magnetic resonance imaging (MRI) in the closed-mouth position demonstrates posterior displacement of the disc (arrow) related to the articular eminence (a) and anterior to the mandibular condyle (c). (**b**) Sagittal proton density-weighted MRI in the open-mouth position demonstrates no reduction of the disc (arrow) between the articular eminence (a) and the mandibular condyle (c)

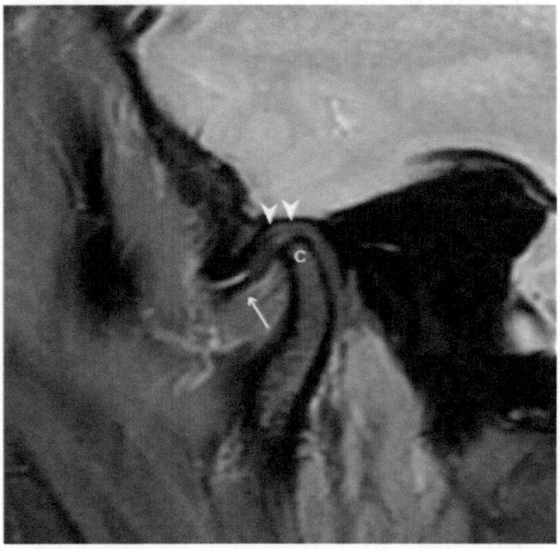

Fig. 13 Pseudo-disc. Sagittal proton density-weighted magnetic resonance imaging (MRI) in the closed-mouth position demonstrates thickening of the posterior attachments (arrowheads) superior to the mandibular condyle (c), seen as "pseudo-disc." Articular disc (arrow) is displaced anteriorly

observed regardless of whether the mouth is open or closed and is likely caused by adhesions. It may occur with or without disc displacement and can lead to pain and joint dysfunction due to limited condylar translation. To accurately diagnose this condition, it is important to image the temporomandibular joint (TMJ) in both open- and closed-mouth positions. Sagittal oblique cine imaging is particularly valuable in assessing the stuck disc [40, 41].

4.5 Perforated Disc

Disc perforation (Fig. 14) occurs in approximately 5–15% of cases involving displaced joints and deranged discs. This occurrence is more frequent in patients with anterior disc nonreducing (ADNR) conditions compared to anterior disc reducing (ADR) conditions, and it is commonly observed in individuals with advanced arthrosis. The prevalence of disc perforation is higher in women than in men, particularly among individuals over 80 years of age. MRI findings associated with disc perforation include disc deformity (100%), disc displacement (81%), condylar bony changes (68%), joint effusion (23%), and nonvisualization of the temporal posterior attach-

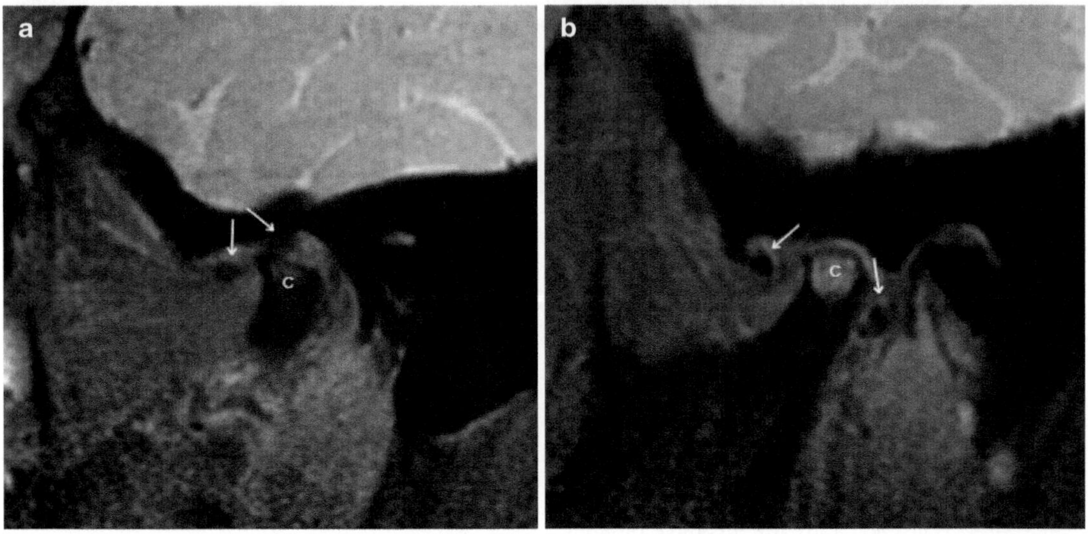

Fig. 14 Perforated disc. (**a**) Sagittal proton density-weighted magnetic resonance imaging (MRI) in the closed-mouth position demonstrates mild disc perforation (arrows) in relation to osteophyte of the mandibular condyle (c). (**b**) Sagittal proton density-weighted MRI in the closed-mouth position demonstrates extensive disc perforation (arrows) with luxation of the disc fragments. Also, there is osseous edema in the mandibular condyle (c)

ment (TPA) of the disc (65–68%). Both conventional and MR arthrograms can aid in diagnosing disc perforation by demonstrating opacification of both joint compartments after injecting a contrast agent into a single lower compartment. To investigate suspected disc perforation, a fat-suppressed T2-weighted MRI can be obtained in the sagittal and coronal planes. Additionally, the absence of stretching or straightening of the posterior temporal disc attachment during mouth opening also suggests the presence of a disc perforation [40–42].

4.6 Joint Effusion and Loose Bodies

Joint effusion refers to an abnormal accumulation of fluid within the joint space and is frequently observed in symptomatic patients (Fig. 15). In asymptomatic individuals, a small amount of joint fluid can be present. The prevalence of effusion is higher in painful joints compared to non-painful joints. Although not all patients with joint pain have effusion, those with large effusions often experience pain and disc displacement [40, 43, 44].

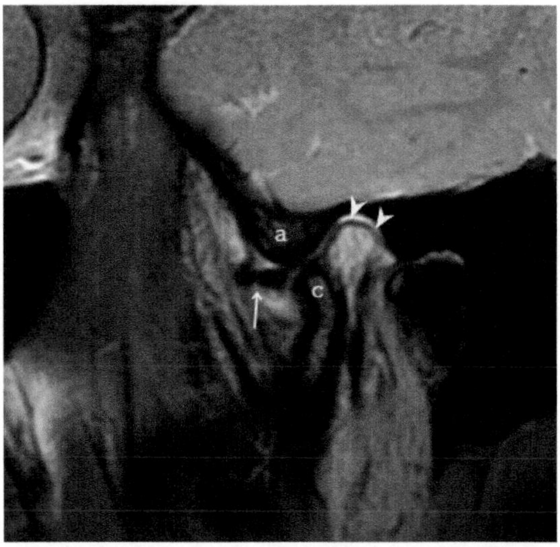

Fig. 15 Joint effusion. Sagittal proton density-weighted magnetic resonance imaging (MRI) in the open-mouth position demonstrates fluidlike signal within the articular space, compatible with joint effusion (arrowheads). Also, there is anterior displacement of the disc (arrow) in relation to the articular eminence (a) and the mandibular condyle (c)

For evaluating joint effusion, T2-weighted MR sequences are considered the most effective. Early-stage effusions typically surround the anterior band, while larger effusions can occupy both the superior and inferior joint spaces. A substantial effusion can provide valuable diagnostic information, as it delineates the disc and may even reveal disc perforation and retrodiscal tissue, creating an "arthrography effect." Gadolinium-enhanced T1-weighted imaging can be useful in differentiating a plain joint effusion from synovial proliferation. In patients with inflammatory arthropathies accompanied by synovial proliferation, the proliferating synovium exhibits enhancement, whereas the effusion does not [9, 43, 45].

Loose bodies within a synovial joint can be classified as primary or secondary synovial chondromatosis (Fig. 16). The primary type occurs when there is spontaneous cartilaginous metaplasia in the synovium, while the secondary type is characterized by the incorporation of osseocartilaginous loose bodies within the synovium, often in the presence of degenerative joint disease. Typical clinical symptoms associated with loose bodies include pain, swelling around the ear, restricted jaw movement, clicking or popping sounds, and deviation of the jaw to one side during mouth opening. Panoramic radiographs of the TMJ may or may not reveal the presence of loose bodies. However, high-resolution CT or MRI imaging can effectively detect small loose bodies within the TMJ space [44–46].

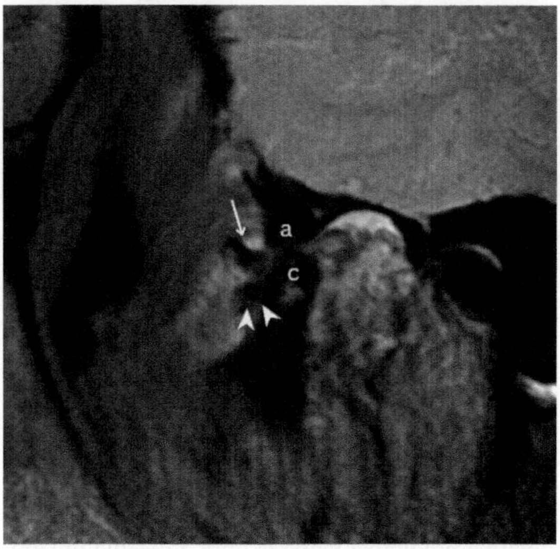

Fig. 16 Loose body. Sagittal proton density-weighted magnetic resonance imaging (MRI) in the open-mouth position demonstrates a loose body (arrowheads) within the joint effusion. Also, there is anterior displacement of the disc (arrow) in relation to the articular eminence (a) and the mandibular condyle (c)

4.7 Thickening of Lateral Pterygoid Muscle Attachment (Double-Disc Sign)

The specific role of the lateral pterygoid muscle (LPM) in TMJ function is still a subject of debate, although it is believed to contribute to generating side-to-side and protrusive jaw forces. Electromyographic studies have shown increased activity in the lower attachment of the LPM in patients with TMJ internal derangement. Various morphological changes in the superior and inferior portions of the LPM have been observed on MRI, including hypertrophy, atrophy, and contractures. These changes have been found to have a significant association with clinical symptoms such as pain or restricted jaw opening in patients with anterior disc nonreducing TMJ conditions. It is suggested that there is a notable connection between anterior disc displacement and attachment of the superior LPM solely to the disc, rather than to the condyle. Radiologists interpreting imaging should be cautious not to mistake a thickened inferior LPM for an anteriorly displaced disc (Fig. 17), a phenomenon known as the "double-disc sign" [16, 17, 20].

4.8 Osteochondritis Dissecans and Avascular Necrosis

Osteochondritis dissecans (OCD) and avascular necrosis (AVN) of the mandibular condyle share similar pathological characteristics and likely represent different stages of the same underlying condition. Common clinical features of OCD/AVN include pain and impaired joint function. Pain is typically localized to the joint area and along the distribution of the trigeminal nerve's third division. Other symptoms may include headache, earache, and muscle spasms in the masticatory muscles. These symptoms can occur with or without limitations in joint movement [42, 47].

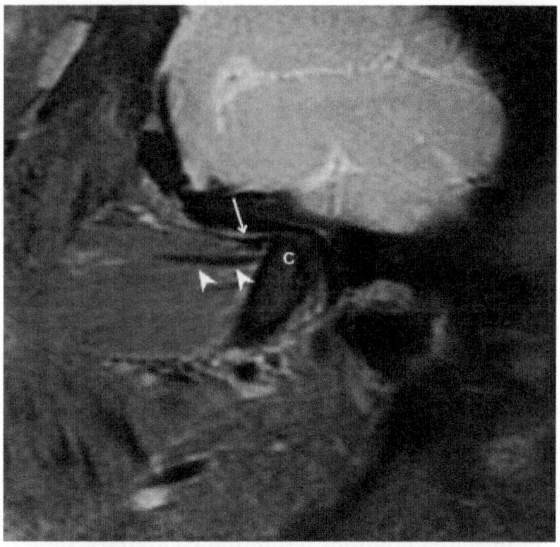

Fig. 17 Double-disc sign (thickening of the lateral pterygoid muscle). Sagittal proton density-weighted magnetic resonance imaging (MRI) in the closed-mouth position demonstrates anterior displacement of the disc (arrow). The thickened lateral pterygoid muscle near the mandibular condylar (c) attachment appears as linear hypointense structure (arrowheads) inferior to the disc in the same orientation giving the appearance of "double disc"

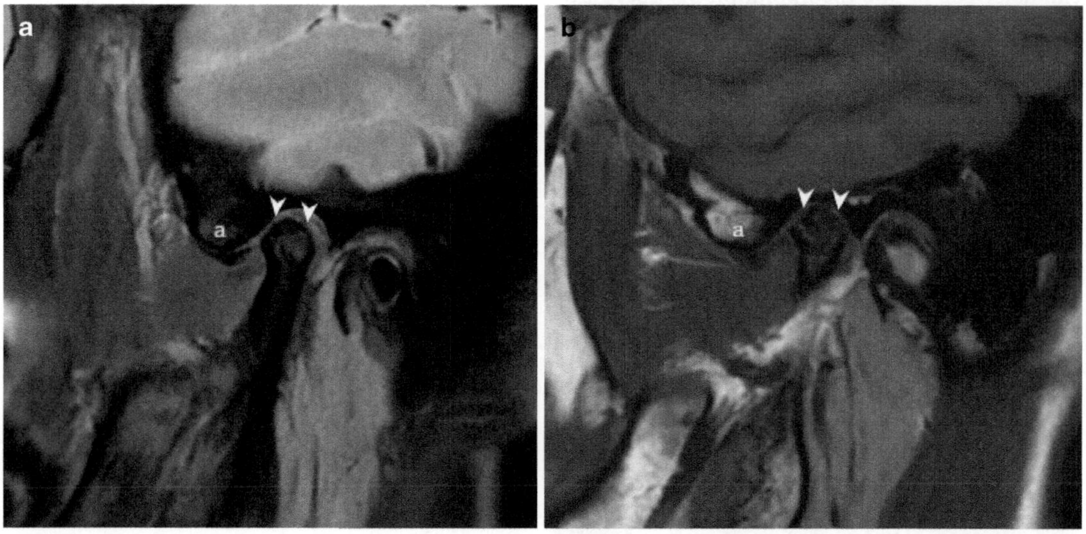

Fig. 18 Avascular necrosis. Sagittal magnetic resonance imaging (MRI) in the closed-mouth position in proton density-weighted (**a**) and on T1-weighted (**b**) images demonstrates high marrow signal intensity in proton density image and low signal intensity in T1-weighted image within the condylar head. Also, there is an area of low signal intensity in both sequences, suggestive of subchondral fracture (arrowheads). Articular eminence (a) has normal signal intensity on both sequences for comparison

MRI is the preferred imaging modality for evaluating OCD/AVN of the mandibular condyle. In cases of AVN, there is a decrease in marrow signal intensity on T1-weighted sequences. T2-weighted sequences exhibit variable signal characteristics depending on the stage of AVN (Fig. 18). Early-stage AVN consistently shows high signal intensity on T2-weighted images, while acute OCD (Fig. 19) typically displays a centrally hypointense fragment surrounded by a zone of higher signal intensity on both T1-weighted and T2-weighted sequences. Although MRI has a sensitivity of 78% and specificity of 84% in diagnosing AVN, the positive predictive value is only 54% due to similar MRI appearances seen in condylar sclerosis secondary to advanced degenerative changes in the TMJ. Radiological changes associated with OCD and AVN of the mandibular condyle often involve joint effusion and internal derangement of the disc [42, 47, 48].

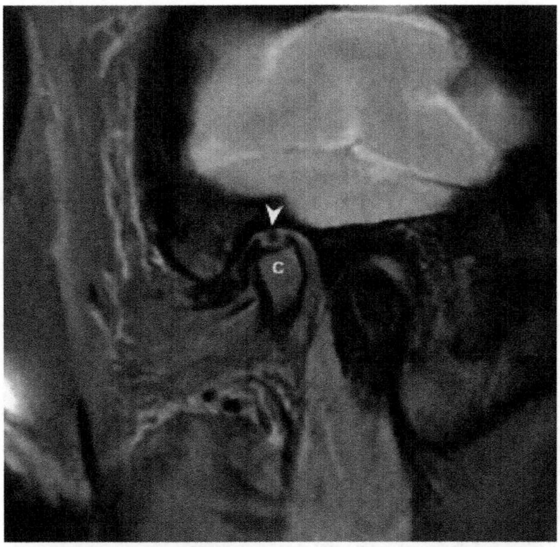

Fig. 19 Osteochondritis dissecans. Sagittal proton density-weighted magnetic resonance imaging (MRI) in the closed-mouth position demonstrates a tiny bone fragment (arrowhead) at the superior aspect of the mandibular condyle (c). It can be noted that there is intermediate/high signal intensity surrounding the bone fragment

4.9 Hypermobility

Patients with a hypermobile temporomandibular joint (TMJ) may have trouble closing their jaw (referred to as an "open lock") following wide jaw opening. This occurs when the condyle translates beyond the boundaries of the anterior attachment of the TMJ capsule. The condyle becomes trapped along the anterior slope of the articular eminence, primarily due to biomechanical constraints related to masticatory muscle activity [1].

In acute cases, imaging studies are typically unnecessary since the open lock can be diagnosed based on clinical signs and a relevant history of wide jaw opening or trauma. However, in chronic cases, MRI can provide valuable information about the height and steepness of the articular eminences, as well as the shape and position of the disc [15, 23].

4.10 Ankylosis

Ankylosis of the TMJ can occur when fibrous adhesions or bony fusion restricts the movement of the jaw (Fig. 20). This condition may develop because of previous infection, trauma, or surgery or in individuals with juvenile idiopathic arthritis or bifid mandibular condyles. MR arthrography is a valuable tool for assessing fibrous adhesions, while a three-dimensional CT scan is necessary for surgical planning when bony fusion is suspected [11, 49].

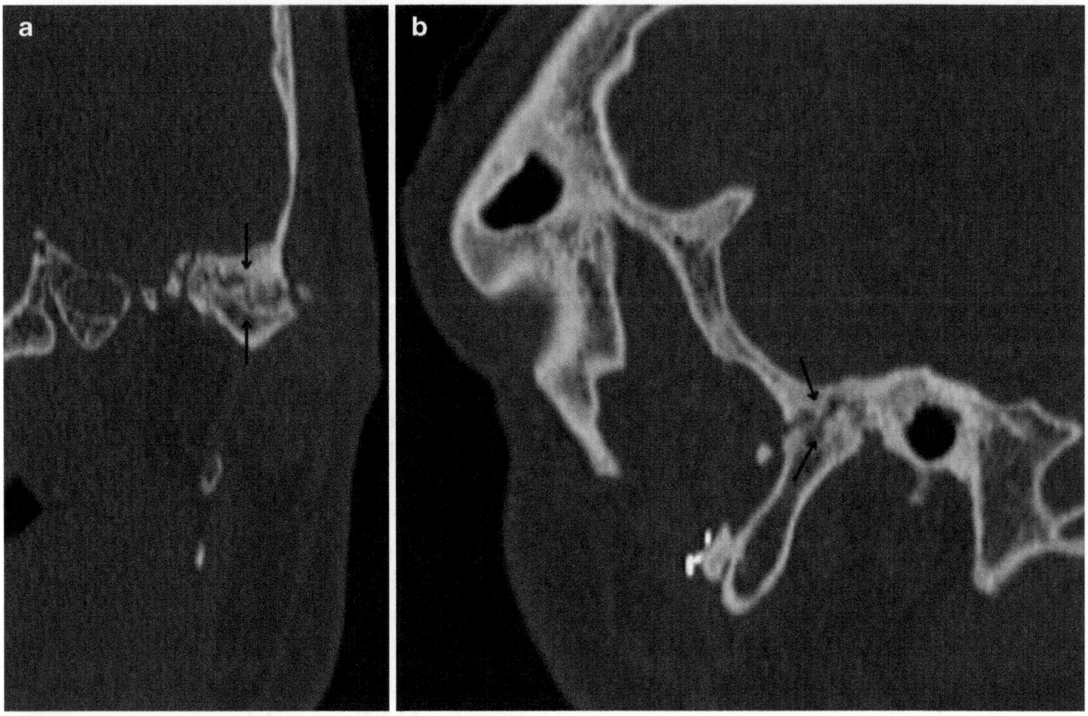

Fig. 20 Ankylosis. Coronal (**a**) and sagittal reformation (**b**) of multislice computed tomography (CT) demonstrates fibrous ankylosis of the left temporomandibular joint (black arrows)

5 TMJ Tumors and Tumorlike Conditions

The temporomandibular joint (TMJ) is one of the most complex joints in the human body. It is responsible for the movement of the lower jaw and plays an important role in mastication, speech, and facial expression. TMJ disorders are a common cause of orofacial pain and dysfunction. Tumors and tumorlike conditions of the TMJ are relatively rare, but they can cause significant morbidity and mortality. This section aims to provide an overview of MRI role in the most common tumors and tumorlike conditions of the TMJ [12].

Magnetic resonance imaging (MRI) is a noninvasive imaging modality that is commonly used in the evaluation of tumors and tumorlike conditions of the temporomandibular joint (TMJ). MRI provides excellent soft tissue contrast and multiplanar imaging capabilities, which make it a valuable tool in the diagnosis and management of these conditions [32].

5.1 MR Features of Tumorlike Conditions

MRI is useful in the evaluation of tumorlike conditions of the TMJ, such as synovial chondromatosis, pigmented villonodular synovitis (PVNS), and osteochondroma. In synovial chondromatosis, MRI typically shows multiple nodular lesions within the synovial membrane and joint space. These nodules are hyperintense on T2-weighted images and hypointense on T1-weighted images. In PVNS, MRI shows diffuse synovial thickening with hypointense areas representing hemosiderin deposition. In osteochondroma, MRI shows a bony protuberance with a cartilaginous cap that is hypointense on T1-weighted images and hyperintense on T2-weighted images [46].

5.2 MR Features of Tumors

MRI is also useful in the evaluation of tumors of the TMJ, such as chondrosarcoma, osteosarcoma, and metastatic tumors. In chondrosarcoma, MRI typically shows a lobulated mass with heterogeneous signal intensity on T1- and T2-weighted images. The mass is usually hypointense on T1-weighted images and hyperintense on T2-weighted images. In osteosarcoma, MRI typically shows a large, lobulated mass with heterogeneous signal intensity on T1- and T2-weighted images. The mass is usually hypointense on T1-weighted images and hyperintense on T2-weighted images. In metastatic tumors, MRI typically shows a mass with heterogeneous signal intensity and variable enhancement [1].

5.3 MR in Evaluation of Tumor Extent

MRI is valuable in the evaluation of tumor extent and involvement of adjacent structures. It can help to determine the involvement of the condyle, articular disc, and adjacent soft tissue structures. MRI can also help to identify the presence of metastases in adjacent bones and soft tissues [50].

5.4 MR in Treatment Planning

MRI is useful in treatment planning for tumors and tumorlike conditions of the TMJ. It can help to determine the extent of surgical resection and to plan for reconstruction of the TMJ. MRI can also help to guide biopsy and to monitor response to therapy [50].

MRI is a valuable tool in the evaluation of tumors and tumorlike conditions of the TMJ. It provides excellent soft tissue contrast and multiplanar imaging capabilities, which make it useful in the diagnosis and management of these conditions. MRI can help to determine the extent of disease, involvement of adjacent structures, and response to therapy. Further research is needed to improve our understanding of the role of MRI in the diagnosis and management of tumors and tumorlike conditions of the TMJ [25, 26].

6 TMJ Arthritis

The TMJ, like other synovial joints in the body, is susceptible to various inflammatory arthritic conditions. In addition to degenerative arthritis, which is a common occurrence in the TMJ, arthritis resulting from crystalline deposition diseases is also prevalent. Furthermore, TMJ arthritis can be secondary to infection or trauma. It is important to discuss arthritis of the TMJ based on the underlying pathophysiological mechanisms involved in its development. By understanding the specific mechanisms at play, clinicians can better diagnose, treat, and manage TMJ arthritis to alleviate symptoms and improve the overall function of the joint [24, 27].

6.1 Degenerative Disease (Osteoarthritis)

Osteoarthritis (OA) is a chronic degenerative disease that primarily affects the articular cartilage of synovial joints. It involves the remodeling of the underlying subchondral bone and can also affect the synovium. Among all joint pathologies, TMJ is commonly affected by osteoarthritis. Interestingly, there is often a discrepancy between radiographic evidence of OA and presence of symptoms, a classic phenomenon in OA, known as clinical-radiological dissociation. Population-based studies have shown that up to 35% of asymptomatic individuals exhibit minimal condylar flattening on radiographs, while approximately 11% of patients experience TMJ symptoms related to OA [51].

The most prevalent symptom of TMJ OA is pain during chewing. Typically, the pain originates from the periarticular soft tissues and masticator muscles, which can be in a protective reflex spasm. Other common symptoms include masticator muscle fatigue, trismus (limited mouth opening), decreased range of motion, difficulty opening the mouth, and joint crepitations [9, 20].

Radiographically, TMJ OA is characterized by specific features such as irregularities in the cortical bone of the articular surface, erosion, and formation of osteophytes (Fig. 21). Erosion refers to focal areas of decreased density along the cortical margin of the mandibular condyle's articular surface and the subchondral region (Fig. 22). Osteophyte formation usually occurs in the later stages of the disease and is an attempt by the joint to stabilize and increase its surface area to better withstand axial loading forces. Various imaging modalities have been utilized to assess TMJ OA, with CT and MRI being the most indicated [24, 51].

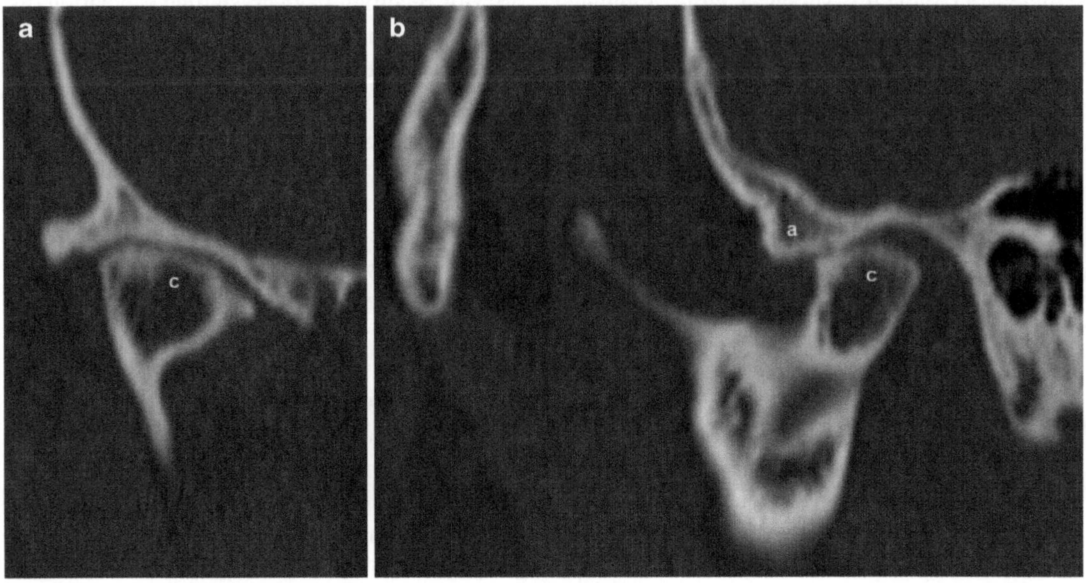

Fig. 21 Degenerative changes. Coronal (**a**) and sagittal reformation (**b**) of multislice computed tomography (CT) demonstrates deformity and osteophytosis of the mandibular condyle (c), subchondral sclerosis of the mandibular condyle and of the articular eminence (a), and asymmetrical loss of joint space

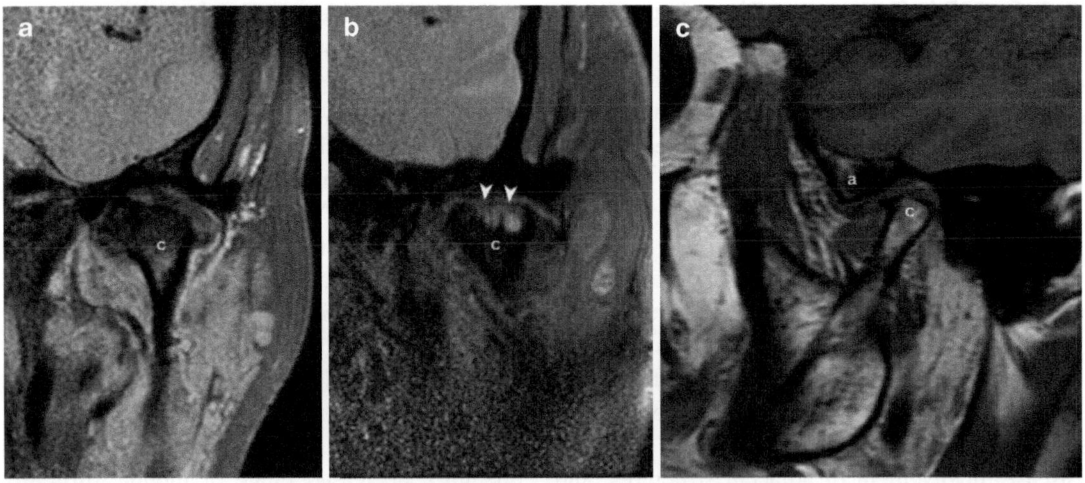

Fig. 22 Degenerative changes. Coronal proton density-weighted (**a**) and (**b**) and sagittal T1-weighted (**c**) magnetic resonance imaging (MRI) of three different patients demonstrates sclerosis and osteophytosis of the mandibular condyle (c), subchondral cysts (arrowheads in **b**) of the mandibular condyle, and loss of joint space

6.2 Inflammatory Arthritis

6.2.1 Juvenile Idiopathic Arthritis

Juvenile idiopathic arthritis (JIA) is the most prevalent rheumatic disease in childhood, affecting girls more frequently than boys. The condition primarily affects synovial joints, and its onset typically occurs in two peaks: the first between 1 and 3 years of age, and the second between 8 and 12 years. TMJ involvement is observed in 17–87% of JIA patients. JIA can manifest as systemic, polyarticular, or periarticular forms, with the TMJ being more commonly affected in those with polyarticular joint involvement. Symptoms of TMJ involvement in JIA often include pain, joint tenderness, crepitation, stiffness, and reduced range of motion. In some cases, late-stage disease may lead to the development of bony ankylosis [49, 52, 53].

Various imaging techniques such as orthopantomography, CT, MRI, and ultrasound have been utilized to evaluate TMJ involvement in JIA. Orthopantomography and CT are particularly useful in detecting bony erosions secondary to TMJ arthritis, but they involve radiation exposure, which can be a concern in young patients. MRI and ultrasound have gained popularity in assessing TMJ involvement in JIA due to their superior soft tissue resolution and the absence of ionizing radiation. These techniques allow for earlier diagnosis of TMJ arthritis without compromising patient safety. Acute TMJ arthritis typically presents with joint effusion and synovial thickening, which are visible on T2-weighted MRI images, without apparent bony changes. However, it is important to note that joint or periarticular tissue enhancement is not a specific sign of acute TMJ arthritis, as abnormal enhancement can also be observed in healthy individuals. Evaluation of condylar resorption, which suggests a more chronic TMJ arthritis, is better achieved using nonfat-suppressed T1-weighted sequences [52–55].

6.2.2 Rheumatoid Arthritis

Rheumatoid arthritis (RA) is a chronic inflammatory condition primarily affecting periarticular tissues such as the synovial membrane, joint capsules, tendons, tendon sheaths, and ligaments. Involvement of the internal joint structures occurs as a secondary effect. The prevalence of RA in the general population is approximately 2–2.5%, with a higher incidence among females. The typical age of onset is between 40 and 60 years, and TMJ involvement is observed in approximately 50–75% of patients with RA [54, 56, 57].

RA is a slowly progressive disease with an insidious onset, leading to the gradual destruction of articular and periarticular soft tissues and adjacent bones, ultimately resulting in joint deformity. TMJ involvement typically occurs at a later stage of the disease (Fig. 23). Symptoms of TMJ involvement in RA include deep, dull aching pain in the preauricular area particularly during chewing, as well as limited range of motion and morning stiffness. As the disease progresses, there is gradual resorption of the mandibular condyle [27, 58, 59].

Radiographically, RA is characterized by specific features such as loss of joint space, destruction of the condyle, flattening with anterior positioning of the condyle, flattening of the articular eminence, and erosion of the glenoid fossa. One distinguishing factor of RA is the presence of synovial proliferation, which is an early pathological process and can be visualized on MRI. Synovial proliferation is a consistent finding in all patients with RA and helps differentiate it from other types of arthritis. Additionally, joint effusion is relatively common in RA cases and can be detected through imaging examinations [24, 56–59].

6.3 Metabolic Arthritis/Crystalline Arthropathies

Calcium pyrophosphate dihydrate deposition disease (CPPD) is a metabolic arthropathy characterized by the accumulation of calcium pyrophosphate dihydrate crystals in and around joints, particularly in the articular and fibrocartilage. TMJ involvement in CPPD can range from asymptomatic calcification of the disc to significant joint destruction with erosive changes in the mandibular condyle and adjacent skull base. Common symptoms include pain, swelling in the

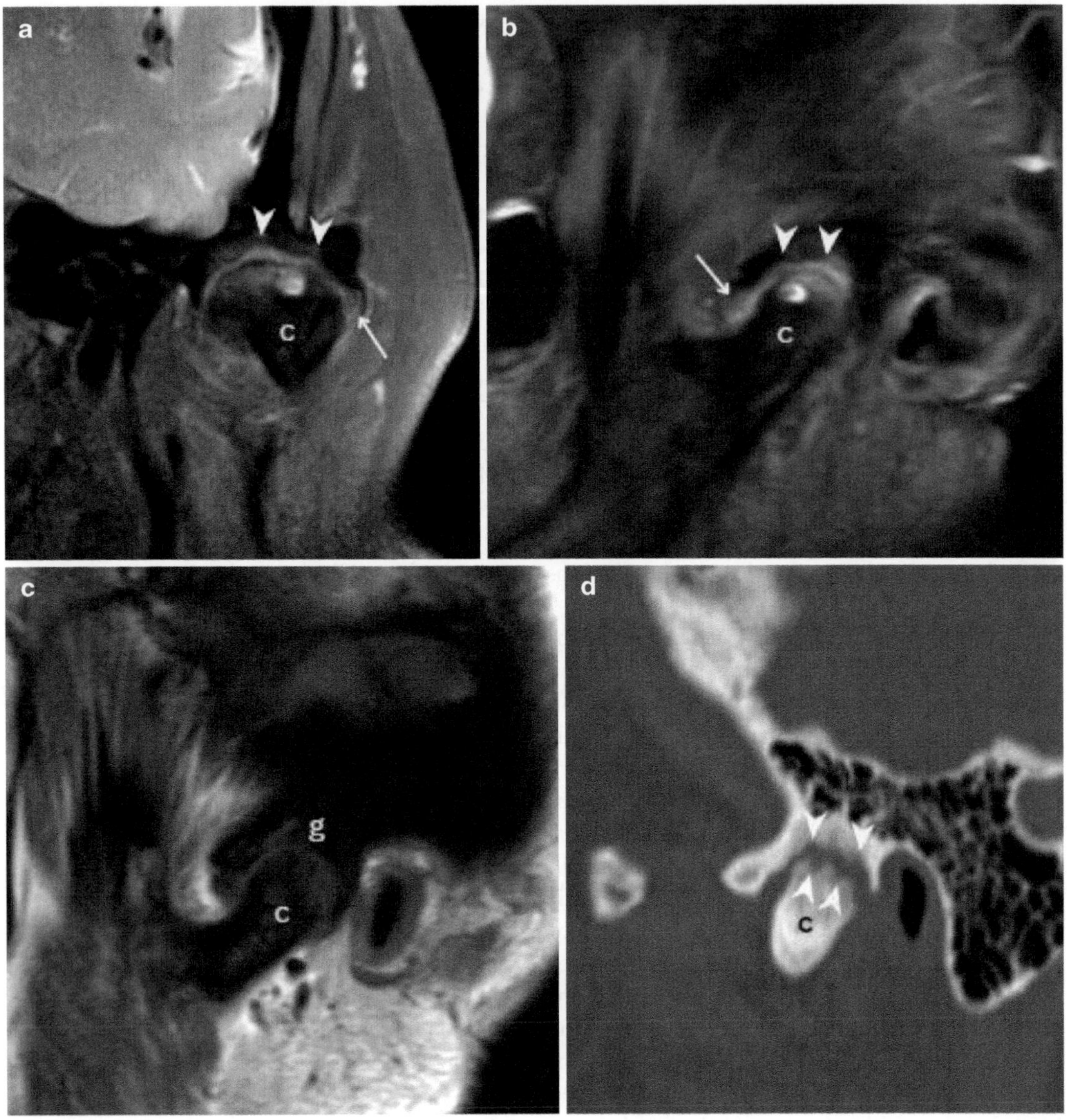

Fig. 23 Coronal proton density-weighted (**a**), sagittal proton density-weighted (**b**), and sagittal T1-weighted (**c**) magnetic resonance imaging (MRI) and sagittal reformation (**d**) of multislice computed tomography (CT) of the same patient demonstrate erosions (arrowheads) of the glenoid fossa (g) and of the mandibular condyle (c). There is also synovial proliferation (arrow in **a** and **b**) in the joint space, associated with bone marrow edema in the mandibular condyle (c)

preauricular area, and occasional hearing loss. Pain can be aggravated by chewing. Less common symptoms may include TMJ clicking, tinnitus, and malocclusion [60].

The radiographic appearance of CPPD can vary. Computed tomography (CT) reveals calcium deposits in the disc or periarticular tissues. On MRI, CPP deposits typically appear as areas of decreased signal intensity on both T1- and T2-weighted sequences (Fig. 24). CT and MRI also show erosions near the condyle and fossa, accompanied by adjacent CPPD deposits. These erosions can extend into the skull base and middle cranial fossa. Involvement of other joints with chondrocalcinosis can provide clues for the diagnosis. Differential diagnoses to consider include synovial chondromatosis, synovial osteochondroma, and osteosarcoma [46, 54].

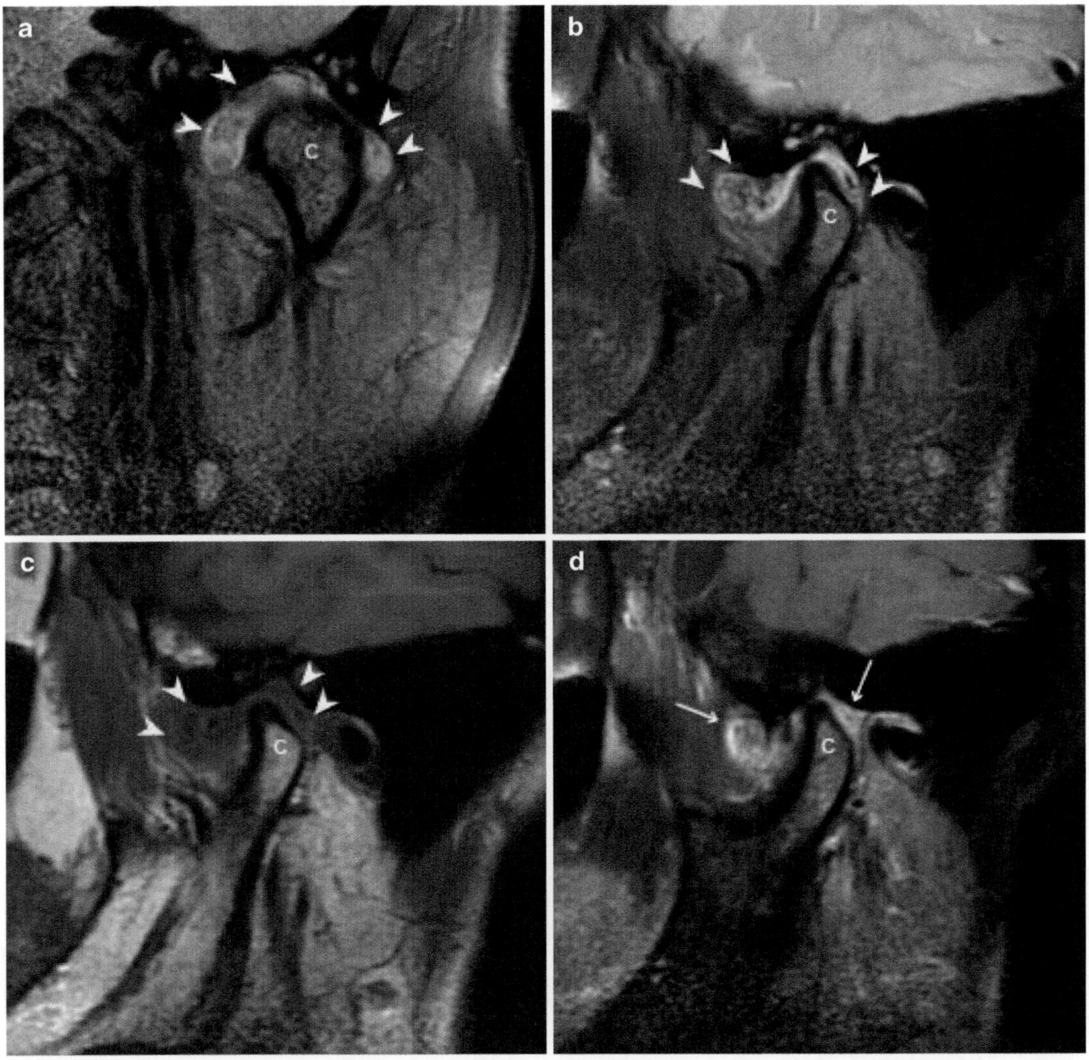

Fig. 24 Coronal proton density-weighted (**a**), sagittal proton density-weighted (**b**), sagittal T1-weighted (**c**), and sagittal T1-weighted FAT SAT post-endovenous gadolinium injection magnetic resonance imaging (MRI) of the same patient demonstrates joint distension with fluid and multiple small foci with low signal intensity in all sequences, compatible with calcifications (arrowheads). There is also exuberant synovitis (arrows in **d**), depicted in the post-contrast image. Mandibular condyle (c)

6.4 Infectious Arthritis

Infections of the TMJ typically occur as a result of the direct spread of infection from nearby tissues into the joint space. Another important mechanism is direct contamination of the articular space, after joint injections. While relatively rare, systemic infections like tuberculosis and syphilis can also affect the TMJ [25].

TMJ infection is more commonly observed in individuals with compromised immune systems and concurrent systemic conditions such as diabetes mellitus, rheumatoid arthritis, or a history of intravenous drug use. These factors increase the susceptibility to TMJ infection and can contribute to the severity and complications associated with the condition.

Therefore, it is crucial to consider these underlying factors when evaluating and managing TMJ infections to ensure appropriate treatment and prevent further complications [54].

6.5 Idiopathic Condylar Resorption

Idiopathic condylar resorption (ICR), also known as progressive condylar resorption or condylar atrophy, is a rare and perplexing condition that primarily affects the TMJ. ICR is characterized by the progressive resorption of the condylar head, leading to significant mandibular deformities and functional disturbances. The etiology of ICR remains unclear, as the condition occurs spontaneously without any apparent triggering factors or underlying systemic diseases. This idiopathic nature makes the diagnosis and treatment of ICR particularly challenging for clinicians [61–63].

ICR typically affects females in their late teens or early adulthood and often presents unilaterally, although bilateral involvement can occur. Patients with ICR may initially complain of mild symptoms such as clicking or popping in the TMJ, joint pain, or limited jaw movement. However, as the condition progresses, patients may experience facial asymmetry, malocclusion, and severe TMJ dysfunction [61, 64].

The radiographic findings typically demonstrate progressive condylar resorption, with the condylar head gradually diminishing in size and shape, leading to a loss of condylar height and structural integrity (Fig. 25) [62–64].

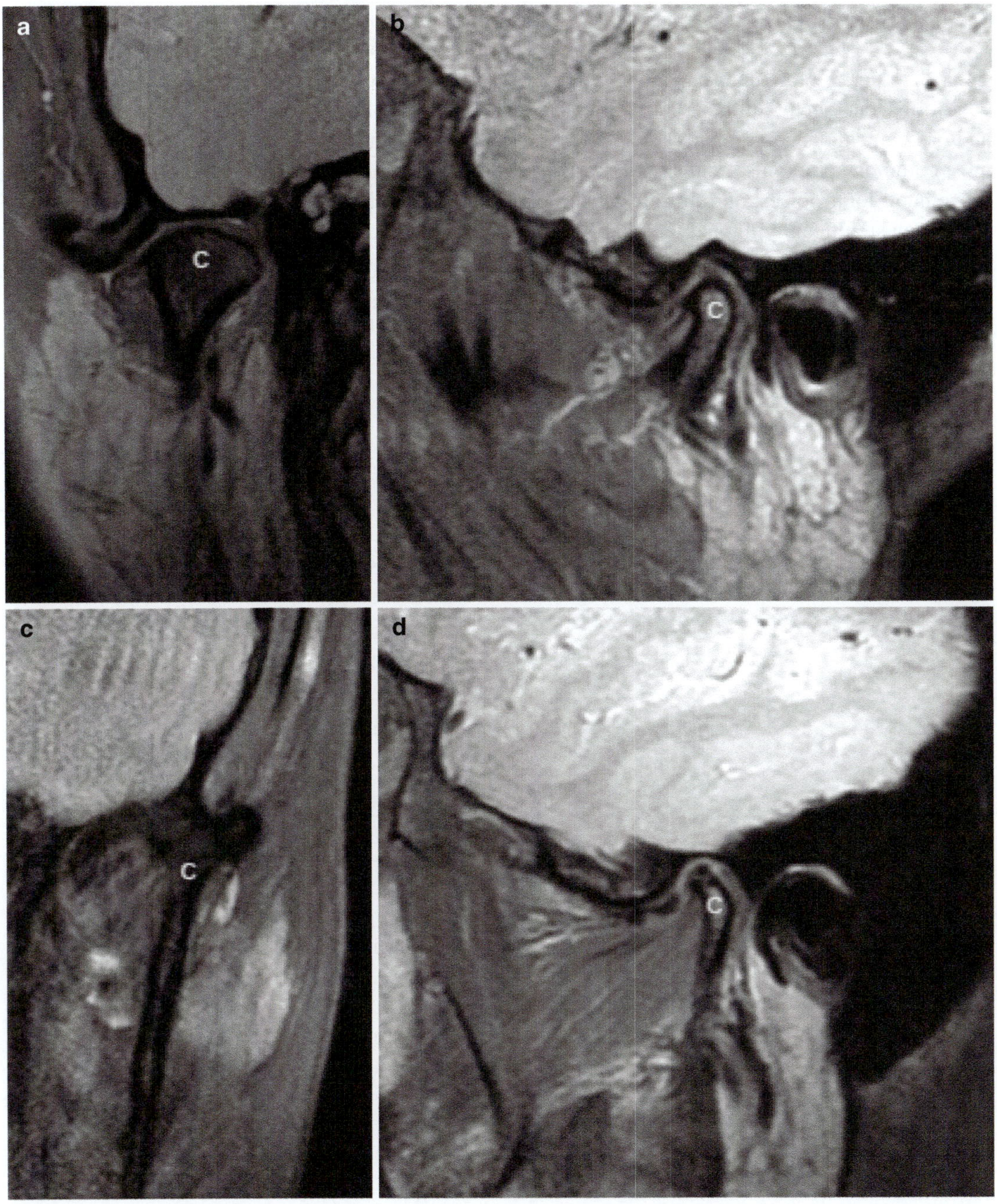

Fig. 25 Coronal proton density-weighted (**a**, **c**) and sagittal proton density-weighted (**b**, **d**) magnetic resonance imaging (MRI) of the same patient demonstrates normal-sized mandibular condyle (c) in (**a**) and (**b**) and typical findings of idiopathic condylar resorption in (**c**) and (**d**)

7 Summary

TMJ disorders are a heterogeneous group of conditions that can affect the articular, muscular, and/or ligamentous components of the joint. The most common symptoms include pain, restricted movement, joint noises, and muscle tenderness, which can significantly impact the quality of life of affected individuals. Although the etiology of TMJ disorders is not fully understood, several factors have been implicated in their pathogenesis, including trauma, malocclusion, parafunctional habits, and systemic diseases such as rheumatoid arthritis. MRI is an imaging modality that is commonly used for TMJ evaluation, especially for assessing the soft tissue components of the joint. MRI is highly sensitive for detecting disc displacement and other soft tissue abnormalities such as joint effusion, synovitis, and muscle edema. Moreover, MRI can provide information about the blood flow and perfusion of the joint, which can be useful for differentiating between inflammatory and noninflammatory conditions.

Appendix. MRI Protocols

Plane	Sequence	Slice thickness	TR	TE	FOV	Mouth position
Axial	T1	2 mm	350	Minimal	250	Closed
Coronal (oblique)	T1	2 mm	350	Minimal	100	Closed
Sagittal (oblique)	PD	2 mm	1500 (350)	Minimal	100	Closed
Sagittal (oblique)	PD	2 mm	1500 (350)	Minimal	100	Open
Sagittal (oblique)	T2	2 mm	2500	70	100	Closed
Plane	**Sequence**	**Slice thickness**	**TR**	**TE**	**FOV**	**Mouth position**
Coronal	T1	3 mm	500	Minimal	250	Closed
Axial	T1	2 mm	500	Minimal	250	Closed
Left sagittal oblique	T2 and PD		3500	Minimal	100	Closed
Right sagittal oblique	T2 and PD		3500	Minimal	100	Closed
Left sagittal oblique	T2 and PD		3500	Minimal	100	Open
Right sagittal oblique	T2 and PD		3500	Minimal	100	Open
Left sagittal oblique	T2		1180	64	100	Dynamic
Right sagittal oblique	T2		1180	64	100	Dynamic
Plane	**Sequence**	**Slice thickness**	**TR**	**TE**	**FOV**	**Mouth position**
Axial	T1	5 mm	300	12	250	Closed
Coronal (oblique)	T1	2 mm	400–500	10–20	100	Closed
Sagittal (oblique)	T2	2 mm	2600	120	100	Closed
Sagittal (oblique)	PD	2 mm	2000	10–14	100	Open
Sagittal (oblique)	T2 GRE	2 mm	600	15	100	Closed
Sagittal	SSFSE PD	3.5 mm	88	12	150	Dynamic
Plane	**Sequence**	**Slice thickness**	**TR**	**TE**	**FOV**	**Mouth position**
Coronal (oblique)	T1	3 mm	300	11	150	Closed
Coronal (oblique)	PD	3 mm	2000	21	150	Closed
Sagittal (oblique)	PD	3 mm	2300	11	150	Closed
Sagittal (oblique)	T2 TSE FS	3 mm	4500	78	150	Closed
Coronal (oblique)	PD	3 mm	2000	20	150	Open
Sagittal (oblique)	PD	3 mm	2300	11	150	Open
Sagittal (oblique)	T2 TSE FS	3 mm	4500	78	150	Open
Plane	**Sequence**	**Slice thickness**	**TR**	**TE**	**FOV**	**Mouth position**
Axial	T1	2 mm	500	Minimal	250	Closed
Coronal (oblique)	T1	3 mm	500	Minimal	100	Closed
Bilateral sagittal oblique	T2 and PD	3 mm	3500	Minimal and 85	100	Closed and open
Bilateral sagittal oblique	T2	3 mm	1180–2000	64	100	Dynamic cine

References

1. Robba T, Tanteri C, Tanteri G. MRI of the temporomandibular joint—correlation between imaging and pathology. Cham: Springer; 2019. https://doi.org/10.1007/978-3-030-25421-6.
2. Vervaeke K, Verhelst P-J, Orhan K, Lund B, Benchimol D, Van der Cruyssen F, De Laat A, Jacobs R, Politis C. Correlation of MRI and arthroscopic findings with clinical outcome in temporomandibular joint disorders: a retrospective cohort study. Head Face Med. 2022;18(1):2. https://doi.org/10.1186/s13005-021-00305-y.
3. Aiken A, Bouloux G, Hudgins P. MR imaging of the temporomandibular joint. Magn Reson Imaging Clin N Am. 2012;20(3):397–412. https://doi.org/10.1016/j.mric.2012.05.002.
4. Vogl TJ, Günther D, Weigl P, Scholtz J-E. Diagnostic value of dynamic magnetic resonance imaging of temporomandibular joint dysfunction. Eur J Radiol Open. 2021;8:100390. https://doi.org/10.1016/j.ejro.2021.100390.
5. Kamel ZSASA, El-Shafey MHR, Hassanien OA, Nagy HA. Can dynamic magnetic resonance imaging replace static magnetic resonance sequences in evaluation of temporomandibular joint dysfunction? Egypt J Radiol Nucl Med. 2021;52:19. https://doi.org/10.1186/s43055-020-00396-8.
6. Nilsson H, Magnusson B, Petersson A. Disk displacement and degenerative changes in the temporomandib-

ular joint: a cross-sectional study. Oral Surg Oral Med Oral Pathol Oral Radiol Endod. 2009;107(3):346–52. https://doi.org/10.1016/j.tripleo.2008.09.020.
7. Azevedo PFM, Patrão PMRC, Torres Rodrigues BM, Ribeiro CFRC, Ribeiro NMP, Silva D, Bacelar MT. MRI of the temporomandibular joint—everything you need to know. ECR. 2018; https://doi.org/10.1594/ecr2018/C-3092.
8. Xiong X, Ye Z, Tang H, Wei Y, Nie L, Wei X, Liu Y, Song B. MRI of temporomandibular joint disorders: recent advances and future directions. J Magn Reson Imaging. 2021;54(4):1039–52. https://doi.org/10.1002/jmri.27338.
9. Suenaga S, Hamamoto S, Kawano K, Higashida Y, Noikura T. Dynamic MR imaging of the temporomandibular joint in patients with arthrosis: relationship between contrast enhancement of the posterior disk attachment and joint pain. AJR Am J Roentgenol. 1996;166:1475–81.
10. Al-Saleh MAQ, Alsufyani NA, Saltaji H, Jaremko JL, Major PW. MRI and CBCT image registration of temporomandibular joint: a systematic review. J Otolaryngol Head Neck Surg. 2016;45(1):30. https://doi.org/10.1186/s40463-016-0144-4.
11. Boccardi A. CT evaluation of chondromatosis of the temporomandibular joint. J Comput Assist Tomogr. 1991;15(5):826–8.
12. Tanaka E, Detamore MS, Mercuri LG. Degenerative disorders of the temporomandibular joint: etiology, diagnosis, and treatment. J Dent Res. 2008;87:296–307.
13. Tomas X, Pomes J, Berenguer J, Quinto L, Nicolau C, Mercader JM, Castro V. MR imaging of temporomandibular joint dysfunction: a pictorial review. Radiographics. 2006;26(3):765–81. https://doi.org/10.1148/rg.263055091.
14. Som PM, Bergeron RT. Head and neck imaging. 2nd ed. St. Louis: Mosby Year Book; 1991.
15. Bag AK, Gaddikeri S, Singhal A, Hardin S, Tran BD, Medina JA, Curé JK. Imaging of the temporomandibular joint: an update. World J Radiol. 2014;6(8):567–82. https://doi.org/10.4329/wjr.v6.i8.567.
16. Yang X, Pernu H, Pyhtinen J, Tiilikainen PA, Oikarinen KS, Raustia AM. MR abnormalities of the lateral pterygoid muscle in patients with nonreducing disk displacement of the TMJ. Cranio. 2002;20:209–21.
17. Taskaya-Yilmaz N, Ceylan G, Incesu L, Muglali M. A possible etiology of the internal derangement of the temporomandibular joint based on the MRI observations of the lateral pterygoid muscle. Surg Radiol Anat. 2005;27:19–24.
18. Chossegros C, Cheynet F, Guyot L, Bellot-Samson V, Blanc JL. Posterior disk displacement of the TMJ: MRI evidence in two cases. Cranio. 2001;19:289–93.
19. Katzberg RW, Westesson P-L. Diagnosis of the temporomandibular joint. 1st ed. Philadelphia: W. B. Saunders; 1993.
20. Poveda-Roda R, Bagan JV, Diaz-Fernandez JM, Hernandez-Bazan S, Jimenez-Soriano Y. Review of temporomandibular joint pathology. Part I: classification, epidemiology and risk factors. Med Oral Patol Oral Cir Bucal. 2007;12(4):E292–8.
21. Tallents RH, Katzberg RW, Murphy W, Proskin H. Magnetic resonance imaging findings in asymptomatic volunteers and symptomatic patients with temporomandibular disorders. J Prosthet Dent. 1996;75:529–33.
22. Schellhas KP, Wilkes CH, Fritts HM, Omlie MR, Heithoff KB, Jahn JA. Temporomandibular joint: MR imaging of internal derangements and postoperative changes. AJR Am J Roentgenol. 1988;150:381–9.
23. Nitzan DW. Temporomandibular joint "open lock" versus condylar dislocation: signs and symptoms, imaging, treatment, and pathogenesis. J Oral Maxillofac Surg. 2002;60:506–11. discussion 512–3
24. Helms CA, Kaban LB, McNeill C, Dodson T. Temporomandibular joint: morphology and signal intensity characteristics of the disk at MR imaging. Radiology. 1989;172:817–20.
25. Dimitroulis G. Condylar resorption of the temporomandibular joint: etiology, diagnosis, and treatment. J Oral Maxillofac Surg. 2005;63(3):379–86.
26. Chang C-L, Wang D-H, Yang M-C, Hsu W-E, Hsu M-L. Functional disorders of the temporomandibular joints: internal derangement of the temporomandibular joint. Kaohsiung J Med Sci. 2018;34(4):223–30. https://doi.org/10.1016/j.kjms.2018.01.004.
27. Eriksen ES, Hellem S, Skartveit L, Brun JG, Bøe OE, Moen K, Geitung JT. Temporomandibular joint pain and associated magnetic resonance findings: a retrospective study with a control group. Acta Radiol Open. 2020;9(9):2058460120938738. https://doi.org/10.1177/2058460120938738.
28. Ribeiro RF, Tallents RH, Katzberg RW, Murphy WC, Moss ME, Magalhaes AC, Tavano O. The prevalence of disc displacement in symptomatic and asymptomatic volunteers aged 6 to 25 years. J Orofac Pain. 1997;11:37–47.
29. Ahmad M, Schiffman EL. Temporomandibular joint disorders and orofacial pain. Dent Clin North Am. 2016;60(1):105–24. https://doi.org/10.1016/j.cden.2015.08.004.
30. Bonjardim LR, Gaviao MB, Pereira LJ, Castelo PM. Anxiety and depression in adolescents and their relationship with signs and symptoms of temporomandibular disorders. Int J Prosthodont. 2005;18(4):347–52.
31. Widmalm SE, Westesson PL, Kim IK, Pereira FJ, Lundh H, Tasaki MM. Temporomandibular joint pathosis related to sex, age, and dentition in autopsy material. Oral Surg Oral Med Oral Pathol. 1994;78:416–25.
32. Tamimi D, Jalali E, Hatcher D. Temporomandibular joint imaging. Radiol Clin North Am. 2018;56(1):157–75. https://doi.org/10.1016/j.rcl.2017.08.011.
33. Gauer RL, Semidey MJ. Diagnosis and treatment of temporomandibular disorders. Am Fam Physician. 2015;91(6):378–86.

34. Paesani D, Westesson PL, Hatala M, Tallents RH, Kurita K. Prevalence of temporomandibular joint internal derangement in patients with craniomandibular disorders. Am J Orthod Dentofacial Orthop. 1992;101:41–7.
35. Larheim TA, Westesson P, Sano T. Temporomandibular joint disk displacement: comparison in asymptomatic volunteers and patients. Radiology. 2001;218:428–32.
36. Cholitgul W, Nishiyama H, Sasai T, Uchiyama Y, Fuchihata H, Rohlin M. Clinical and magnetic resonance imaging findings in temporomandibular joint disc displacement. Dentomaxillofac Radiol. 1997;26:183–8.
37. Katzberg RW, Westesson PL, Tallents RH, Anderson R, Kurita K, Manzione JV, Totterman S. Temporomandibular joint: MR assessment of rotational and sideways disk displacements. Radiology. 1988;169:741–8.
38. Rammelsberg P, Pospiech PR, Jager L, et al. Variability of disc position in asymptomatic volunteers and patients with internal derangements of the TMJ. Oral Surg Oral Med Oral Pathol Oral Radiol Endod. 1997;83(3):393–9.
39. de Leeuw R, Boering G, Stegenga B, de Bont LG. TMJ articular disc position and configuration 30 years after initial diagnosis of internal derangement. J Oral Maxillofac Surg. 1995;53:234–41. discussion 241–242
40. Kuribayashi A, Okochi K, Kobayashi K, Kurabayashi T. MRI findings of temporomandibular joints with disk perforation. Oral Surg Oral Med Oral Pathol Oral Radiol Endod. 2008;106:419–25.
41. Yura S, Nobata K, Shima T. Diagnostic accuracy of fat-saturated T2-weighted magnetic resonance imaging in the diagnosis of perforation of the articular disc of the temporomandibular joint. Br J Oral Maxillofac Surg. 2012;50:365–8.
42. Schellhas KP, Wilkes CH. Temporomandibular joint inflammation: comparison of MR fast scanning with T1- and T2-weighted imaging techniques. AJR Am J Roentgenol. 1989;153:93–8.
43. Rudisch A, Innerhofer K, Bertram S, Emshoff R. Magnetic resonance imaging findings of internal derangement and effusion in patients with unilateral temporomandibular joint pain. Oral Surg Oral Med Oral Pathol Oral Radiol Endod. 2001;92:566–71.
44. Westesson PL, Brooks SL. Temporomandibular joint: relationship between MR evidence of effusion and the presence of pain and disk displacement. AJR Am J Roentgenol. 1992;159:559–63.
45. Xiang S, Rebellato J, Inwards CY, Keller EE. Malocclusion associated with osteocartilaginous loose bodies of the temporomandibular joint. J Am Dent Assoc. 2005;136:484–9.
46. van Ingen JM, de Man K, Bakri I. CT diagnosis of synovial chondromatosis of the temporomandibular joint. Br J Oral Maxillofac Surg. 1990;28:164–7.
47. Schellhas KP, Wilkes CH, Fritts HM, Omlie MR, Lagrotteria LB. MR of osteochondritis dissecans and avascular necrosis of the mandibular condyle. AJR Am J Roentgenol. 1989;152:551–60.
48. Mesgarzadeh M, Sapega AA, Bonakdarpour A, Revesz G, Moyer RA, Maurer AH, Alburger PD. Osteochondritis dissecans: analysis of mechanical stability with radiography, scintigraphy, and MR imaging. Radiology. 1987;165:775–80.
49. Güven O. A clinical study on temporomandibular joint ankylosis. Auris Nasus Larynx. 2000;27:27–33.
50. DaSilva AF, Shaefer J, Keith DA. The temporomandibular joint: clinical and surgical aspects. Neuroimaging Clin N Am. 2003;13:573–82.
51. Hussain AM, Packota G, Major PW, Flores-Mir C. Role of different imaging modalities in assessment of temporomandibular joint erosions and osteophytes: a systematic review. Dentomaxillofac Radiol. 2008;37:63–71.
52. Cannizzaro E, Schroeder S, Müller LM, Kellenberger CJ, Saurenmann RK. Temporomandibular joint involvement in children with juvenile idiopathic arthritis. J Rheumatol. 2011;38:510–5.
53. Twilt M, Mobers SM, Arends LR, ten Cate R, van Suijlekom-Smit L. Temporomandibular involvement in juvenile idiopathic arthritis. J Rheumatol. 2004;31:1418–22.
54. Smith HJ, Larheim TA, Aspestrand F. Rheumatic and nonrheumatic disease in the temporomandibular joint: gadolinium-enhanced MR imaging. Radiology. 1992;185:229–34.
55. Weiss PF, Arabshahi B, Johnson A, Bilaniuk LT, Zarnow D, Cahill AM, Feudtner C, Cron RQ. High prevalence of temporomandibular joint arthritis at disease onset in children with juvenile idiopathic arthritis, as detected by magnetic resonance imaging but not by ultrasound. Arthritis Rheum. 2008;58:1189–96.
56. Konttinen YT, Ainola M, Valleala H, Ma J, Ida H, Mandelin J, Kinne RW, Santavirta S, Sorsa T, López-Otín C, et al. Analysis of 16 different matrix metalloproteinases (MMP-1 to MMP-20) in the synovial membrane: different profiles in trauma and rheumatoid arthritis. Ann Rheum Dis. 1999;58:691–7.
57. Koh ET, Yap AU, Koh CK, Chee TS, Chan SP, Boudville IC. Temporomandibular disorders in rheumatoid arthritis. J Rheumatol. 1999;26:1918–22.
58. Yoshida A, Higuchi Y, Kondo M, Tabata O, Ohishi M. Range of motion of the temporomandibular joint in rheumatoid arthritis: relationship to the severity of disease. Cranio. 1998;16:162–7.
59. Kretapirom K, Okochi K, Nakamura S, Tetsumura A, Ohbayashi N, Yoshino N, Kurabayashi T. MRI characteristics of rheumatoid arthritis in the temporomandibular joint. Dentomaxillofac Radiol. 2013;42:31627230.
60. Matsumura Y, Nomura J, Nakanishi K, Yanase S, Kato H, Tagawa T. Synovial chondromatosis of the

temporomandibular joint with calcium pyrophosphate dihydrate crystal deposition disease (pseudogout). Dentomaxillofac Radiol. 2012;41:703–7.
61. Wolford LM, Cottrell DA, Henry CH. Idiopathic condylar resorption: diagnosis, treatment protocol, and outcomes. Am J Orthod Dentofacial Orthop. 2006;129(6):S9–S24.
62. Lobo ML, Amado FM, Almeida LE, et al. Idiopathic condylar resorption: systematic review of clinical features. J Oral Maxillofac Surg. 2014;72(7):1361–78.
63. Mercuri LG. Idiopathic condylar resorption. J Oral Maxillofac Surg. 2011;69(3):645–55.
64. Hakim SG, Eulert J, Reinhart E. Idiopathic condylar resorption of the temporomandibular joint: pathogenesis, diagnosis, and therapy. Oral Maxillofac Surg Clin North Am. 2015;27(1):39–50.

Basic Clinical Management of Temporomandibular Disorders (TMDs)

Cyril Pandarakalam

1 Introduction

Temporomandibular disorders (TMDs) are a group of diseases that affect temporomandibular joint (TMJ), masticatory muscles, and associated structures [1]. The success of treatment of TMD largely depends on a proper diagnosis. An accurate diagnosis depends on proper history taking and thoroughness of the exam with appropriate imaging. Early intervention can prevent a reversible condition from becoming irreversible.

The initial treatment strategy should mainly involve measures to eliminate pain and provide proper education to patients to reduce recurrence or progression of the disorder. The primary location of the source of pain should be identified, which can be either within the joints, at the preauricular region, or associated with muscles of mastication and cervical muscles. Practitioners should be able to differentiate between locations of the source of pain and site of pain. Treating the referred pain location which is often the site of pain rather than the source of pain will not help with the condition and its symptoms.

Elimination of etiological factors is the key to the long-term management of TMD. Etiological factors can be parafunctional habits, psychological factors, or extension of pain from disorders of surrounding structures. Identification of historical factors like falls, motor vehicle accidents, sports accidents, and recent traumatic or extended dental appointments is also important. For some patients, occlusal disturbances can be a causative factor of symptoms.

Initial management of TMD should be directed towards whether the condition is acute or chronic. Acute symptoms require immediate strategies to mitigate pain. Chronic symptoms may need strategies that may require inclusion of methods to address the emotional aspects of pain. Acute conditions have the potential to become chronic if not addressed on time.

2 Patient Education

Patient education is one of the key factors in the successful treatment of many diseases including TMD [2–5]. An anatomical model will be very helpful for this purpose (Fig. 1). It would be beneficial to give an anatomical comparison between TMJ and other joints. This will help patients understand better about TMJ and surrounding structures since most patients do not think that TMJ is a type of joint like shoulders, hip, or knee.

Additionally, educate patients that teeth are not supposed to touch each other unless they are eating. Identify if there is a habit of daytime clenching. The resting tongue-jaw position should be taught and reinforced. The tongue is supposed to rest on the anterior part of the palate

C. Pandarakalam (✉)
Division of Maxillofacial Surgery, Department of Plastic and Reconstructive Surgery, Kaiser Permanente Medical Center, Santa Clara, CA, USA
e-mail: Cyril.X.Pandarakalam@kp.org

B. C. Stack Jr. et al. (eds.), *Craniofacial Pain*, https://doi.org/10.1007/978-3-031-57563-1_7

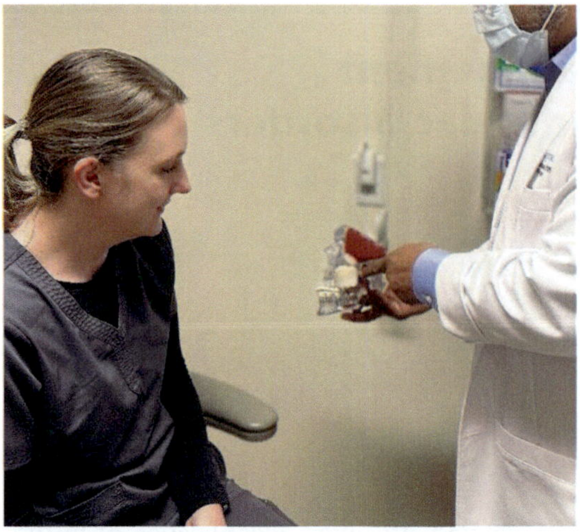

Fig. 1 Practitioner educating patient with the help of anatomical model

behind the upper teeth. When keeping the tongue at that position, make sure that the tongue needs to be placed there rather than pressing against the palate or the upper anterior teeth. With the lips closed, the jaw should be dropping or hanging from the joints rather than carrying the jaw, in the same way as hanging or dropping the arms from the shoulder. This mandibular resting position should be carried out during the whole day, and patients should be advised to keep reminders and alarms. These measures need to be maintained during bedtime before sleeping.

Initial management should include resting the joint and muscles. Try to give comparison to the knee or shoulder which are the joints that may become painful. Explain and make the patient aware of the things that they would do if these joints were tender, painful, or swollen. First and foremost, resting the joint is required. For knee, shoulder, or any other joint, resting the joint is easy: just sit down or lie down. These joints can be unused or minimally used for days or weeks if needed. But it is difficult to stop using TMJ and chewing muscles. These structures move while talking, eating, laughing, singing, etc. Resting is the most difficult task regarding TMJ-related disorders. Make the patient aware of this difficulty, and advise them to eat soft food and to eat slowly. Also advise them not to open their mouth wide. If you explain the difficulty by comparing a similar situation with other joints, patients are most likely to understand, and they are more likely to follow what you advised them.

3 Avoidance Therapy

Another important step is to identify a patient's parafunctional habits and educate them to reduce microtraumas to the joint structures [6]. Bruxism (daytime or nighttime) is the most common habit you might identify. Other habits are chewing gums, nail biting, lip and cheek chewing, and chewing objects like pen or pencil. As discussed earlier, daytime clenching needs to be identified [7]. Also observe during the office visit if they are biting lips, biting nails, or biting or chewing the cheeks or tongue. Identify and make sure that they understand, and advise to avoid these habits. Avoid poor head and neck posture while working and using the phone. If a patient has clicking or popping, educate them to avoid clicking or popping as much as possible. Mostly they can avoid clicking by limiting the wide opening of the mouth. Advise them to open gently to avoid loud clicking while they open their mouths.

4 Psychological Factors

Psychological disorders have a significant role in the development of TMD in a portion of patients. Identify anxiety, stress, depression, or other psychiatric disorders, and facilitate with appropriate referrals for the management of these disorders [8–10]. For patients presenting with psychological diagnoses, there are some antipsychotic and antidepressant medications that can induce bruxism in patients. Identify these medications while informing the patient and their providers that their substitution or elimination could benefit the management of TMD.

5 Obstructive Sleep Apnea

Identify if your patient has any risk for obstructive sleep apnea (OSA). OSA and TMD do coexist [11]. Excessive daytime sleeping, snoring, witnessed apnea, being unrefreshed upon waking, and sleepy after a meal or while watching television are some of the indicators. OSA might induce bruxism. Use Epworth Sleepiness Scale or STOP-BANG questionnaire. Continuous positive airway pressure (CPAP) is the gold standard and most efficacious for treating OSA. Mandibular advancement device (MAD, oral sleep appliance) can be used if a patient is intolerant to CPAP [12, 13]. When you identify a patient with OSA using the questionnaires listed above, refer the patient for a sleep study. MAD is an option for OSA, but make sure to educate patients about its possible side effects [14, 15]. Be aware that it is common for some patients to request for MAD after a short and inadequate trial of CPAP usage.

6 Examination

A thorough examination will tell you whether the pain is primarily from the muscles (Fig. 2) or the temporomandibular joint (Fig. 3). Tenderness to palpation of the preauricular region indicates joint inflammation. Consider imaging in these cases. A panoramic radiograph is a good place to start. A CBCT is ideal to see a three-dimensional image. If there is painful click or lock with difficulty opening mouth, an MRI with TMJ protocol (closed mouth and open mouth) should be considered to confirm the historical and clinical diagnosis.

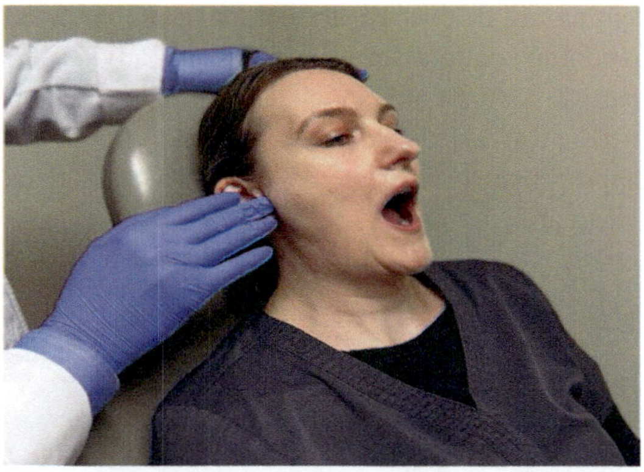

Fig. 3 Examination of temporomandibular joint at the preauricular region

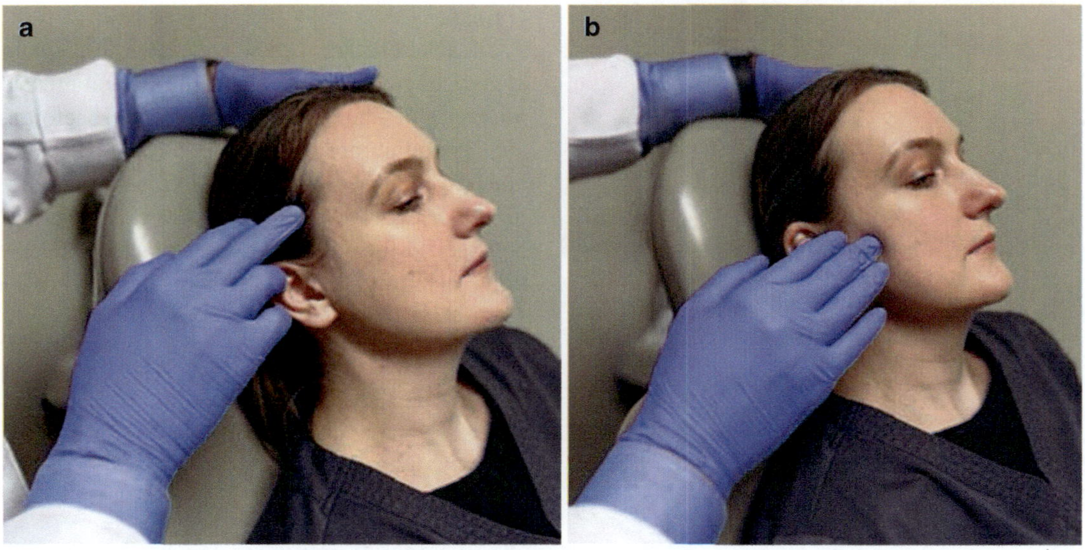

Fig. 2 Examination of (**a**) masseter and (**b**) temporalis muscle

7 Thermal Application

Cold and heat compresses are very useful for successful management of TMD [16–18]. Generally, a cold compress is beneficial if there is inflammation and pain (Fig. 4). Heat is beneficial for muscle tightness and aches. Whether the pain source is TMJ or muscle, generally for acute symptoms cold application is recommended and for chronic symptoms heat application is advised. If these recommendations are insufficient, advise the patient to try cold and heat compresses alternately for 2–4 weeks to assess and choose the appropriate thermal method which is beneficial for their symptoms.

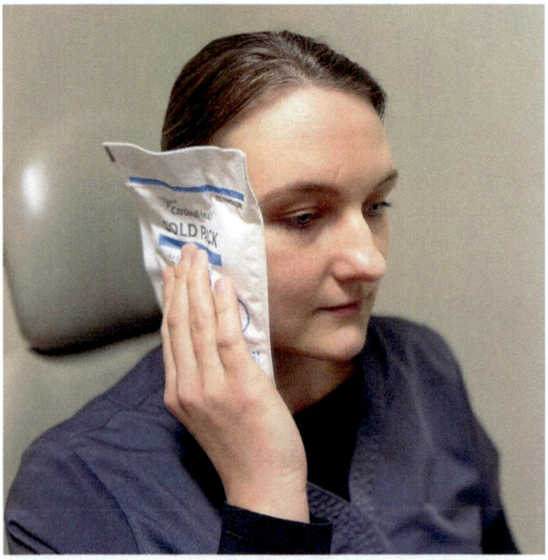

Fig. 4 A patient applying thermal (cold) compress

8 Pharmacologic Management

If you suspect acute joint inflammation, an NSAID (ibuprofen) can be prescribed even though these are also beneficial for select cases of muscular pain conditions [19–21]. The choice of anti-inflammatory depends on the practitioner, but make sure that you know the half-life of the medication. For example, ibuprofen needs to be taken every 6–8 h, and naproxen needs only a 12-h interval. Since the TMJ and associated structures cannot be rested like other joints, it would be wise to take these medications for a few days in a regimen (10–14 days) without break. Generally, the use of oral NSAIDS should be limited to 1–2 months.

Avoid oral NSAIDs for elderly patients, pregnant patients, and patients with gastric issues and kidney problems. Use Tylenol instead even though it is a weak anti-inflammatory medication. Alternatives include topical medications. There are several over-the-counter topical pain relievers like Voltaren (TM) gel, Aspercreme (TM), and Biofreeze (TM). You can also discuss with a pharmacist for compounded topical pain options.

Muscle relaxants can be considered if the pain is myogenous in nature. There are several muscle relaxants of choice: cyclobenzaprine, baclofen, and tizanidine are the most common. They are not proven to be good for TMD for more than a month or two. Any medication prescribed should be checked for interaction with existing medications taken by patients. Other medications to be considered are tricyclic antidepressants like nortriptyline, serotonin norepinephrine reuptake inhibitors, selective serotonin reuptake inhibitors, and anticonvulsant medications [22–24]. These medications should be prescribed by their primary physician or psychiatrist.

9 Physical Therapy

Office-based and home-based physical therapy are great tools in the management of TMJ. Even though physical therapy exercises can be utilized for acute conditions like closed lock (disc displacement without reduction), they are specifically suitable for chronic cases of TMD. A physical therapist trained in the management of TMD is ideal to treat these patients. They can do office-based physical therapy and reinforce patients to do certain exercises at home. Physical therapy may not give immediate relief of the symptoms, and the success of the treatment depends on the adherence and consistency of performing the exercises (Fig. 5). These exercises involve massaging palpable muscles, isometric jaw-strengthening exercises, and active or passive stretching exercises [25–27]. For most of the patients, regular self-reminders and reinforcement by practitioners are required for adherence to instructions.

10 Acupuncture

Several studies have shown that acupuncture is effective for patients with TMD and is generally used as an adjunctive therapy [28–32]. Though acupuncture has been shown to help reduce symptoms, TMD therapy needs a multidimensional approach which often requires identification and elimination of its causes.

11 Occlusal Stabilization Splints (Night Guards or Bite Splints)

There are several philosophies about the design of night guard or bite splints. There are several brands of over-the-counter (OTC) night guards available with varying degrees of thickness, hardness, and design. These are generally used to protect the teeth if a patient thinks that they have a habit of bruxism or if their dentist mentions it to them. Without TMD, these are basically enough to be a night guard. These OTC night guards are also beneficial for patients with TMD, but preferably it is used only for a short period of time until a custom-made night guard or bite splint is fabricated. A custom-made full-coverage night guard (or bite splint) with even occlusion is the most widely used, with least risk of complications, if

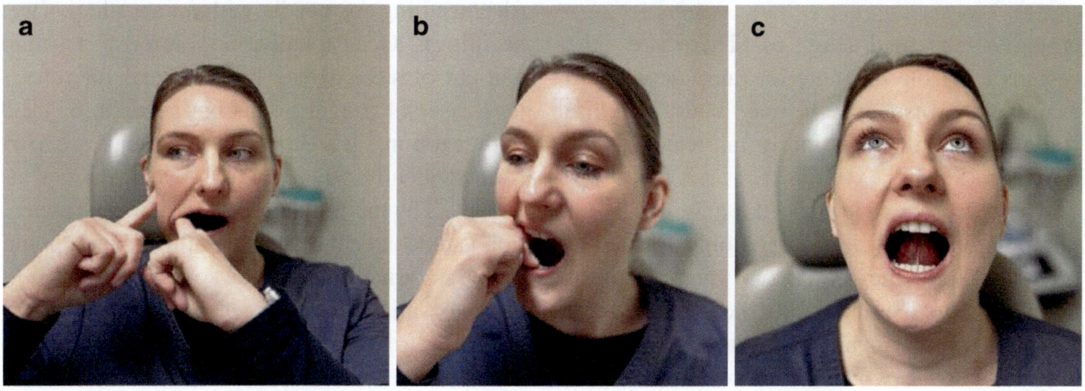

Fig. 5 Physical therapy exercises: (**a**) self-massage, (**b**) passive stretching, (**c**) active stretching

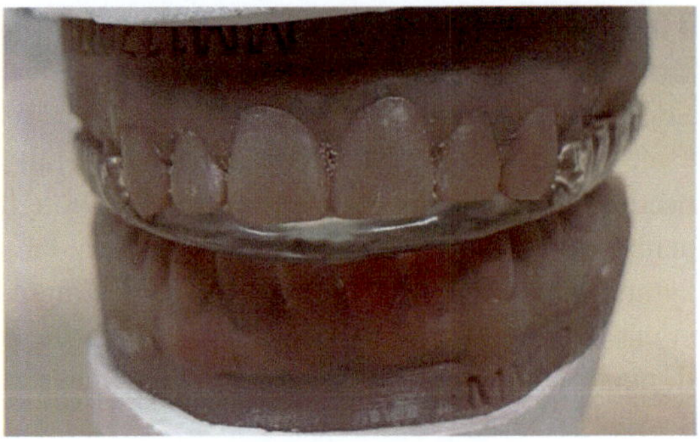

Fig. 6 A study model with a maxillary bite splint

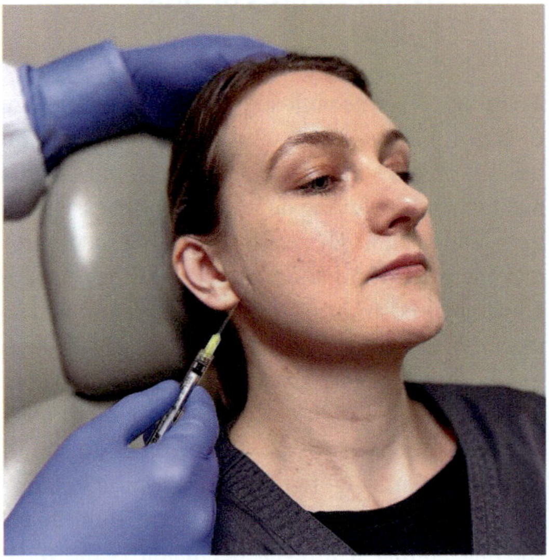

Fig. 7 Trigger-point injection to the masseter muscle

properly fabricated (Fig. 6). There are other designs available like anterior ramp devices, for example NTI-tss, which may cause occlusal complications if not properly fabricated or followed up [33–36].

There are other devices like anterior repositioning splints, which are used only for a short term to relieve the joint from compression or trauma if injured or inflamed. These are also used for disc displacement. These appliances need close follow-ups to minimize occlusal complications.

As mentioned before, MADs are options to manage sleep apnea if the patient is intolerant to CPAP. Learn about different MAD designs, discuss with a lab about their designs, and choose 2–3 and know their indications. Certain MADs are good for bruxers, some are good for esthetics, and others are good for mouth breathers. When making an MAD, make sure that you mention to the patient that there is a high chance of bite changes that will happen over time. Reinforce them to do morning exercises regularly to restore the position of the jaw to minimize permanent occlusal changes.

12 Injections

There are several injection techniques indicated for TMD. For acute closed lock, meaning the disc dislocation is preventing translation of the condyle, a joint injection with anesthetic with or without steroid can help manually (self or practitioner assisted) reduce the disc from the locked position allowing translation of the condyle. TMJ steroid injection can also be used for acute joint inflammation caused by trauma and flare-up of arthritis [37, 38].

Another group of injections are muscle injections used for myofascial pain. As discussed, myofascial pain is characterized by trigger points with radiating and referring pain to distant regions. Trigger-point injections are given to break the taut bands of the muscle tissue, which are referred to as trigger points. These injections are performed with a needle without any solution (dry needling) or needle with an anesthetic (wet needling). Occasionally, addition of a small amount of steroid may be beneficial for refractory cases of trigger points but needs to be used with caution. Trigger-point injections are performed ideally with a 6- to 8-week interval as needed. The main function of trigger-point injection is mechanical disruption of the trigger point, which in turn eliminates the source of pain [39].

Botox injections have recently become a very common treatment modality for TMD. These injection vials contain botulism toxin, initially approved for movement disorders. They are used off-label for myofascial pain disorder, and injection with Botox needs training. The main skill depends on knowing the anatomy of each masticatory muscle. Masseter and temporalis muscles

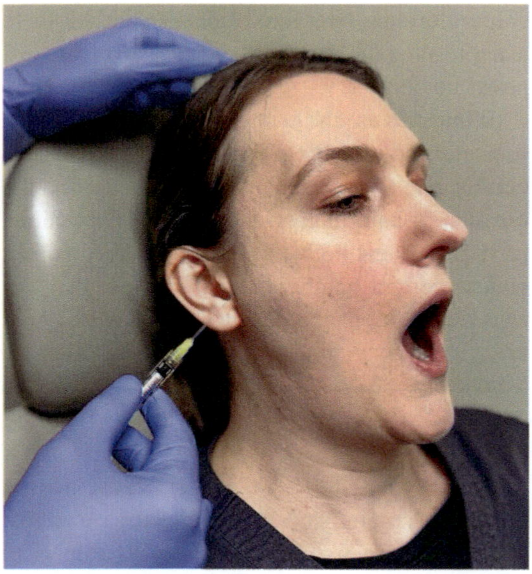

Fig. 8 Steroid injection to the temporomandibular joint

are easy to identify and palpate (Fig. 7). Pterygoids are not easy to isolate for injection, but these muscles can also be injected with the help of an electromyography (EMG) machine by a trained specialist [40, 41].

Another injection technique utilizes hyaluronic acid which lubricates the joints. These are commonly used for other larger joints, most commonly for knees. These agents can also be injected into the TMJ in small quantities (Fig. 8). These are used to reduce joint sounds and have also shown to reduce inflammation [42].

13 Chronic Pain Management

Occasionally, some patients do not respond to general conservative management strategies. For these patients, we may need to refer them to a pain psychologist, or pain management programs, which may include specialized methodologies including cognitive behavioral therapy (CBT) and biofeedback. These referrals can be facilitated by the patient's primary care physician. In these circumstances, identifying the need and proper communication with the physician are very important for the success of management of TMD [43].

14 Referrals

There are situations where patients present with ear symptoms with or without symptoms of TMD (jaw pain or joint noises). When your patient presents with ear symptoms, evaluate their ear with an otoscope or, if not comfortable, send the patient to an otolaryngologist to rule out any primary ear disorder. When using an otoscope, you are checking for any signs of infection, inflammation, or bleeding in the external auditory canal. Also, you may see cerumen impaction. If you find severe arthritis or structural changes of the joints, a referral to their physician or rheumatologist may be warranted to rule out inflammatory arthritis.

Sometimes, a patient with TMD presents with unusual symptoms like numbness, paresthesia, headaches, and migraines. Therefore, it is very important to get information from the patient about the location of pain, quality or type of pain, and severity of pain. It would be beneficial to perform cranial nerve exam, at least for the fifth cranial nerve. These patients may need a neurology evaluation to rule out primary headache disorders, migraine, or intracranial causes of pain.

Patients who are refractory to any procedures even after multiple specialist evaluations may need referral to the pain medicine department for interventional pain management methods like sphenopalatine nerve block and infusions with lidocaine or ketamine.

15 Surgical Management

For certain patients, surgical management may be necessary. Those are patients who are resistant to conservative management with persistent joint inflammation, severe joint noises, severe arthritic changes of the joints, skeletal malocclusion, etc. Arthrocentesis is the least invasive surgical procedure that involves flushing of the TMJ with saline to remove inflammatory exudates, adhesions, and bony particles or "joint mice" from breakdown of articular surfaces as part of arthritic process. There are other surgical techniques utilized based on the severity of TMD, which include arthroscopy, arthroplasty, modified condylotomy, and total joint replacement [44].

16 Initial Consultation

When a patient comes with jaw pain and TMD is suspected, the initial step is to take a thorough history. It is important to gather details of the signs and symptoms since the onset. Another important information needed is about parafunctional habits like teeth grinding and clenching (day- or nighttime), gum chewing, pen and pencil chewing, ice cube or crushed ice chewing, and cheek or lip biting.

Next, examine TMJ region, which is the preauricular area in front of the ear, and external muscles of mastication (masseter and temporalis) and cervical muscles, mainly the sternocleidomastoid and trapezius muscles. Also take measurements of maximum mouth (interincisal) opening without pain and with pain separately. You need to record any joint sounds while opening the mouth during exams and their mouth opening pathway which can be straight, deviated (transiently deviates from the midline), or deflected (off to an angle). The next step is to examine intraorally for any dental or periodontally related diseases, soft and hard tissue diseases, and malocclusion. A mylar strip (shim stock) would be beneficial to check occlusion between each tooth.

Initial observation should be to determine whether it is primary TMD or secondary TMD disorder related to other causes like dental or periodontal pain. Once TMD is suspected, the next step is to determine whether the symptoms are from the TMJ or muscles by palpating these areas and observing the patient's response.

If one suspects the primary source is from the joint from the response of the patient on exam, a panoramic radiograph can be used to screen for arthritic changes, fractures, or tumors. The most common tumor associated with mandibular condyle is osteochondroma. A cone beam computed tomography (CBCT), if available, can also be used to assess bony structures three dimensionally. It is beneficial to attend one of the CBCT courses offered by a maxillofacial radiologist to learn to read TMJ and other bony structures of head and neck.

If muscles are the primary source of pain, perform a thorough palpation of the masseter, temporalis, and temporalis tendon to exactly find the location of pain in each muscle and, if possible, include cervical muscles. Identify trigger points, which are taut bands of muscle tissue, that can cause referred pain to distant sites on palpation.

17 Pain

If it is determined that the primary cause of pain is within the joint, and any emergency cause like fracture has been ruled out, the next step is to control the pain.

17.1 Primary Joint Pain

Almost always joint pain is from inflammation. The pain could be from a flare-up of arthritis or inflammation of the retrodiscal tissue from trauma. The trauma can be from a fall or biting on a hard object (nuts, etc.). Inflammation of retrodiscal tissue is most likely because of displacement of the articular disc. The articular disc, which is supposed to act as a cushion between the articular surface of the condyle and the temporal bone, when displaced can cause retrodiscal tissue, which is highly vascular and innervated, prone to injury.

As we discussed earlier, the initial measure to control pain is achieved by resting the joint (soft diet, slower chewing, smaller bites) and not opening mouth wider. Instruct patients to take an anti-inflammatory medication, like ibuprofen or naproxen. In patients who cannot tolerate NSAIDs, Tylenol or a topical NSAID can be given. Patients should also be advised to use cold compresses several times a day to reduce inflammation. A custom-made or a short-term OTC night guard should be considered to reduce joint loading.

Patients should be advised to follow these instructions for 1–2 weeks before re-evaluation. If pain persists, the next step is to give a steroid (cortisone) injection. The injection technique requires a thorough knowledge about the anatomy, and it is beneficial to attend a hands-on training to master the technique. If not comfortable, send the patient to a maxillofacial surgeon to perform arthrocentesis (lavage of the joint).

If the articular disc, which is the cushion (shock absorber) within the joint, is dislocated in closed-mouth position, it may reduce or go back to the normal position on mouth opening causing a clicking sound (disc dislocation with reduction) or it may not go back leading to closed lock (disc dislocation without reduction) leading to inability to open mouth wider. The TMJ has an initial hinge (rotational) movement followed by gliding (translational) movement. A hinge movement is enough to open the mouth up to about 25–30 mm, and translational movement is required for wider mouth opening. This situation can happen unilaterally or bilaterally. If there is unilateral locking, the jaw will deflect to the affected side on mouth opening. Disc dislocation without reduction (closed lock) can also cause pain in the joint, and the treatment is the same as for joint inflammation described above.

17.2 Primary Muscle Pain

If it is determined that the primary source of pain is the muscles of mastication or cervical muscles, identify the location of pain in each muscle. Identify if the source of pain is a trigger point. A trigger point is a tight band of muscle tissue that when palpated radiates or refers pain to distant sites. If you can identify trigger points, injections can be performed to eliminate these sources of pain. An orofacial pain specialist or a trained acupuncturist can perform these injections. There are training courses available.

If there is absence of trigger points and the muscle pain is diffuse and an aching kind of pain, general instructions can be given as previously explained which include resting the muscles, avoidance of parafunctional habits, and thermal applications. A short regimen of muscle relaxant can also be considered. A referral to a physical therapist would be beneficial.

If bruxism is identified, a custom-made night guard should be fabricated. For long-term care, these night guards need to be checked every 6–12 months.

17.3 Open Lock (TMJ Dislocation)

An open lock of TMJ is often confused with closed lock. Closed lock is caused by disc dislocation, leading to inability to open the mouth. Open lock is caused by dislocation of the condyle in front of the articular eminence. An open lock can be self-reducible or reduced by a practitioner using finger pressure on the unrelaxed patient or under sedation.

18 Summary

There are many treatment modalities that have been used by many practitioners for TMD which were reviewed above and in other parts of this text. Surgical referral is entertained if the diagnosis suggests an internal derangement of the TMJ. Additionally, occlusal rehabilitation and neuromuscular therapy are some of the popular methodologies. The evidence behind these methods is controversial and not conclusive. There are other modalities such as ultrasound therapy, laser therapy, and chiropractic therapy. Any treatment that relieves pain and other symptoms of the patient is acceptable, if the treatment is not harmful to the patient.

References

1. Schiffman E, Ohrbach R, Truelove E, Look J, Anderson G, Goulet JP, List T, Svensson P, Gonzalez Y, Lobbezoo F, Michelotti A, Brooks SL, Ceusters W, Drangsholt M, Ettlin D, Gaul C, Goldberg LJ, Haythornthwaite JA, Hollender L, Jensen R, John MT, De Laat A, de Leeuw R, Maixner W, van der Meulen M, Murray GM, Nixdorf DR, Palla S, Petersson A, Pionchon P, Smith B, Visscher CM, Zakrzewska J, Dworkin SF, International RDC/TMD Consortium Network, International association for Dental Research; Orofacial Pain Special Interest Group, International Association for the Study of

Pain. Diagnostic Criteria for Temporomandibular Disorders (DC/TMD) for clinical and research applications: recommendations of the International RDC/TMD Consortium Network* and Orofacial Pain Special Interest Group†. J Oral Facial Pain Headache. 2014;28(1):6–27. https://doi.org/10.11607/jop.1151. PMID: 24482784; PMCID: PMC4478082.
2. Albano MG, d'Ivernois JF, de Andrade V, Levy G. Patient education in dental medicine: a review of the literature. Eur J Dent Educ. 2019;23(2):110–8. https://doi.org/10.1111/eje.12409. Epub 2019 Jan 9. PMID: 30556294.
3. Management of temporomandibular disorders. National Institutes of Health technology assessment conference statement. J Am Dent Assoc. 1996;127(11):1595–1606.
4. Dimitroulis G. Temporomandibular disorders: a clinical update. BMJ. 1998;317(7152):190–4.
5. Xu L, Cai B, Lu S, Fan S, Dai K. The impact of education and physical therapy on oral behaviour in patients with temporomandibular disorder: a preliminary study. Biomed Res Int. 2021;2021:6666680. https://doi.org/10.1155/2021/6666680. PMID: 33564681; PMCID: PMC7850854.
6. Ohrbach R, Sharma S. Behavioral therapy for temporomandibular disorders. Front Oral Maxillofac Med. 2021;3:37.
7. Glaros AG, Hanson AH, Ryen CC. Headache and oral parafunctional behaviors. Appl Psychophysiol Biofeedback. 2014;39(1):59–66. https://doi.org/10.1007/s10484-014-9242-0. PMID: 24519847.
8. Sójka A, Stelcer B, Roy M, Mojs E, Pryliński M. Is there a relationship between psychological factors and TMD? Brain Behav. 2019;9(9):e01360. https://doi.org/10.1002/brb3.1360. Epub 2019 Jul 24. PMID: 31339236; PMCID: PMC7649956.
9. Fillingim RB, Ohrbach R, Greenspan JD, Knott C, Diatchenko L, Dubner R, Bair E, Baraian C, Mack N, Slade GD, Maixner W. Psychological factors associated with development of TMD: the OPPERA prospective cohort study. J Pain. 2013;14(12 Suppl):T75–90. https://doi.org/10.1016/j.jpain.2013.06.009. PMID: 24275225; PMCID: PMC3855656.
10. Jung W, Lee KE, Suh BJ. Influence of psychological factors on the prognosis of temporomandibular disorders pain. J Dent Sci. 2021;16(1):349–55. https://doi.org/10.1016/j.jds.2020.02.007. Epub 2020 Mar 31. PMID: 33384819; PMCID: PMC7770244.
11. Sanders AE, Essick GK, Fillingim R, Knott C, Ohrbach R, Greenspan JD, Diatchenko L, Maixner W, Dubner R, Bair E, Miller VE, Slade GD. Sleep apnea symptoms and risk of temporomandibular disorder: OPPERA cohort. J Dent Res. 2013;92(7 Suppl):70S–7S. https://doi.org/10.1177/0022034513488140. Epub 2013 May 20. PMID: 23690360; PMCID: PMC3706181.
12. Ilea A, Timuş D, Höpken J, Andrei V, Băbţan AM, Petrescu NB, Câmpian RS, Boşca AB, Şovrea AS, Negucioiu M, Mesaros A. Oral appliance therapy in obstructive sleep apnea and snoring—systematic review and new directions of development. Cranio. 2021;39(6):472–83. https://doi.org/10.1080/08869634.2019.1673285. Epub 2019 Oct 5. PMID: 31588866.
13. Rossi A, Lo Giudice A, Di Pardo C, Valentini AT, Marradi F, Vanacore N, Grippaudo C. Clinical evidence in the treatment of obstructive sleep apnoea with oral appliances: a systematic review. Int J Dent. 2021;2021:6676158. https://doi.org/10.1155/2021/6676158. PMID: 34035815; PMCID: PMC8124002.
14. Al-Jewair T, Shibeika D, Ohrbach R. Temporomandibular disorders and their association with sleep disorders in adults: a systematic review. J Oral Facial Pain Headache. 2021;35(1):41–53. https://doi.org/10.11607/ofph.2780. PMID: 33730126.
15. Merrill RL. Temporomandibular disorder pain and dental treatment of obstructive sleep apnea. Dent Clin North Am. 2012;56(2):415–31. https://doi.org/10.1016/j.cden.2012.01.004. PMID: 22480811.
16. Furlan RM, Giovanardi RS, Britto AT, Oliveira e Britto DB. The use of superficial heat for treatment of temporomandibular disorders: an integrative review. Codas. 2015;27(2):207–12. English, Portuguese. PMID: 26107088. https://doi.org/10.1590/2317-1782/20152014148.
17. Wieckiewicz M, Boening K, Wiland P, Shiau YY, Paradowska-Stolarz A. Reported concepts for the treatment modalities and pain management of temporomandibular disorders. J Headache Pain. 2015;16:106. https://doi.org/10.1186/s10194-015-0586-5. Epub 2015 Dec 7. PMID: 26644030; PMCID: PMC4671990.
18. Freesmeyer WB, Fussnegger MR, Ahlers MO. Diagnostic and therapeutic-restorative procedures for masticatory dysfunctions. GMS Curr Top Otorhinolaryngol Head Neck Surg. 2005;4:Doc19. Epub 2005 Sep 28. PMID: 22073067; PMCID: PMC3201006.
19. Ouanounou A, Goldberg M, Haas DA. Pharmacotherapy in temporomandibular disorders: a review. J Can Dent Assoc. 2017;83:h7. PMID: 29513209.
20. Hersh EV, Balasubramaniam R, Pinto A. Pharmacologic management of temporomandibular disorders. Oral Maxillofac Surg Clin North Am. 2008;20(2):197–210, vi. PMID: 18343325. https://doi.org/10.1016/j.coms.2007.12.005.
21. Chan NHY, Ip CK, Li DTS, Leung YY. Diagnosis and treatment of myogenous temporomandibular disorders: a clinical update. Diagnostics (Basel). 2022;12(12):2914. https://doi.org/10.3390/diagnostics12122914. PMID: 36552921; PMCID: PMC9776546.
22. Tran C, Ghahreman K, Huppa C, Gallagher JE. Management of temporomandibular disorders: a rapid review of systematic reviews and guidelines. Int J Oral Maxillofac Surg. 2022;51(9):1211–25. https://doi.org/10.1016/j.ijom.2021.11.009. Epub 2022 Mar 23. PMID: 35339331.

23. Dammling C, et al. The use of pharmacologic agents in the management of temporomandibular joint disorder. Front Oral Maxillofac Med. 2022;4:17.
24. Mujakperuo HR, Watson M, Morrison R, et al. Pharmacological interventions for pain in patients with temporomandibular disorders. Cochrane Database Syst Rev. 2010:CD004715.
25. Shimada A, Ishigaki S, Matsuka Y, Komiyama O, Torisu T, Oono Y, Sato H, Naganawa T, Mine A, Yamazaki Y, Okura K, Sakuma Y, Sasaki K. Effects of exercise therapy on painful temporomandibular disorders. J Oral Rehabil. 2019;46(5):475–81. https://doi.org/10.1111/joor.12770. Epub 2019 Feb 19. PMID: 30664815.
26. Macías-Hernández SI, Morones-Alba JD, Tapia-Ferrusco I, Vélez-Gutiérrez OB, Hernández-Diaz C, Nava-Bringas TI, Cruz-Medina E, Toro LC, Soria-Bastida MLA. A home-based exercise program for temporomandibular joint osteoarthritis: pain, functionality, and joint structure. J Korean Assoc Oral Maxillofac Surg. 2022;48(1):50–8. https://doi.org/10.5125/jkaoms.2022.48.1.50. PMID: 35221307; PMCID: PMC8890964.
27. Al-Moraissi EA, Conti PCR, Alyahya A, Alkebsi K, Elsharkawy A, Christidis N. The hierarchy of different treatments for myogenous temporomandibular disorders: a systematic review and network meta-analysis of randomized clinical trials. Oral Maxillofac Surg. 2022;26(4):519–33. https://doi.org/10.1007/s10006-021-01009-y. Epub 2021 Oct 21. Erratum in: Oral Maxillofac Surg. 2021 Nov 5. PMID: 34674093.
28. Cho SH, Whang WW. Acupuncture for temporomandibular disorders: a systematic review. J Orofac Pain. 2010;24(2):152–62. PMID: 20401353.
29. Jung A, Shin BC, Lee MS, Sim H, Ernst E. Acupuncture for treating temporomandibular joint disorders: a systematic review and meta-analysis of randomized, sham-controlled trials. J Dent. 2011;39(5):341–50. https://doi.org/10.1016/j.jdent.2011.02.006. Epub 2011 Feb 25. PMID: 21354460.
30. Dietrich L, Rodrigues IVS, Assis Costa MDM, Carvalho RF, Silva GRD. Acupuncture in temporomandibular disorders painful symptomatology: an evidence-based case report. Eur J Dent. 2020;14(4):692–6. https://doi.org/10.1055/s--0040-1716631. Epub 2020 Oct 1. PMID: 33003235; PMCID: PMC7536091.
31. Şen S, Orhan G, Sertel S, Schmitter M, Schindler HJ, Lux CJ, Giannakopoulos NN. Comparison of acupuncture on specific and non-specific points for the treatment of painful temporomandibular disorders: a randomised controlled trial. J Oral Rehabil. 2020;47(7):783–95. https://doi.org/10.1111/joor.12952. Epub 2020 Mar 9. PMID: 32077514.
32. de Salles-Neto FT, de Paula JS, Romero JGAJ, Almeida-Leite CM. Acupuncture for pain, mandibular function and oral health-related quality of life in patients with masticatory myofascial pain: a randomised controlled trial. J Oral Rehabil. 2020;47(10):1193–201. https://doi.org/10.1111/joor.13055. Epub 2020 Jul 31. PMID: 32668487.
33. Al-Moraissi EA, Farea R, Qasem KA, Al-Wadeai MS, Al-Sabahi ME, Al-Iryani GM. Effectiveness of occlusal splint therapy in the management of temporomandibular disorders: network meta-analysis of randomized controlled trials. Int J Oral Maxillofac Surg. 2020;49(8):1042–56. https://doi.org/10.1016/j.ijom.2020.01.004. Epub 2020 Jan 22. PMID: 31982236.
34. Poorna TA, John B, E K J, Rao A. Comparison of the effectiveness of soft and hard splints in the symptomatic management of temporomandibular joint disorders: a randomized control study. Int J Rheum Dis. 2022;25(9):1053–9. https://doi.org/10.1111/1756-185X.14379. Epub 2022 Jul 4. PMID: 35785423.
35. Bilir H, Kurt H. Influence of stabilization splint thickness on temporomandibular disorders. Int J Prosthodont. 2022;35(2):163–73. https://doi.org/10.11607/ijp.6923. PMID: 35507529.
36. Conti PC, dos Santos CN, Kogawa EM, de Castro Ferreira Conti AC, de Araujo Cdos R. The treatment of painful temporomandibular joint clicking with oral splints: a randomized clinical trial. J Am Dent Assoc. 2006;137(8):1108–14. https://doi.org/10.14219/jada.archive.2006.0349. PMID: 16873326.
37. Moldez MA, Camones VR, Ramos GE, Padilla M, Enciso R. Effectiveness of intra-articular injections of sodium hyaluronate or corticosteroids for intracapsular temporomandibular disorders: a systematic review and meta-analysis. J Oral Facial Pain Headache. 2018;32(1):53–66. https://doi.org/10.11607/ofph.1783. Epub 2017 Dec 15. PMID: 29244893.
38. Torres D, Zaror C, Iturriaga V, Tobias A. Intra-articular corticosteroids for treatment of temporomandibular joint internal disorders: protocol for systematic review and network meta-analysis. BMJ Open. 2020;10(9):e034327. https://doi.org/10.1136/bmjopen-2019-034327. PMID: 32895260; PMCID: PMC7476463.
39. Aksu Ö, Pekin Doğan Y, Sayıner Çağlar N, Şener BM. Comparison of the efficacy of dry needling and trigger point injections with exercise in temporomandibular myofascial pain treatment. Turk J Phys Med Rehabil. 2019;65(3):228–35. https://doi.org/10.5606/tftrd.2019.1802. PMID: 31663071; PMCID: PMC6797918.
40. Delcanho R, Val M, Guarda Nardini L, Manfredini D. Botulinum toxin for treating temporomandibular disorders: what is the evidence? J Oral Facial Pain Headache. 2022;36(1):6–20. https://doi.org/10.11607/ofph.3023. PMID: 35298571.
41. Anwar H, Attard A, Green J, Elledge ROC. Botulinum toxin in the management of myalgia in temporomandibular disorders: are all injections equal? Br J Oral Maxillofac Surg. 2023;61(1):89–93. https://doi.org/10.1016/j.bjoms.2022.11.279. Epub 2022 Nov 29. PMID: 36522255.
42. Goiato MC, da Silva EV, de Medeiros RA, Túrcio KH, Dos Santos DM. Are intra-articular injections

of hyaluronic acid effective for the treatment of temporomandibular disorders? A systematic review. Int J Oral Maxillofac Surg. 2016;45(12):1531–7. https://doi.org/10.1016/j.ijom.2016.06.004. Epub 2016 Jun 30. PMID: 27374020.
43. de Barros Pascoal AL, de Freitas RFCP, da Silva LFG, Oliveira AGRC, Dos Santos Calderon P. Effectiveness of counseling on chronic pain management in patients with temporomandibular disorders. J Oral Facial Pain Headache. 2020;34(1):77–82. https://doi.org/10.11607/ofph.2163. Epub 2019 Apr 12. PMID: 30978270.
44. Dimitroulis G. Management of temporomandibular joint disorders: a surgeon's perspective. Aust Dent J. 2018;63(Suppl 1):S79–90. https://doi.org/10.1111/adj.12593. PMID: 29574810.

Review of TMJ Surgery for Non-surgeons

Ioannis Gkikas

1 Introduction

The temporomandibular joint (TMJ) is a ginglymoarthrodial joint (Figs. 1 and 2), with a high degree of anatomical precision. Under normal conditions, the TMJ performs coordinated movements as a single functional unit with sliding surfaces and anatomical structures that cooperate in perfect harmony with its associated neuromuscular structures. The integrity of the structural elements of TMJ (articular surfaces, articular disc, muscles, and ligaments) supports basic functions such as chewing, breathing, speech, and development of the craniofacial complex.

The TMJ can be affected by various pathological conditions, which cause dysfunctional disorders with a wide range of clinical symptoms and severity. In summary, the pathological conditions that may affect the anatomical area of TMJ are the following:

1. Masticatory muscle disorders (extra-articular disorder)
2. Disc TMJ pathology (internal derangement)
3. Osteoarthritis (inflammatory and noninflammatory)
4. Functional disorders mainly affecting mandibular mobility (subluxation/dislocation/ankylosis)
5. Soft and/or hard tissue trauma
6. Benign and malignant (primary or metastatic) neoplasms
7. Congenital and developmental disorders (TMJ agenesia, condylar hypoplasia)

The role of surgery in the treatment of the above-listed pathological conditions of the TMJ is sometimes distinct and is the only way to correct and restore the functionality of the joint. This occurs specifically in cases where the joint is affected by neoplasia, ankylosis, or congenital

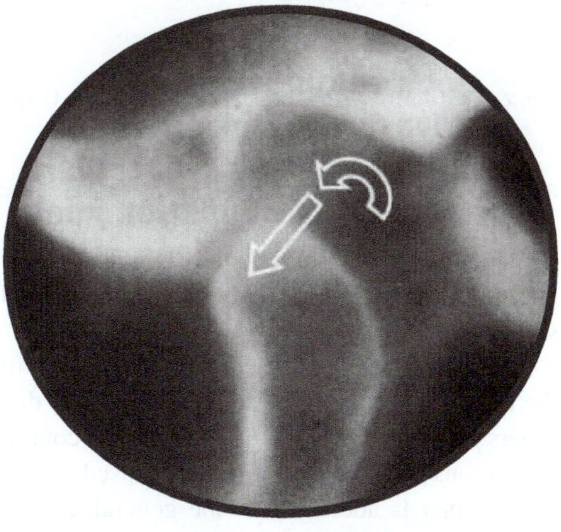

Fig. 1 TMJ is a ginglymoarthrodial joint that allows both hinge and gliding movements

I. Gkikas (✉)
Department of Maxillofacial Surgery, Southern Illinois University School of Dental Medicine, Alton, IL, USA
e-mail: igkikas@siue.edu

B. C. Stack Jr. et al. (eds.), *Craniofacial Pain*, https://doi.org/10.1007/978-3-031-57563-1_8

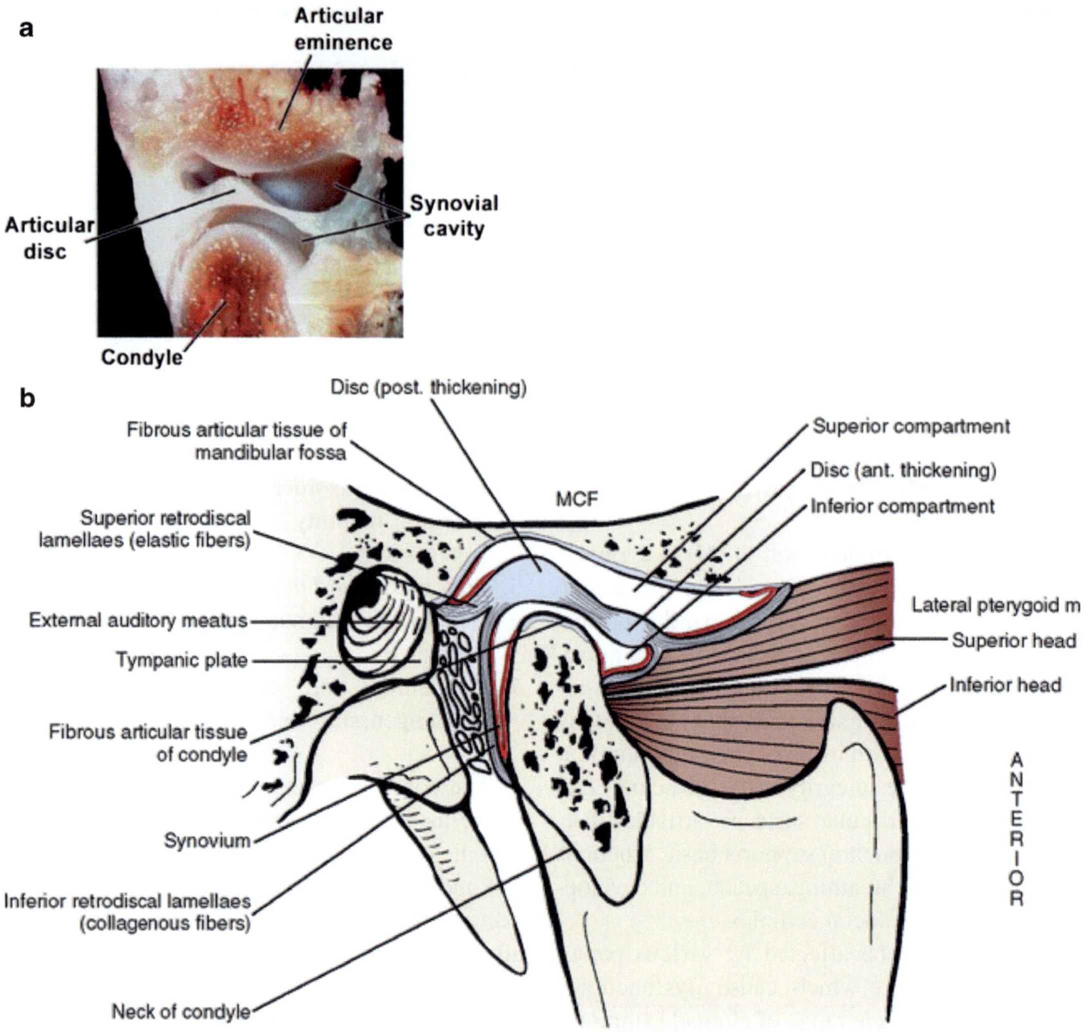

Fig. 2 TMJ anatomy. (**a**) Gross TMJ anatomy. (**b**) Diagram of TMJ anatomy

and developmental disorders. However, for the most common diseases associated with osteoarticular damage and functional disorders of the articular disk (internal derangement), the role of surgery is less clear.

The aim of this chapter is the presentation of the role for surgery in the treatment of TMJ disorders by highlighting the indications and contraindications of surgical procedures used today. The chapter is addressed to the general dentist, the health provider who most often meets patients with TMJ functional disorders. Therefore, dentists must have a comprehensive and structured knowledge of both pathology and available therapeutic modalities, including surgery, that are currently available to offer the maximum benefit for patients.

2 Surgical intervention of TMJ

Surgical intervention of TMJ disorders has a long history. The first attempts to surgical treatment of symptomatic patients assumed that symptoms are mainly due to a disturbed position of the structural anatomical elements of the joint and more specifically the articular disc. These open TMJ procedures, from a technical point of view, combined removal or reposition the articular disc in combination with arthroplasty of boney articular surfaces. In addition, extra-joint interventions (condylotomy) were adopted to further improve the anatomical disc relationship. These procedures, usually associated with a significant rate of intraoperative and postoperative complications. The initial enthusiasm for clinical results in improving symptomatic patients, has waned over time.

With the introduction and application of TMJ arthroscopy in the mid-1980s and later arthrocentesis, the landscape of surgical intervention of TMJ disorders was changed dramatically. Arthroscopy gave to TMJ surgeons the opportunity to have a precise picture of internal pathology in a surgically undisrupted joint. In addition, information that was collected from TMJ arthroscopy prompted further research into the true etiology of TMJ dysfunction disorders.

From a surgical point of view, arthroscopy and arthrocentesis contributed substantially to the treatment of symptomatic patients while ensuring fewer complications, improved healing potential, and a shorter recovery period. Today, the controversy with surgical interventions of patients with TMJ disorders, although significantly mitigated, still exists. This is contributed by the absence of strict surgical protocols that determine when a patient with a TMJ disorder is a good candidate for surgical intervention, and, if so, what is the appropriate technique for each case so that maximal results are achieved with the fewest complications. Criteria that should always be considered during the process of investigating candidates for TMJ surgery are the following:

1. TMJ should be the cause of the patient's dysfunctional symptoms.
2. Previous nonsurgical treatments have failed to resolve patient's symptoms.
3. The clinical X-ray examination proves that symptoms are due to intra-articular TMJ damage.

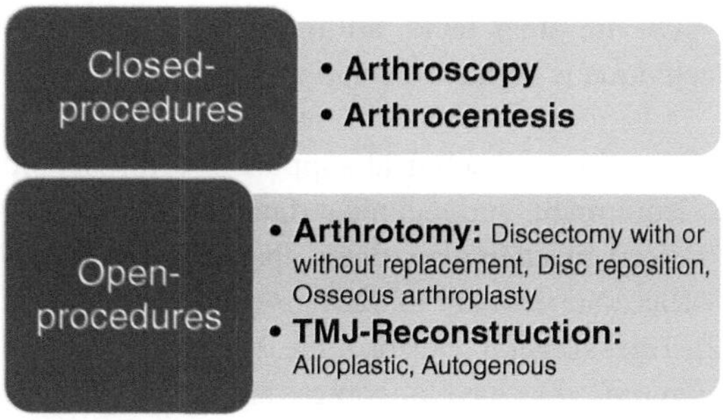

Fig. 3 Closed vs. open TMJ procedures

Today, the procedures we apply for surgical treatment of TMJ disorders are the following (Fig. 3):

3 TMJ Arthroscopy (Diagnostic)

TMJ arthroscopy is a surgical technique in which the surgeon can directly survey the internal structures of the TMJ through the insertion of a specially designed arthroscope. A key feature of arthroscopy, which makes it particularly popular in relation to existing open procedures, is the investigation of the joint and the possibility of performing specific surgical procedures without open-access of the TMJ. Benefits for the patient, are less postoperative complications and faster postoperative rehabilitation. In addition, during arthroscopy, it is possible to review the internal structure of the TMJ both in a state of relaxation of the lower jaw and during its wide excursions. Consequently, it is possible to diagnose intra-articular problems in real time due to observation of movement.

The introduction of arthroscopy as a minimally invasive procedure has greatly changed the rationale by which surgeons approach TMJ disorders, especially disorders due to internal derangements. Clinically, it has been proven that a less invasive surgery when applied in a timely manner and targeted to the appropriate patient, is accompanied by satisfactory results such as pain reduction and painless opening of the mouth.

On the other hand, arthroscopy as a surgical technique is demanding and requires:

1. Continuous technical support of arthroscopic equipment and technical data: This technique takes place in a restricted space (upper articular compartment of TMJ).
2. The surgeon performing the operation is required to have ongoing training and knowledge of TMJ's pathophysiology.

According to the American Association of Oral and Maxillofacial Surgeons, the following five are the main indications for this technique:

1. Internal derangement of the TMJ (Wilkes stages 2–4) (Table 1)
2. Degenerative joint disease-osteoarthritis
3. Inflammation of the synovial membrane
4. Painful hypermobility or recurrent luxation of the disc
5. Hypermobility because of intra-joint adherence (acute or chronic closed lock)

Contraindications to the application of TMJ arthroscopy are active inflammation of the preauricular region, intra-articular malignant tumors, ankylosis, as well as special anatomical conditions (i.e., resorption of glenoid fossa). TMJ arthroscopy, in its simplest form, includes investigation of the upper articular cavity through an arthroscope, diagnosis of pathological conditions, rinsing of the articular cavity, and introduction of pharmaceutical substances (diagnostic arthroscopy).

During the diagnostic arthroscopy, the surgeon after appropriate demarcation of the arthroscope (Figs. 4 and 5) begins a systematic examination of the upper articular space, where a large number of pathological disorders is noted. The arthroscopic anatomical regions examined in sequence, are the following (Fig. 6):

1. Medial synovial drape
2. Pterygoid shadow
3. Retrodiscal synovial and posterior ligament
4. Posterior slope of the articular eminence and glenoid fossa
5. Articular disc
6. Intermediate zone
7. Anterior recess

Table 1 Wilkes staging classification for internal derangement of TMJ

Stage	Clinical findings	Radiographic findings
I	Adequate range of motion Painless clicking	Normal disc
II	Occasional painful clicking Joint locking Few episodes of symptomatic TMJ	Mild disc deformity
III	Restriction of motion Closed locks Frequent pain Persistent symptoms	No osseous changes Disc displacement without reduction
IV	Restriction of motion History of chronic pain	Disc displacement without reduction Degenerative changes
V	Chronic restriction of motion Crepitus Episodic joint pain	Joint deformity Severe disc displacement Perforation of the disc Degenerative arthritis changes Presence of osteophyte

The investigation of the lower articular space is not a routine during arthroscopy. In cases of disc perforation, however, its examination can be achieved by inserting the arthroscope through the perforation. With the above arthroscopic examination, which is performed in parallel with movements of the jaw, the surgeon can diagnose a large part of pathological conditions, such as:

- Synovial inflammation (Fig. 7)
- Degenerative changes of the articular cartilage of the fossa and eminence (Fig. 8)
- Presence of adhesions (fibrous tissue between disc and fossa) (Fig. 9)

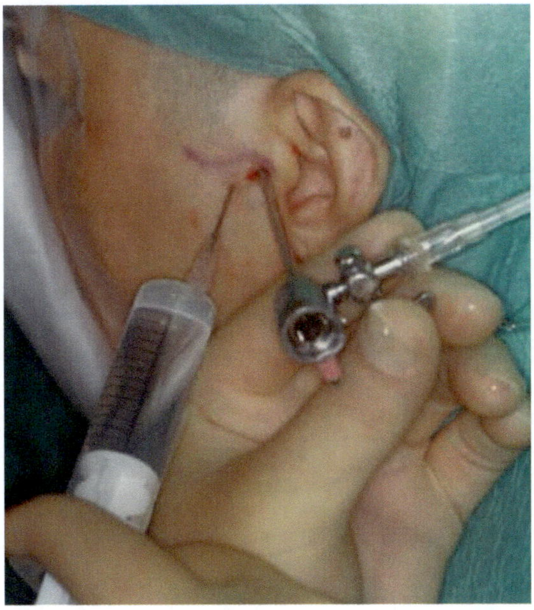

Fig. 4 Diagnostic TMJ arthroscopy

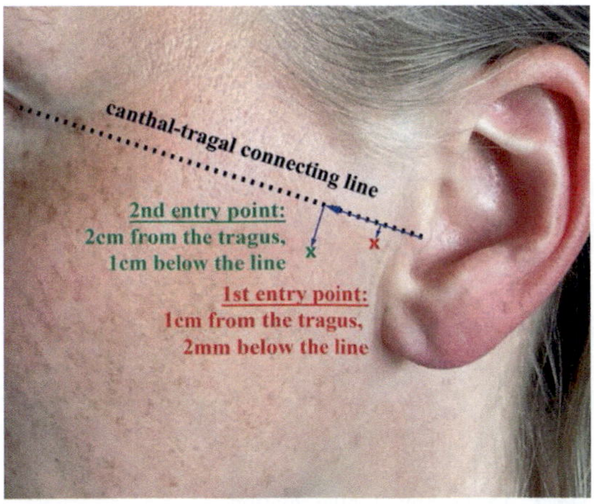

Fig. 5 Landmarks for orientation during approaching TMJ (entry points)

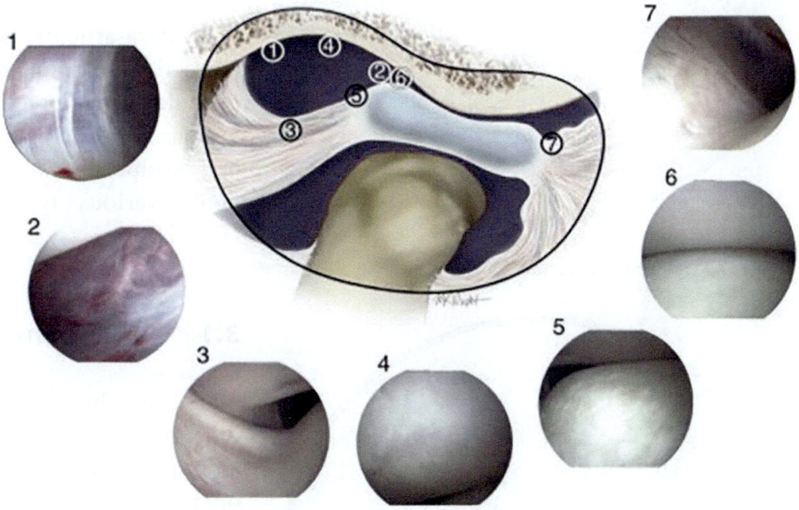

Fig. 6 TMJ arthroscopic anatomic regions

- Identify disc integrity (disc perforation) (Fig. 10)
- Movement of TMJ during procedure allows also the identification of restricted movement of the disc

The final step of the diagnostic arthroscopy is completed by moving the arthroscope to the anterior part of the upper articular space. When lysis of adhesions is required, it is accomplished by sweeping the arthroscope or the irrigation cannula through the adhesions and lysing them. At the end of the process, the synovial space is irrigated to remove debris, blood clots, and inflammatory products. In this final phase, the surgeon has the option to inject various drugs such as:

Corticosteroids (TMJ arthritis, psoriasis, RA)

Sodium hyaluronate (degenerative joint disease)

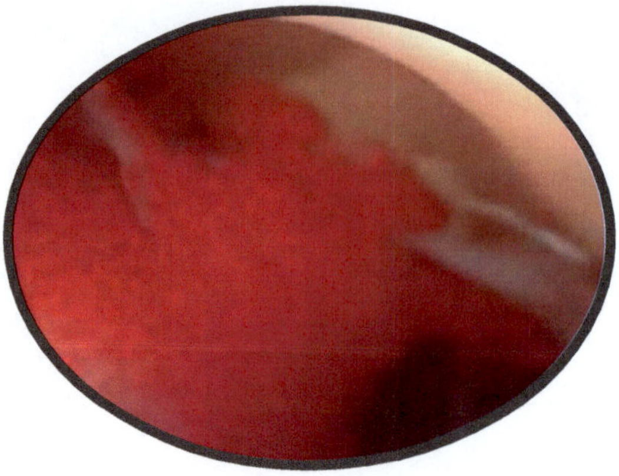

Fig. 7 TMJ synovial inflammation

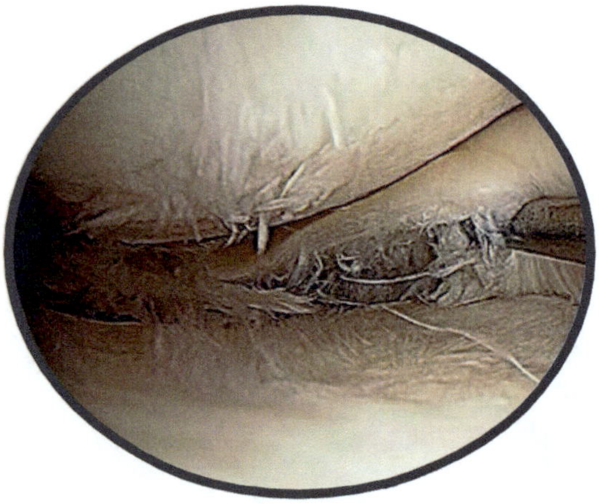

Fig. 8 TMJ degenerative changes

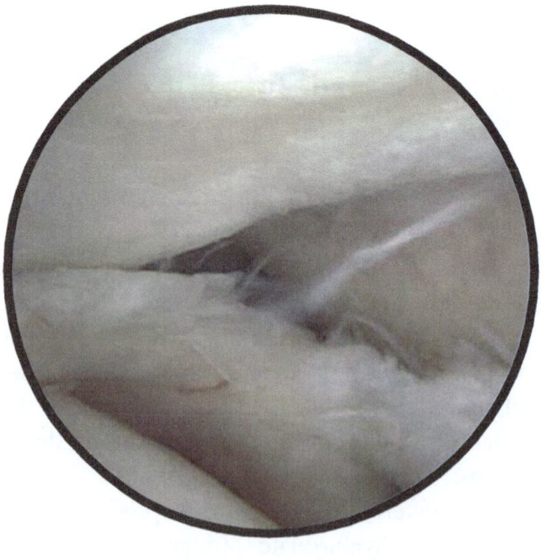

Fig. 9 TMJ adhesions

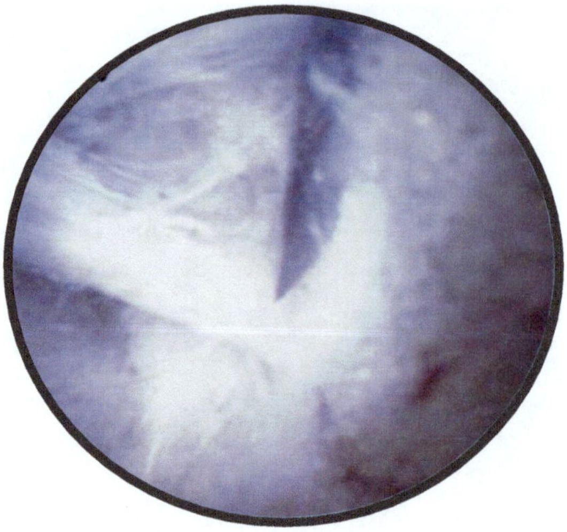

Fig. 10 TMJ disc perforation

Plasma rich in growth factors (anterior disc displacement and osteoarthritis)

Opioids (postoperative pain control)

At the end of the diagnostic arthroscopy, and if an intra-articular problem requiring surgical correction, the surgeon through an additional cannula (articular eminence portal) can insert various tools (palpators, forceps, scissors, scrapers, scalpels, and motorized terminals) and apply various types of surgical techniques (Fig. 11).

3.1 TMJ Arthroscopy (Surgical)

Surgical arthroscopy is more demanding than diagnostic arthroscopy and requires experience and special training. Using coblation devices or shaver-cutting devices (Fig. 12), the surgeon can bring about lysis of the adhesions that are often seen in anterior disc displacement, synovitis disc perforation, and bone osteoarthrosis. With the use of Ho:YAG (holmium:yttrium aluminum garnet) lasers or coblation, one can achieve anterior disc release. Coblation of the retrodiscal tissues including all the areas with synovitis and the most lateral and posterior joint capsule must be conducted to stabilize the disc. Disc perforations are often found in the junction of the retrodiscal tissues and the disc.

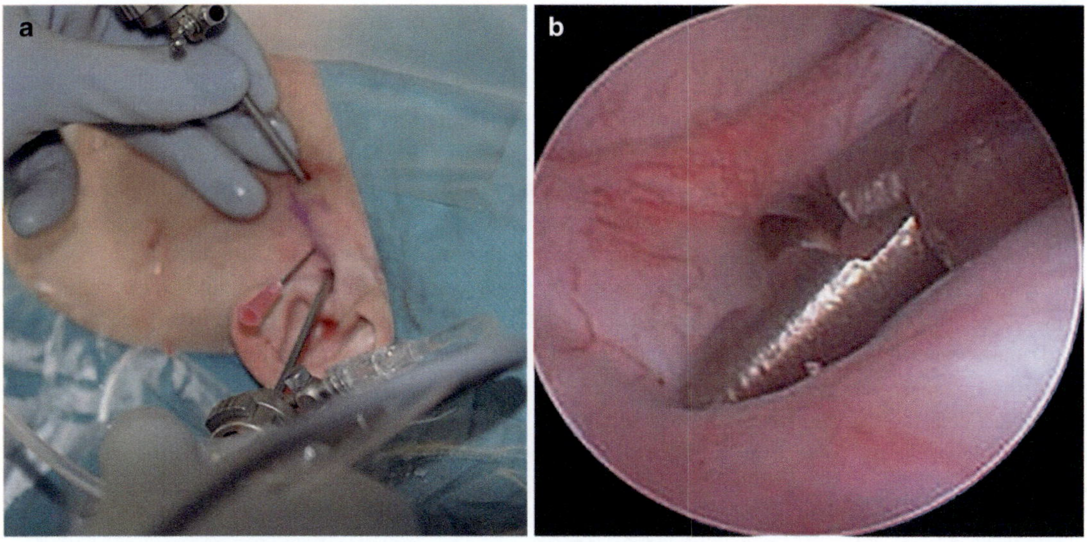

Fig. 11 Surgical TMJ arthroscopy. (**a**) Scope insertion. (**b**) Intra-articular endoscopic view

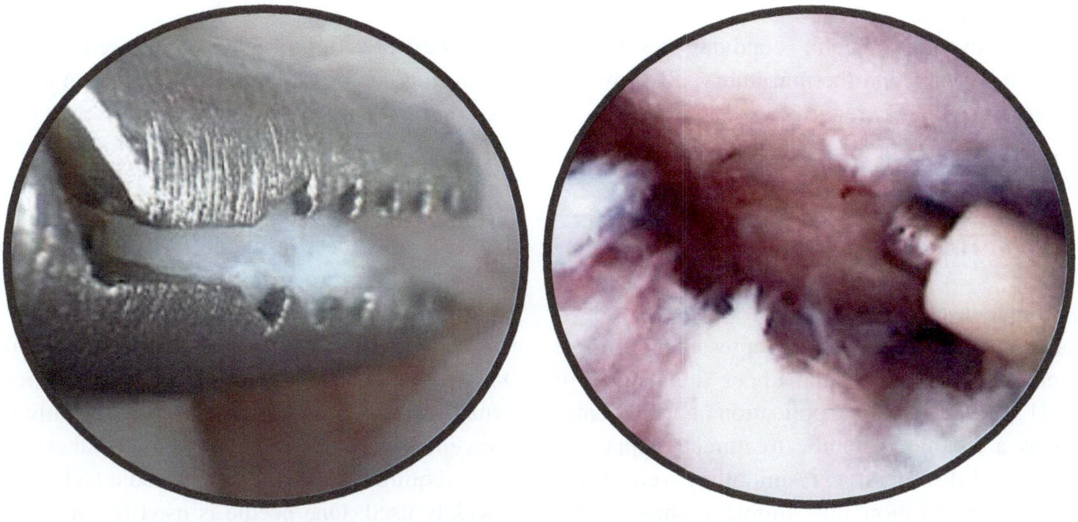

Fig. 12 Coblation, shaver/cutting devices used in arthroscopic TMJ surgery

Arthroscopic surgery also includes coblation of the retrodiscal tissues with the debridement of the disc perforation borders.

In patients diagnosed with synovial chondromatosis, arthroscopic surgery contributes to the removal of loose bodies formed inside the articular cavity representing metaplastic cartilaginous nodules. Coblation of the lateral and posterior capsule is the surgical procedure of choice in cases of painful hypermobility or recurrent luxation of the disc.

Today, TMJ arthroscopy is a safe and minimally invasive surgical procedure covering a wide spectrum of TMJ pathology. As a surgical procedure, it can develop complications both during the operation and postoperatively. To date, the most common complications that have been reported are:

- Damage of articular surfaces or articular discs during the insertion of the trocar.
- The breakage of thin dimensional tools inserted for the performance of arthroscopy.
- Intraoperative extra-articular bleeding secondary to injury of the superficial temporal vessels.
- Transient nerve injury of the zygomatic branch of the facial nerve (VII), the auriculotemporal nerve (V3), the masseter nerve (V3), or other branches of the third division of the trigeminal nerve (V3).
- Otologic complications such as lacerations of the external auditory canal or tympanic membrane.
- TMJ or infratemporal space infection.
- Otitis media.
- Arteriovenous fistula, condylar resorption, skin atrophy, and thermal injury, all of which have been rarely reported.

4 TMJ Arthrocentesis

Arthrocentesis is the least invasive surgical approach to TMJ and represents a simple method for lavage of the upper joint space of TMJ. The concept and application of arthrocentesis as a technique for the treatment of patients with TMJ disorders, were initially based on the clinical observation that simple rinsing of the articular cavity through arthroscopy was possible to reduce pain and improve mandibular mobility in patients diagnosed with acute disc displacement without reduction. Its exact mode of action is not fully understood. It is believed that the rinsing of the upper articular space results in the removal of inflammatory products that are responsible for causing pain. In addition, pressure rinsing in combination with mobilization of the lower jaw during the procedure is believed to result in resolution of the inflammatory adhesions that have been created between the disc and the articular surfaces, thus improving disc position as observed in cases of anterior disc displacement.

Arthrocentesis, although not a panacea, can be considered a safe and a rational first approach on patients suffering from internal derangement and in whom conservative treatment has not worked. It is applied to patients with pain and mobility disorder of the lower jaw due to anterior disc displacement with or without disc reduction. Satisfactory results seem to have been achieved in terms of reducing symptoms in patients with disc adhesions within the glenoid fossa as well as in patients with a nonreducing disc. It has also been applied as a palliative method in cases of degenerative osteoarthritis of TMJ as well as a diagnostic and therapeutic modality for patients with inflammatory arthritis. Finally, it has been used as a diagnostic and therapeutic approach of hemarthrosis of the TMJ following mandibular trauma.

Abscess or cellulitis at the site of needle insertion during this procedure is considered an absolute contraindication as well as the presence of a malignant tumor. The history of previous surgeries in the area (discectomy) as well as the reduced opening of the mouth due to fibrous or osseous ankylosis must be considered additional contraindications of arthrocentesis.

Arthrocentesis as a technique is simple; however, it requires that the surgeon be experienced. One of its main advantages is that it can be performed under local anesthesia with or without intravenous (IV) sedation. General anesthesia is rarely required. Today, the two-needle technique is widely used. One needle is used for injection and the second for aspiration of the injected solution. After properly preparing and draping the surgical site, a line is drawn from the middle of the tragus to the outer canthus. Then two points are drawn to indicate the location of the needle entry. The first point is 10 mm from the middle tragus and 2 mm below the line. The second point is located 10 mm farther along the line and 10 mm below it (Fig. 13). The goal is to rinse the upper articular compartment. For this reason, the final position of the needle entry points is confirmed by asking the patient to perform movements of the lower jaw in all directions

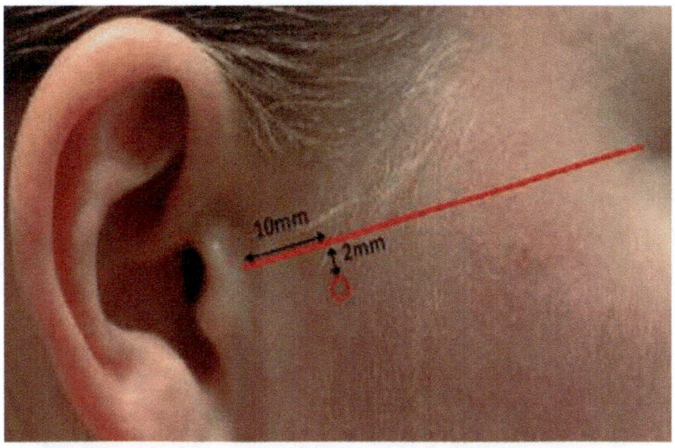

Fig. 13 Anatomic orientation of the upper joint space in TMJ arthrocentesis

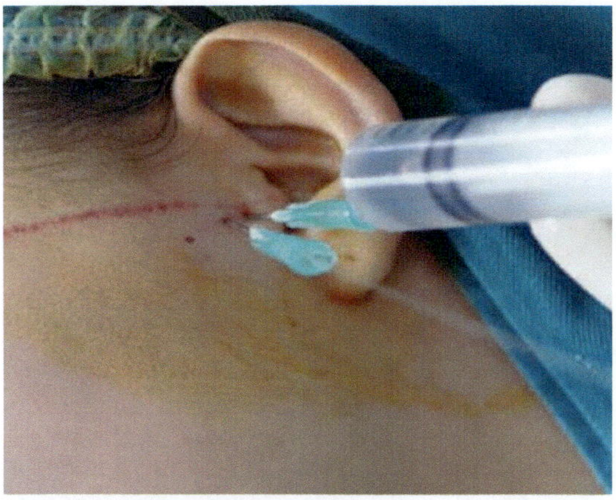

Fig. 14 Injection of Ringer's solution into upper joint space during arthrocentesis

while surgeon palpates the anatomical elements of the joint.

This is followed by the numbing of the area and the insertion of the first needle of 19 gauge size, at the first entry point. The needle is attached to a syringe containing approximately 1 mL of Ringer's solution. This amount of the solution is injected into the joint and immediately aspirated, which confirms the correct position of the needle. This is followed by an injection of 1.5–2 mL of anesthetic solution to dilate the articular spaces. After inserting the second needle, the surgeon begins to rinse the upper articular compartment. Usually, the total amount of Ringer's lactate solution used is 150–500 mL. (Fig. 14). The injection is performed with controlled pressure as the patient performs movements of the lower jaw. At the end of the procedure, the second needle is removed, and the surgeon has the ability, through the first needle, to administer corticosteroids, analgesics, or hyaluronic acid.

The complications that accompany this operation are relatively rare and of short duration. The most common complication is swelling due to perfusion of Ringer's solution as well as temporary upper facial paralysis caused by extravasation of the anesthetic solution.

5 TMJ Arthrotomy

Arthrotomy means direct surgical exposure of the TMJ. TMJ arthrotomy includes a wide range of surgical procedures that mainly aim to reduce pain and restore normal TMJ function in patients with osteoarthritis and advanced stages of internal derangement. In a large percentage of these patients, any conservative treatment to improve symptoms and dysfunction hae failed. The rationale of most of the interventions included by TMJ arthrotomy is based on the elimination or modification of the mainly intra-articular elements of the joint with the goal of improving the anatomical relationship between the disc and the articular surfaces, recognizing that mechanical interference is the main factor in internal derangements.

The widespread application of TMJ arthroscopy as a less invasive TMJ surgery has significantly limited both the frequency and the range of indications for TMJ arthrotomy.

Currently acceptable interventions for TMJ arthrotomy are:

1. Discectomy with replacement
2. Discectomy without replacement
3. Disc repositioning with various plication techniques
4. Osseous arthroplasty, usually in conjunction with disc surgeries

All the above interventions share the same chance of surgical access. In all cases, the aim is the unhindered opening of the articular cavity so that the surgeon can assess the condition of both the soft elements of the joint and the hard articular surfaces. After exposure of the joint capsule, the TMJ is entered, and the surgeon an systematicly:

1. Evaluate the disc position
2. Determine whether the disc or posterior attachment is perforated
3. Evaluate soft tissues for signs of synovitis and fibrillation of the articular cartilage
4. Evaluate the pathologic changes of the bony surfaces in cases of osteoarthritis

After evaluation of the joint's hard and soft tissues, the surgeon can choose the appropriate operation for each damaged element.

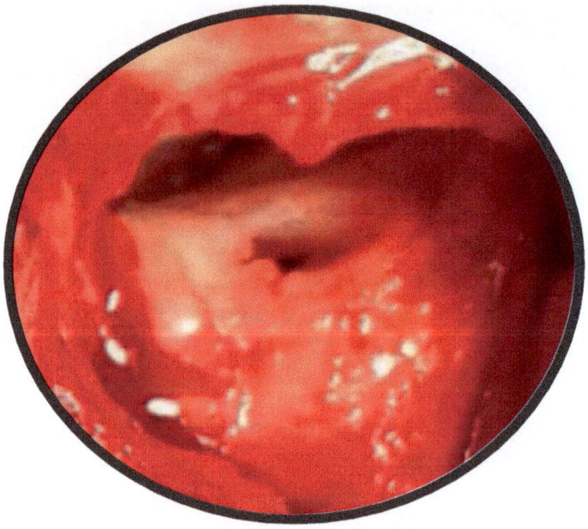

Fig. 15 Disc damage

5.1 Discectomy

In some cases, the disc is so severely damaged (Fig. 15) that the remnants of disc tissue must be removed (Fig. 16). This is generally indicated in cases where the damaged disc acts as a mechanical obstacle causing pain and limited mouth opening. This usually happens with anterior disc displacement without reduction and more rarely in posterior or lateral disc displacements.

Although discectomy has been practiced for years, its therapeutic effects are characterized by a high degree of heterogeneity. Discectomy was most often accompanied by minimal bone recontouring of the articular bone to ensure a wider articular space after surgery. It has been reported that joint noises (crepitus) tend to increase after discectomy. In addition, degenerative structural articular surface changes of the condyle and glenoid fossa tend to occur radiographically following discectomy.

The above observations led the surgeons to the fact that the removed disc should be restored to avoid any pathological contact with the articular surfaces and dampen the stresses exerted during the function of the joint. The initial silastic sheet placement did not bring the desired results, and in addition, it led to intensive inflammation reaction to silicone/silastic material. For this reason, autogenous grafts were used. The following autogenous grafts have been successfully used:

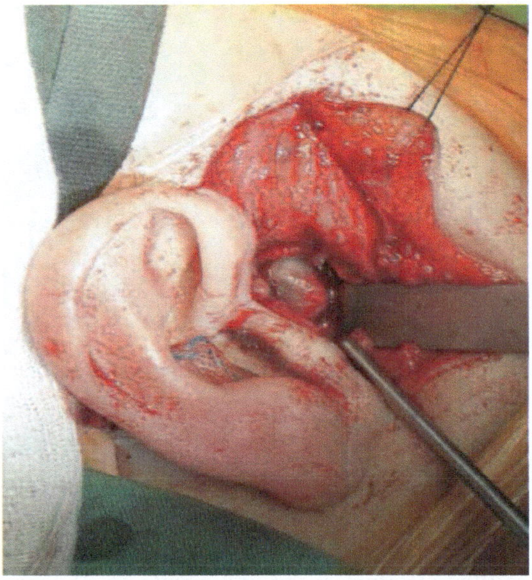

Fig. 16 Discectomy

1. Temporalis muscle/fascia
2. Myofascial flaps
3. Dermis with or without the fat of abdominal fat alone
4. Auricular cartilage

According to the literature, no ideal material satisfies all the criteria for replacing a missing disc following discectomy.

5.2 Disc Repositioning

This technique is used to correct anterior disc displacement in patients with persistent painful clicking or closed locking. A basic requirement is the integrity of the disc and the possibility of repositioning it without tension. In this operation, the displaced disc is identified and repositioned into a more normal position by removing a wedge of tissue from the posterior attachment of the disc. In some cases, when the surgeon judges, he/she recontours the disc, articular eminence, and mandibular condyle. Currently, the most common methods used to stabilize the articular disc are:

1. Suturing the disc directly to the retrodiscal tissues (Fig. 17).
2. Suturing the disc directly to the condyle through an intraosseous implant anchor (MiTek anchor), a technique that to ensure greater stability of the disc (Fig. 18).

5.3 Arthroplasty

Arthroplasty means reshaping of articular surfaces to remove osteophytes and bone surface erosions. Arthroplasty procedures are taken either as individual procedures (condyloplasty, eminoplasty, condylectomy) or in combination with intra-articular procedures that mainly involve the removal or repositioning of the disc.

In *condyloplasty*, what is sought is the removal of osteophytic areas by contouring the head of the condyle. Although condyloplasty can sometimes become beneficial in removing osteophytes, the fibrocartilage is damaged during the procedure, and further degenerative changes can occur secondary to the procedure. A *high condylar shave* is another condylar head technique which involves the removal of part of the anterior-superior slope of the condyle. Exposure to the underlying marrow in the condylar head can lead to progressive sclerosis and degenerative changes.

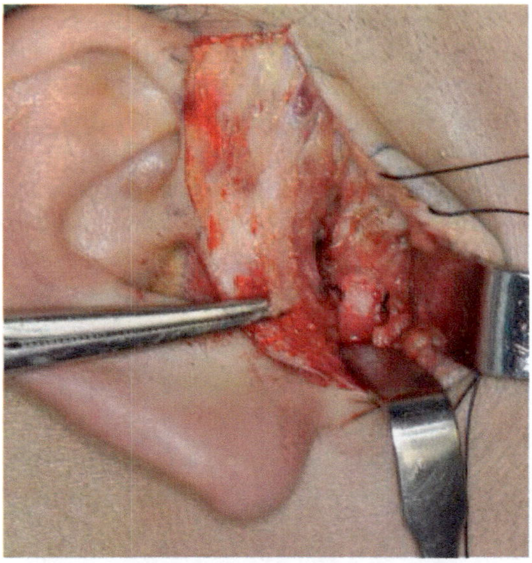

Fig. 17 Suturing a repositioned disc

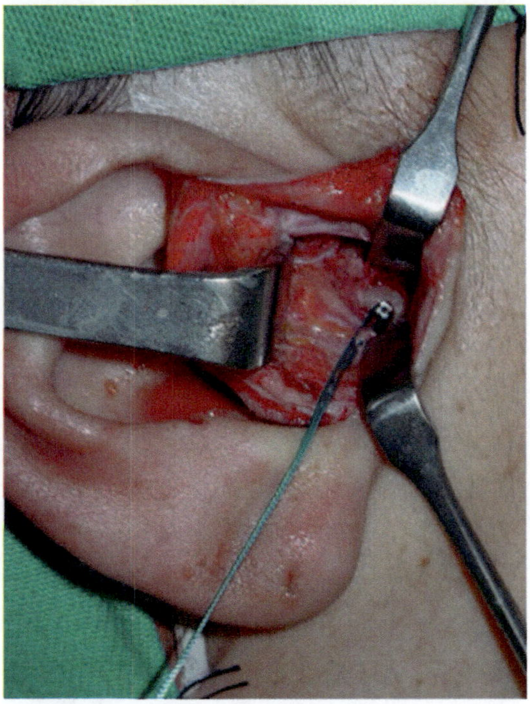

Fig. 18 Suturing a repositioned disc directly to the condyle

Eminoplasty can also be used as an adjunct in the surgical correction of internal derangement or it can be used alone for the treatment of recurrent dislocation (Fig. 19). *Eminectomy* eliminates articular eminence and can be combined with other types of arthroplasty procedures (Fig. 20). The main goal of eminectomy procedure is to eliminate mechanical interference by the TMJ disc and it is interposition anteromedially between the condyle and the eminence.

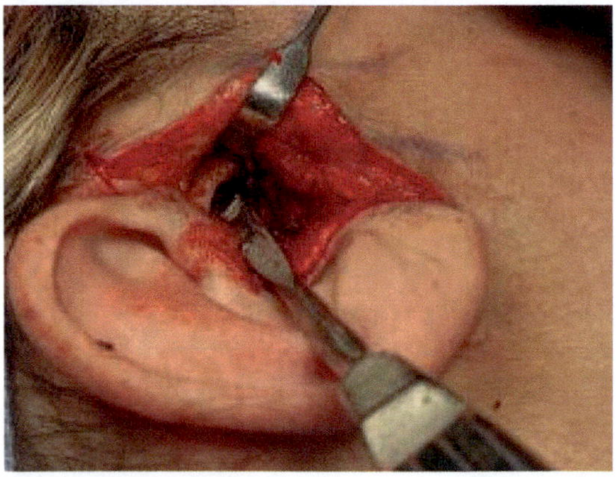

Fig. 19 Eminoplasty

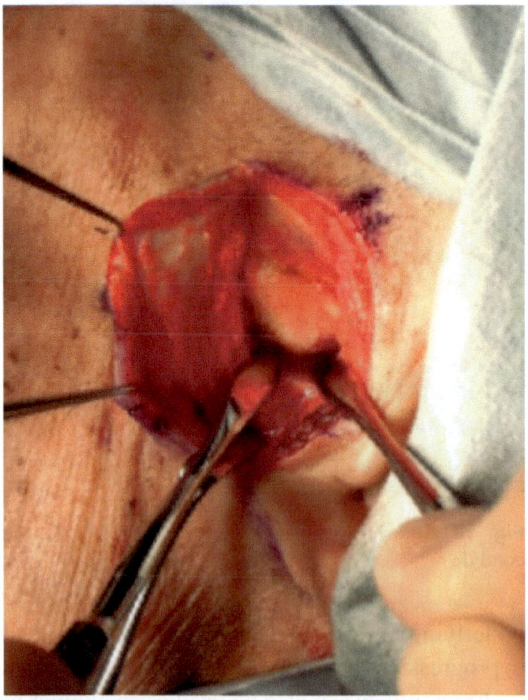

Fig. 20 Eminectomy

Regardless of the diagnosis, arthrotomy procedures have a group of common potential complications, including:

1. Damage to adjacent structures (nerves, vessels, ear, parotid gland, base of the skull, middle cranial fossa)
2. Infections
3. Ankylosis
4. Functional disorders and increased postoperative pain

6 Reconstruction of TMJ (TMJR)

TMJR is the total reconstruction and replacement of TMJ articular elements in those cases where they have suffered irreversible damage. Patients with irreversible TMJ lesions show severe symptoms which depend on the type of condition that caused the damage and the length of time the cause has affected the area. In any case, the need to restore TMJ is deemed necessary when important functions such as airway control, speech, and swallowing have been disturbed. The goal of reconstruction is now well established and includes the restoration of mandibular function and form, reduction of further disability, control or elimination of disease progression, avoidance of repeat surgeries, and, in the case of growing children, providing for normal development of the facial skeleton.

Indications for TMJR can be summarized as follows:

1. Bony ankylosis
2. Failed previous TMJR (alloplastic or autogenous)
3. Need for TMJR after tumor-ablative surgery
4. Developmental abnormalities that indirectly or directly affect the anatomical region of TMJ
5. Severe inflammatory conditions that have failed to respond to conservative treatment

In the pediatric population, indications for TMJR mainly concern cases of developmental deformities, trauma, and neoplastic tumors or odontogenic cysts with extension to TMJ that cause irreversible damage to the area, such as:

Congenital deformities

Hemifacial microsomia

Treacher Collins syndrome

Bilateral craniofacial microsomia

Congenital TMJ ankylosis

TMJ pathology (tumors, cysts)

TMJ trauma

Juvenile idiopathic arthritis

Progressive condylar resorption

The options of TMJR can be considered as alloplastic or autogenous. The role of autogenous reconstruction in adults has diminished considerably and presently is limited to those patients who have a significant contraindication or cannot afford the cost of alloplastic reconstruction. However, in children, autogenous reconstruction remains the method of choice during the period of skeletal growth.

Alloplastic TMJR

In the past, several types of prosthetic joint replacement have been available. Unfortunately, long-term results of prosthetic joints placed back in the mid-1990s have been disappointing due to a variety of engineering and biological problems. Systems containing Proplast, Teflon, and Silastic have been removed from the market due to foreign-body giant cell reactions.

6.1 Joint Prostheses

Newer generation joint prosthesis has been improved in many of their key features such as engineering, biocompatibility, and wear resistance. Past failures in TMJ's restoration materials have highlighted the basic requirements that a TMJ prosthesis must meet:

- Any TMJ prosthesis should be able to imitate the translation movements of the condyle without restricting the movements of the uninvolved or non-replaced contralateral TMJ.
- The material of the implant must meet basic mechanical specifications mainly reducing stress during joint operation and minimizing the chances of bone resorption or prosthesis loosening.
- TMJ prosthesis components should promote osseointegration
- Biological parameters of TMJ prosthesis such as biocompatibility, corrosion resistance, and low wear rates should characterize their materials.

Today, there are two basic types of TMJ prostheses:

1. *Stock prosthesis* (Biomet Microfixation TMJR System) is composed of a polyethylene fossa component and a chromium alloy mandibular component, which comes in three lengths and with an offset of the condylar head. It is a rehabilitation system ready for immediate use with metal-on-polyethylene articulation with good osseointegration. From a technical point of view, it is considered a reliable rehabilitation system; it is not a first choice in those cases where simultaneous correction of dentofacial deformity and TMJR is required (Fig. 21).
2. *Custom-fitted prosthesis* (TMJ Concepts): This prosthesis is mounted on a 3D stereolithic model constructed with virtual surgical planning (VSP). The fossa component is composed of a pure titanium shell fitted to the fossa with the shell covered in a titanium mesh. The mandibular component is made of

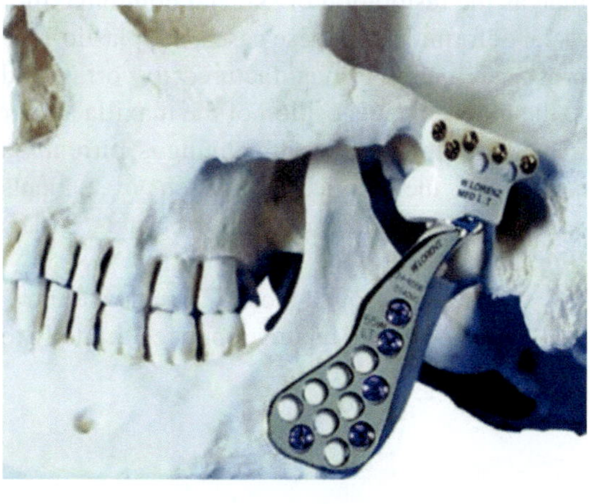

Fig. 21 Biomet microfixation system prosthesis

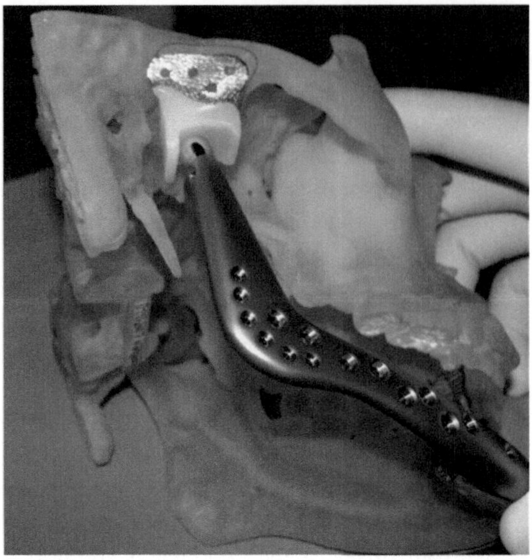

Fig. 22 TMJ concept prosthesis fitted on the patient's stereolithographic model

titanium alloy, and the condylar head is chromium cobalt alloy. The choice of this prosthesis, although it satisfies to a great extent the anatomical and functional peculiarities of each case separately, is a surgically demanding technique with high cost (Fig. 22).

The possibility of using the above alloplastic prostheses has completely changed the landscape of the total rehabilitation of TMJ mainly with the widening of the pathological conditions of TMJ that can be restored. A typical example of the expanded use of TMJR today is the possibility of restoring the joint in combination at the same time as the restoration of skeletal craniomaxillofacial deformities. In these cases, alloplastic TMJ prosthesis must be manufactured to correspond to the planned new position of the maxilla and/or mandible. Virtual surgical planning is currently a routine in the surgical approach of patients requiring orthognathic surgery and TMJR (Fig. 22).

Patients' data from a facial CT scan and intraoral scan are merged and manipulated digitally to create a new jaw position and occlusion. The next step is the creation of a stereolithographic model with the new anatomical data of the maxillofacial complex as rendered. The stereolithographic model is also used to construct the prosthesis that will meet the new anatomical data to give the patient the maximum possible functionality.

6.2 Autogenous TMJR

For many years, the primary method for TMJR was to use autogenous tissue grafts. Indications for using autogenous bone grafting as a "condylar replacement" include the following:

- Minimize TMJ surgeries
- Provide a good vascular bed for free grafts after tumor-ablative surgery
- Cover large soft and hard tissue defects
- Growth center transplant
- Cost and patient preference
- Allergy (documented) to metals in total joint prostheses

Autogenous TMJR offers several advantages such as availability, biocompatibility, and potential for growth in children. The main disadvantage is the variability of biological responses (resorption, ankylosis, excessive growth). Autogenous tissues used to reconstruct TMJ include costochondral grafts (Fig. 23), iliac crest, and sternoclavicular grafts. The use of costochondral grafts in pediatric and adult patients has been extensively documented in the literature. As a graft is more adaptable to the TMJ because of its native dimensions, it is the preferred method of reconstruction in the pediatric patient. In the adult population, autogenous TMJR is accomplished with the use of vascularized bone grafts, especially in patients undergoing tumor resection that requires postoperative radiation treatment.

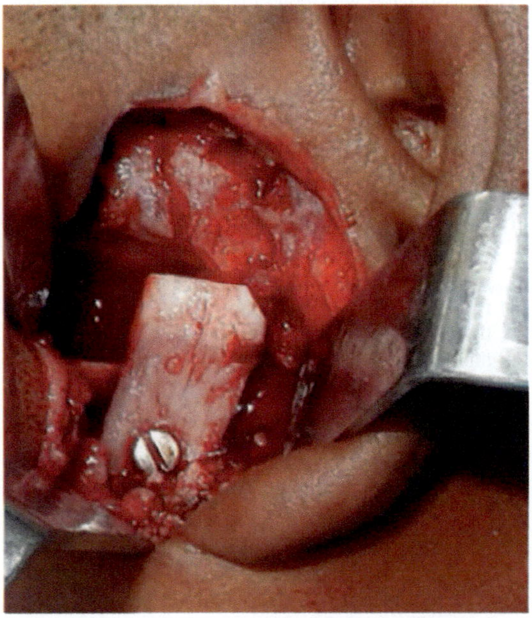

Fig. 23 Costochondral graft in place

7 Summary

Not all of the patients diagnosed with temporomandibular disorders (TMD) are good candidates for TMJ surgery. Only 3–5% of the patients with TMJ disorders may actually benefit from surgical intervention. There have been no long-term clinical trials to study the safety and effectiveness of TMJ surgery, at least for the most common TMJ disorders. Furthermore, there are no standards to identify patients who would most likely benefit from surgery. Failure to respond to conservative treatments, for example, is not an absolute indication for surgery. Successful treatment of patients with TMDs depends on an accurate diagnosis.

The application of less invasive procedures, like arthroscopy, has enabled patients with frequent TMDs to be treated with minimum complications compared with open surgeries, providing them better healing and faster recovery. The evolution of the prosthetic TMJ has created a safer ground in cases where total joint reconstruction is indicated. In addition, it expanded the range of rehabilitation to patients simultaneously undergoing corrective surgery (orthognathic surgery) and TMJ surgery.

Highlighting the importance of immediate physiotherapy after every TMJ operation is an integral part of surgical rehabilitation, ensuring both the surgical result and a faster healing. Dentists must be informed about new developments in the field of TMJ disorders and, in collaborating with a specialized maxillofacial surgeon, should offer the best treatment options to these patients.

Suggested Readings

1. Wilkes CH. Internal derangements of the temporomandibular joint. Pathological variations. Arch Otolaryngol Head Neck Surg. 1989a;115:469–77.
2. Auerbach SM, Laskin DM, Frantsve LM, Orr T. Depression, pain, exposure to stressful life events, and long-term outcomes in temporomandibular disorder patients. J Oral Maxillofacial Surg. 2001;59:628–33.
3. Armijo-Olivo S, Pitance L, Singh V, et al. Effectiveness of manual therapy and therapeutic exercise for temporomandibular disorders: systematic review and meta-analysis. Phys Ther. 2016;96:9–25.
4. Graff-Radford SB, Abbott JJ. Temporo-mandibular disorders and headache. Oral Maxillofac Surg Clin N Am. 2016;28:335–49.
5. Laskin DM. Temporomandibular disorders: a term whose time has passed! J Oral Maxillofac Surg. 2020;78:496–7.
6. Dolwick MF, Sanders B. TMJ internal derangement and arthrosis—surgical atlas. St. Louis: CV Mosby Co; 1985.
7. Dym H, Bowler D, Zeidan J. Pharmacologic treatment for temporomandibular disorders. Dent Clin N Am. 2016;60:367–79.
8. Sanders B. Arthroscopic surgery of the temporomandibular joint: treatment of internal derangement with persistent closed lock. Oral Surg. 1986;62:361.
9. Murakami KI, Segami N, Okamoto M. Outcome of arthroscopic surgery for internal derangement of the

temporomandibular joint: long term results covering 10 years. J Craniomaxillofac Surg. 2000;28:264.
10. McCain JP. Principles and practice of temporomandibular joint arthroscopy, vol. 4253. St Louis: Mosby; 1996. p. 12865.
11. Gonzalez-Garcia R, Rodríguez-Campo FJ. Arthroscopic lysis and lavage versus operative arthroscopy in the outcome of temporomandibular joint internal derangement: a comparative study based on Wilkes stages. J Oral Maxillofac Surg. 2011;69:2513.
12. McCain JP, Hossameldin RH, Srouji S, et al. Arthroscopic discopexy is effective in managing temporomandibular joint internal derangement in patients with Wilkes Stage II and III. J Oral Maxillofac Surg. 2015;73:391–401.
13. Nitzan DW, Dolwick MF, Martinez GA. Temporomandibular joint arthrocentesis: a simplified treatment for severe, limited mouth opening. J Oral Maxillofac Surg. 1991;49:1163–7.
14. Nitzan DW. The process of lubrication impairment and its involvement in temporomandibular joint disc displacement: a theoretical concept. J Oral Maxillofac Surg. 2001;59:36–45.
15. Nitzan DW, Svidovsky J, Zini A, et al. Effect of arthrocentesis on symptomatic osteoarthritis of the temporomandibular joint and analysis of the effect of preoperative clinical and radiologic features. J Oral Maxillofac Surg. 2017;75:260–7.
16. Malachovsky I, Statelova D, Stasko J, et al. Therapeutic effects of arthrocentesis in treatment of temporomandibular joint disorders. Bratisl Lek Listy. 2019;120:235–9.
17. Vaira LA, Raho MT, Soma D, et al. Complications and post-operative sequelae of temporomandibular joint arthrocentesis. Cranio. 2018;36:264–7.
18. Nogueira EFC, Lemos CAA, Vasconcellos RJH, et al. Does arthroscopy cause more complications than arthrocentesis in patients with internal temporomandibular joint disorders? Systematic review and meta-analysis. Br J Oral Maxillofac Surg. 2021;59:1166.
19. Holmlund A, Lund B, Weiner CK. Discectomy without replacement for the treatment of painful reciprocal clicking or catching and chronic closed lock of the temporomandibular joint: a clinical follow-up audit. BJOMS. 2013;51:211–4.
20. Miloro M, McKnight M, Han MD, et al. Discectomy without replacement improves function in patients with internal derangement of the temporomandibular joint. J Craniomaxillofac Surg. 2017;45:1425–31.
21. Renapurkar SK. Discectomy versus disc preservation for internal derangement of the temporomandibular joint. Oral Maxillofac Surg Clin N Am. 2018;30:329–33.
22. Dimitroulis G. The use of dermis grafts after discectomy for internal derangement of the temporomandibular joint. J Oral Maxillofac Surg. 2005;63:173–8.
23. Dimitroulis G. Condyler morphology after temporomandibular joint discectomy with interpositional abdominal dermis-fat graft. Oral Maxillofac Surg. 2011;69:439–46.
24. Mehra P, Wolford LM. The Mitek mini anchor for TMJ disc repositioning: surgical technique and results. Int J Oral Maxillofac Surg. 2001;30:497–503.
25. Wolford LM, Mercury LG, Schneiderman ED, Mogahed R, Allen W. Twenty-year follow-up study on a patient-fitted temporomandibular joint prosthesis: the Techmedica/TMJ concepts device. J Oral Maxillofac Surg. 2015;73:952–60.
26. Wolford LM. Computer-assisted surgical simulation for concomitant temporomandibular joint custom-fitted total joint reconstruction and orthognathic surgery. Atlas Oral Maxillofac Surg Clin N Am. 2016;24:55–66.
27. Mercuri LG. Prevention and detection of TMJ prosthetic joint infections update. Int J Oral Maxillofac Surg. 2019;48:217–24.

Arthrocentecis and Arthroscopy

Anis Tebyanian

1 Introduction

TMJ disorders and associated pain and dysfunction are increasingly prevalent in the modern age, largely due to parafunctional habits such as bruxism. These habits stem from psychological stressors and manifest physically through unconscious clenching and grinding of the teeth. The substantial masticatory force exerted during these actions can have detrimental effects on the related muscles and the TMJ itself, leading to pain, limited mouth opening, and inability to chew food properly. These symptoms can significantly impact one's quality of life, causing discomfort and difficulty in performing daily activities related to eating and speaking. Other causes of TMD are trauma, arthritis, dentofacial deformity all of which can result in alteration or destruction of TMJ and related structures.

1.1 Internal derangement of TMJ

Refers to abnormal position of the articular disk in relation to the condylar head within the glenoid fossa. This condition is considered a progressive disorder with symptoms that can vary depending on the severity of the derangement. As the internal derangement (ID) progresses, several changes can occur including posterior ligament elongation, disk deformation or perforation, and complete displacement of the disc out of glenoid fossa.

The most famous classification system for internal derangement is Wilkes classification and shows five stages of disease progression based on clinical, radiographic, and pathological features.

There are several treatment modalities available for TMJ disorders, and the choice of treatment depends on the severity and specific symptoms experienced by the patient. Here is a review of office-based Arthrocentesis and a brief overview of Arthroscopy.

(A) Arthrocentesis is a minimally invasive procedure that can be safely performed in office setting for the treatment of symptomatic internal derangements such as disc displacement without reduction. Arthrocentesis has shown successful results in treating patients with Wilkes classification of I–III (Fig. 1). This procedure involves irrigation and lavage of the joint to reduce inflammatory mediators responsible for pain and to break soft adhesions that limit the mobility of the disc.
(B) Arthroscopy is similar to arthrocentesis, but the scope provides direct visualization of the joint structures like the medial synovial drape, pterygoid shadow, retro-discal synovium, articular disc, and anterior recess. Studies have demonstrated that arthroscopy

A. Tebyanian (✉)
Olney Center for Oral and Maxillofacial Surgery, Olney, MD, USA
e-mail: dr.tebyanian@olneyoralfacialsurgery.com

B. C. Stack Jr. et al. (eds.), *Craniofacial Pain*, https://doi.org/10.1007/978-3-031-57563-1_9

Stage I	Painless clicking, no restriction on opening	Slight anterior disc displacement with reduction
Stage II	First few episodes of pain, Temporal headache, increase in clicking intensity	Mild to moderate anterior disc displacement with reduction, Slight deformity of the disk
Stage III	Multiple episodes of pain, Restricted motion, headache, Locking, pain with function	Moderate to severe anterior disc displacement without reduction, oderate disc deformity, no changes in bony contours
Stage IV	Chronic pain, restricted motion, locking, crepitus	Significant disc deformity and displacement, moderate changes in osseous contour
Stage V	Chronic variable pain, crepitus, grinding, grating, chronic restriction on motion, and function	Gross deformity of disc and osseous anatomy, osteophyte formation

Fig. 1 Wilkes classification. (Adapted from Wilkes CH. Internal derangements of the temporomandibular joint: pathological variations. Arch Otolaryngol Head Neck Surg 1989;115:469–7)

is more effective than arthrocentesis in lysing adhesions and increasing joint mobility.

There are three levels of arthroscopic procedures performed based on initial diagnosis and operator skill level.

- **Level I** is arthrocentesis with visual diagnostics. It uses a single puncture entry for the scope and one anterior needle for outflow of the irrigant. Once the scope is inside the joint, a systematic sweep from anterior to posterior recess will readily show the anatomy and involved pathology of the joint for proper diagnosis. The rest of the procedure is similar to arthrocentesis (Fig. 2).
- **Level II** uses two puncture points, one for the scope and the other for a working cannula. The working cannula port will allow lasers, coblation, rotary instruments, and other mechanical instruments to reduce and better mobilize the disc and break the more prominent adhesions.
- **Level III**, also called advanced or operative arthroscopy, is more surgically invasive and uses two or more puncture points to use cannulas along with the scope to perform endoscopic debridement, myotomy of lateral pterygoid muscle for anterior release of the disc, disc reduction, and rigid disc fixation. Advanced arthroscopy is a very sensitive technique and requires further training enabling clinicians to perform open surgical procedures endoscopically (Fig. 3).

Arthrocentesis involves flushing and irrigating the superior joint space to push the disc apart from the glenoid fossa, remove inflammatory byproducts and debris, and improve joint mobility by breaking down adhesions. While it may not be suitable for advanced cases, it serves as a preferred initial surgical option for the

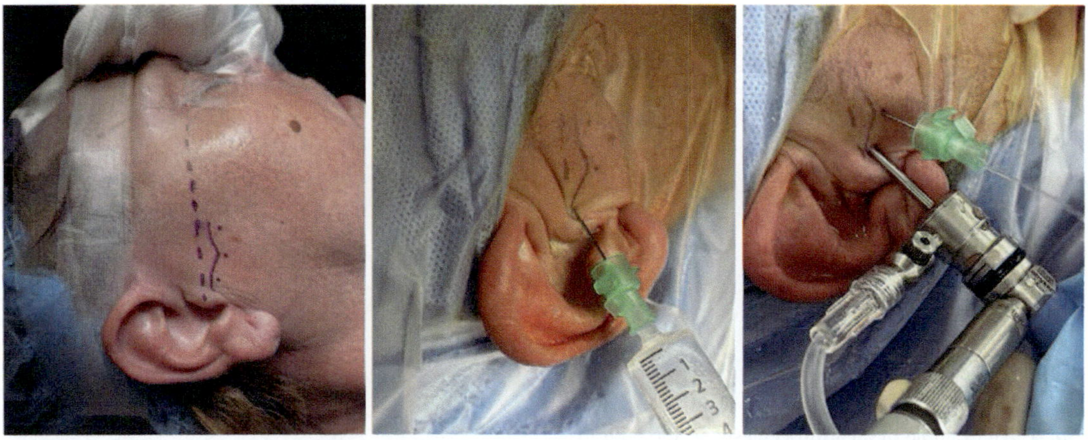

Fig. 2 Level I arthroscopy. (Verde et al. Approach to TMJ Intermediate Space by Triangulation. J Oral Maxillofac Surg 2023)

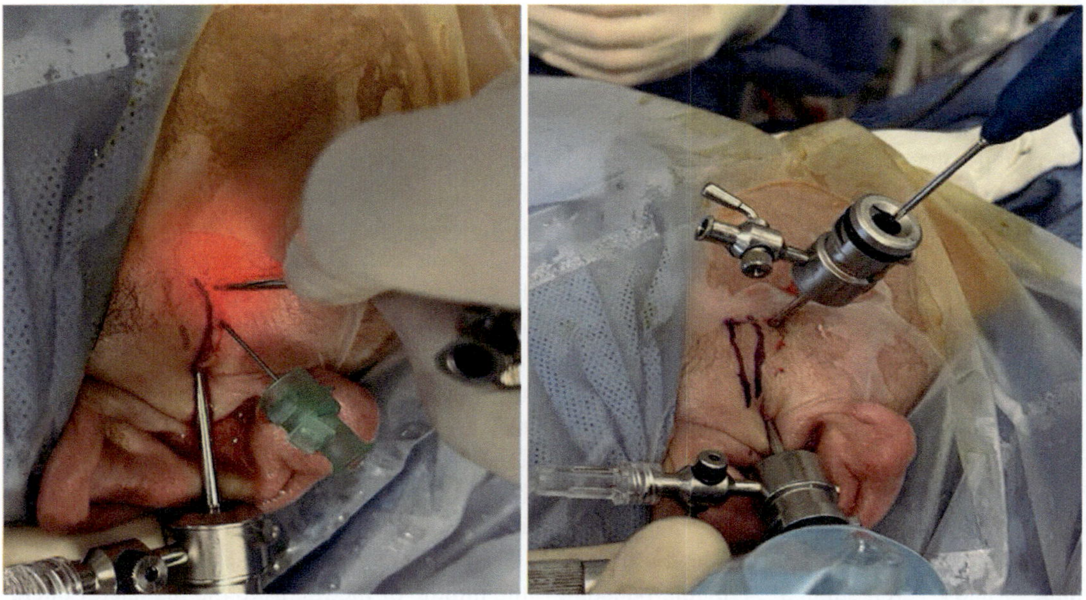

Fig. 3 Level III arthroscopy. (Verde et al. Approach to TMJ Intermediate Space by Triangulation. J Oral Maxillofac Surg 2023)

majority of cases that do not respond to conservative treatments. The indications for arthrocentesis include failed conservative treatment, anterior disc displacement without reduction, TMJ trauma with associated hemarthrosis, symptomatic arthropathies such as osteoarthritis or rheumatoid arthritis, and situations where patients opt against more invasive surgical procedures. Arthrocentesis is contraindicated in the presence of tumor, degenerative bone osteophytes, disc perforation, overlying skin infection, and condylar ankylosis.

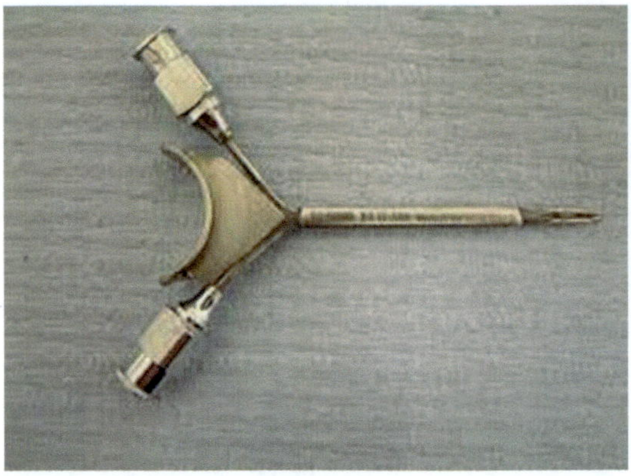

Fig. 4 An example of an arthrocentesis needle with irrigation and suction ports

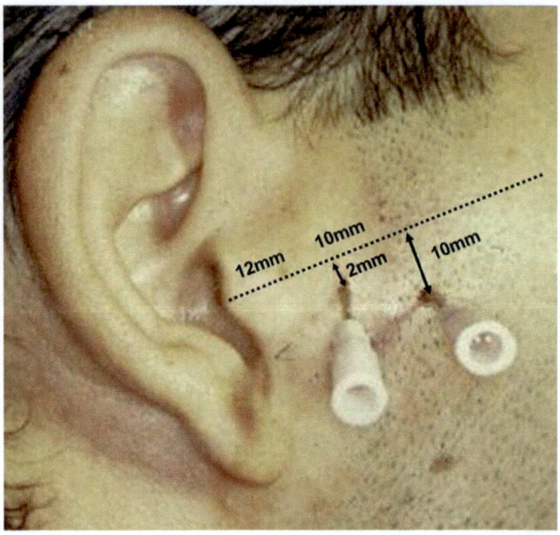

Fig. 5 External anatomical landmarks. (Nitzan, D.W., Naaman, H.L., (2022) Arthrocentesis; What, When, and Why. *Atlas Oral Maxillofacial Surg Clin N Am 30*, 137–145)

2 Techniques

The two commonly used techniques for arthrocentesis are as follows:

(A) Single-puncture technique: In this approach, a single needle cannula with two lumens (one for inflow and the other for outflow) is inserted into the joint. The irrigation and lavage of the joint will be performed through this single puncture site (Fig. 4).
(B) Double-puncture technique: In this method, two needles are placed into the joint at two separate sites. One needle is used for inflow, while the other is used for outflow during the irrigation and lavage process.

In this chapter, we will review the more common and well-studied double-puncture technique.

3 Preparation

Arthrocentesis can be performed under local anesthesia or IV sedation depending on clinician and patient preferences. Patients should be positioned in a semi-reclined position, and their hair should be secured away from surgical field using sterile towels and antibiotic ointment. External auditory canal should be protected from fluid and blood with soft cotton. Subsequently, the surgical field is prepared using Betadine solution. Aside from the surgeon, who will wear a sterile gown and gloves, two additional surgical assistants will be required, but they will not need to wear sterile gloves. One of the assistants will be responsible for handling and stabilizing the mandible during the procedure, wearing non-sterile gloves for this task. The other assistant's role will involve pushing the fluid into the joint under appropriate hydraulic pressure and suctioning the outflow irrigant.

The operator draws a canthal-tragal line from the middle of the tragus to the ipsilateral lateral canthus. This topography avoids injury to upper branches of the facial nerve. The first puncture point (A) will be marked at 10–12 mm anterior to mid-tragus, 2 mm inferior to this line. This is the posterior extent of glenoid fossa and should be palpated by fingertip with mandible placed in protrusion. The second point (B) will estimate the height of the articular eminence and will be marked 20 mm anterior to mid-tragus and 10 mm below the canthal-tragal line. These two points will be a good estimate landmark for inflow-outflow needle position (Figs. 5 and 6).

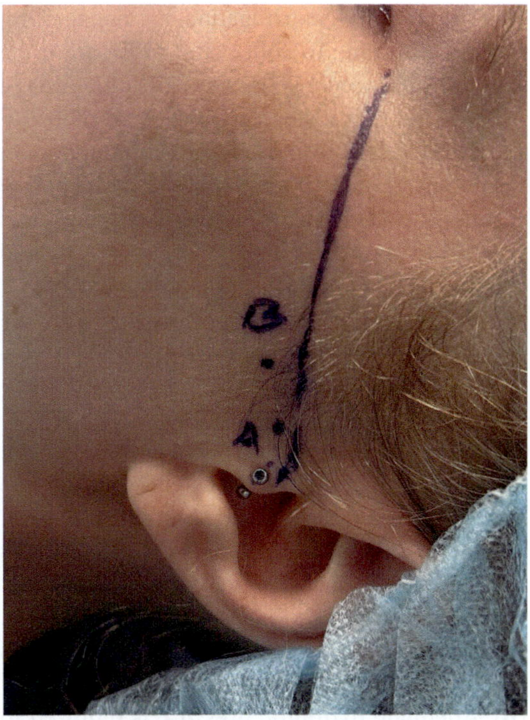

Fig. 6 Anatomical landmarks marked on patient

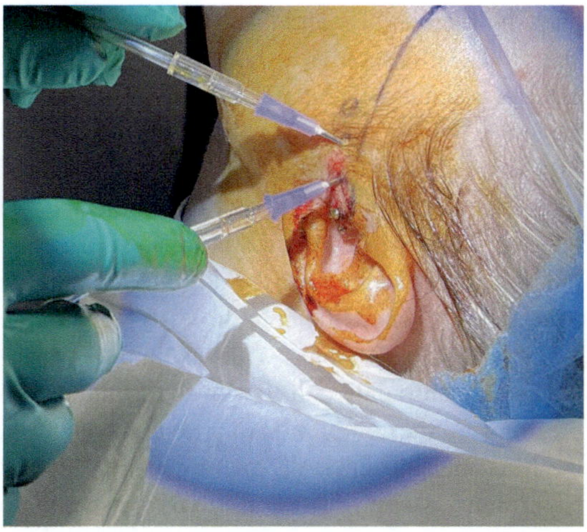

Fig. 7 Inflow and outflow access for irrigation and lavage

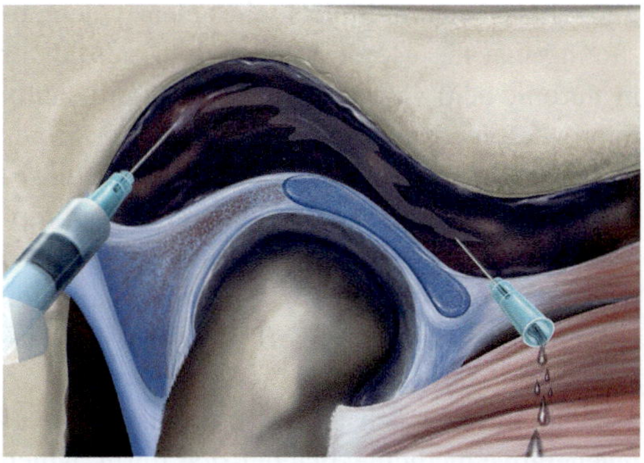

Fig. 8 Joint lavage with adequate pressure and volume, with proper outflow stream of the irrigant. (Adopted from Nitzan, D.W., Naaman, H.L., (2022) Arthrocentesis; What, When, and Why. *Atlas Oral Maxillofacial Surg Clin N Am 30*, 137–145)

4 Procedure

Auriculotemporal block and local infiltration into the joint will be done with 1–2 carpules 2% lidocaine with 1:1,000,000 epinephrine. Superior joint space will then be entered at point A with 18G needle directed in anterior–medial–inferior 45° angle. One easy and safe technique is to touch the tip of the needle to the zygomatic arch and slowly walk the needle into the superior joint space. Then the joint will be insufflated with 2–5 cc of LR via a syringe connected to the 18G needle. With the needle held in place, the syringe will be detached and IV irrigation line will be attached to the needle. A second needle previously attached to IV irrigation line will be placed into the joint capsule anteriorly at point B while the assistant holding the mandible in protrusion. The second needle will serve as outflow line (Fig. 7). The joint will be irrigated with 250 cc of LR drawn in 60 cc syringes and is pushed under moderate to high pressure by the assistant while outflow can be let to drip in kidney basin held away from the surgical field.

During the lavage, it is very important to pay attention to the position of the two needles to prevent their dislocation, which can block the outflow or potentially penetrate through the thin surrounding bony walls. As long as the outflow is consistent with the inflow fluid volume, the needles should be properly positioned and held in place by the operator and lavage continued to the end (Fig. 8). After the lavage is completed, the anterior needle will be removed, and using the posterior needle, adjuncts like steroid, liquid PRF, or PRP can be injected into the superior joint space and then the posterior needle will be removed. This will conclude the sterile portion of the procedure. Then using the dominant hand, the operator will open the mandible to almost the maximum extent along with excursive movements to manipulate and loosen the joints multiple times. At the completion of joint manipulation, the Maximal Intraincisal Opening (MIO) should be around 40 mm with minimal resistance to opening.

5 Additives

There have been multiple studies clearly demonstrating that the use of adjuncts like steroids or hyaluronic acid with arthrocentesis significantly improves outcome. Long-acting corticosteroids like triamcinolone acetonide or methylprednisolone acetate have robust anti-inflammatory properties that last weeks to months and helps reduce pain and improve function by suppressing the inflammatory cytokines like TNF-alpha, interleukins, or interferon-gamma.

With the new advancements in the field of regenerative medicine, platelet-rich fibrin, which is a second generation of platelet concentrate with longer growth factor bioavailability, has shown to promote healing, reduce inflammation, and potentially improve the condition of the joint and surrounding tissue. Platelet-rich fibrin (PRF) provides a concentrated collection of growth factors including platelet-derived growth factor (PDGF), transforming growth factor beta (TGF-beta), and vascular endothelial growth factor (VEGF), and it can be obtained in either solid or liquid form. Liquid PRF, also known as injectable PRF (i-PRF), consists of liquid fibrinogen mixed with growth factors. Once injected, fibrinogen transforms into fibrin and takes on a gel-like solid state. The process of creating i-PRF involves using a horizontal centrifuge and specific liquid PRF tubes. The centrifugation is conducted at 300 *g* for 5 min. To collect the i-PRF from the tube, an 18G needle is used to penetrate through the tube lid. Approximately, 0.5–1 cc of i-PRF can be harvested from each tube. It is important to administer i-PRF promptly into the joint before clotting occurs to maximize its effectiveness (Fig. 6). This author uses 40 mg Kenalog and 2 cc of i-PRF as additives with arthrocentesis.

6 Clinical Pearls

(a) Multiple studies have investigated irrigant volume required to sufficiently reduce the pro-inflammatory proteins from the joint. Most studies have concluded that 200 cc is sufficient to achieve statistically significant reduction in pro-inflammatory mediators. This author's protocol uses 250 cc of LR as irrigation volume for arthrocentesis.

(b) Adequate hydraulic pressure is required to stretch the joint space and break down the adhesions between the disc and glenoid fossa that limit the joint mobility. It has been reported that 40 KPa (kilopascal units) is sufficient to achieve this goal. Using an irrigation pump is one way to ensure that the irrigant is being flushed into the joint under sufficient pressure, but this requires additional equipment. Instead, the clinician can roughly estimate the adequate pressure to inject the fluid by observing the outflow stream to stay continuous during the lavage.

7 Complications

A potential complication may arise if one or both needles are misplaced outside of the joint during the procedure causing the fluid to infiltrate the surrounding tissue. This can be identified by rapid swelling of the surrounding tissue. If such an occurrence happens, the lavage process should be halted immediately, and needles should be repositioned to ensure proper outflow and prevent further tissue infiltration. The extravasated fluid will be either drained through the skin pores or absorbed naturally over the course of the next several days. Other complications can be injury to the branches of facial nerve, injury to the eighth cranial nerve or tympanic disruption, perforation of the glenoid fossa, and communication with middle cranial fossa and subsequent cerebrospinal fluid leak, skin hematoma or hemarthrosis, and postoperative infection and pain.

8 Post-op Care

The patient will be prescribed postoperative antibiotics such as Keflex to prevent infection. Pain management will involve the use of nonsteroidal anti-inflammatory medication like ibuprofen 800 mg TID with food and/or mild strength narcotics like tramadol. As a prophylactic measure, this author typically has patients start the antibiotic 1 h prior to the surgery. To aid in the healing process, the patient will be put on a non-chew diet for 3–4 weeks. Additionally, they will be instructed to perform mouth opening and excursive movement exercises multiple times a day.

References

Alkan A, Kilic E. A new approach to arthrocentesis of the temporomandibular joint. Int J Oral Maxillofac Surg. 2009;38:85–6.

Dolwick MF, et al. A randomized, double-blind-placebo-controlled study of the efficacy of steroid supplementation after temporomandibular joint arthrocentesis. J Oral Maxillofac Surg. 2020;78:1088–99.

Gonzalez-Garcia R. The current role and the future of minimally invasive temporomandibular joint surgery. Oral Maxillofac Surg Clin N Am. 2015;27:69–84.

Grossmann E, Poluha RL. Comparison between TMJ arthrocentesis techniques with different needle positions: a randomized single-blind controlled clinical trial. J Cranio-Maxillo-Facial Surg. 2021;49:368–72.

Iskik G, et al. Does the use of injectable platelet-rich fibrin after arthrocentesis for disc displacement without reduction improve clinical outcomes? J Oral Maxillofac Surg. 2023;81:689–97.

Kaneyama K, et al. The ideal lavage volume for removing bradykinin, interleukin-6, and protein from temporomandibular joint by arthrocentesis. J Oral Maxillofac Surg. 2004;62:657–61.

Nitzan DW, Naaman HL. Arthrocentesis; what, when, and why. Atlas Oral Maxillofac Surg Clin N Am. 2022;30:137–45.

Nitzan DW, Price A. The use of arthrocentesis for the treatment of osteoarthritic temporomandibular joints. J Oral Maxillofac Surg. 2001;59:1154–9.

Verde L, et al. Temporomandibular Joint: Approach to the Intermediate Space by Triangulation With Transillumination Reference. J Oral Maxillofac Surg 2023;81:684–88.

Wilkes CH. Internal Derangement of Temporomandibular Joint, Pathological Variation. Arch Otolarnygol Head Neck Surg. 1989;115:469–77.

Yura S, Totsuka Y. Relationship between effectiveness of arthrocentesis under sufficient pressure and conditions of temporomandibular joint. J Oral Maxillofac Surg. 2005;63:225–8.

Yura S, Totsuka Y, Yoshikawa T. Can arthrocentesis release intracapsular adhesions? Arthroscopic findings before and after irrigation under sufficient hydraulic pressure. J Oral Maxillofac Surg. 2003;61:1253–6.

Part II

Advanced Topics

The Neurological Aspects of the Trigeminal Cranial Complex and Its Role in the TMJ Dysfunction and Multiple Movement Disorders

Anthony B. Sims

Abbreviations

ABCFP	American Board of Craniofacial Pain
DHS	Doctor of Humanitarian Services
IMD	Integrative Medical Doctor
WONM	World Organization of Natural Medicine

1 Introduction

Aside from the brain, the masticatory system plays a major role in the functions and physiology of the head. The principal nerve to this masticatory system is the trigeminal nerve (cranial nerve (CN) 5). Since CN 5 is embryologically developed from the neural crest cells and the neural tube, as are the brain and spinal cord structures, it too should be considered a major component in the influence of the latter. CN 5 has a very intricate and complex integration with almost all the cranial nerves, the structures that developed from the mesencephalon, metencephalon, and myelencephalon, along with the craniofacial complex of the maxilla, mandible, and temporomandibular joint (TMJ).

The term "movement disorders" is described as neurological syndromes in which there is either an excess of movement (hyperkinesias) or a paucity of voluntary and automatic movements unrelated to weakness or spasticity (hypokinesias) [1]. Some movement disorders are thought to be associated with pathological changes in the basal ganglia (i.e., Parkinson's disease [PD], idiopathic torsion dystonia, Tourette syndrome [TS], and essential tremor [ET]). ET is the most common movement disorder followed by idiopathic PD and dystonia. The greatest attention to movement disorders concentrates on PD with all others being secondary. Diagnosing a patient with movement disorders involves (1) the probable etiology of the disorder, (2) understanding whether it is isolated or associated with another neurological disorder, and (3) understanding the pattern of the disorder (see Table 1). Illustrative cases are contained in Chap. 14.

What is not usually considered is that the trigeminal cranial complex, though originating from neural embryonic tissue, could be a factor in the disturbances known as movement disorders. Through commonly known anatomical and physiological principles, definitions of neurological diagnoses, diagnostic examinations, evaluations, and treatments, it may be that the trigeminal cranial nerve holds an answer to some of the disorders that have previously been attributed to disorders of the brain, cerebellum, and/or basal ganglia. This chapter shows relevant content both anatomically and physiologically as to why the CN 5 system should not be ignored when diagnosing and/or treating those with movement disorders.

A. B. Sims (✉)
Columbia, MD, USA

B. C. Stack Jr. et al. (eds.), *Craniofacial Pain*, https://doi.org/10.1007/978-3-031-57563-1_10

Table 1 Evaluation of movement disorders

Neurologic physical exam			
	Brain		
		Cerebellum	
		Cranial nerves	
		Mental status exam	
		Reasoning and cognition	
	Spine/periphery		
		Motor/strength	
		Sensation	
			Dysesthesias
		Reflex testing	
Nerve conduction testing			
	Visual evoked response (VER)		
	Auditory evoked response (ABR or BAER)		
Muscle testing			
	Electromyography		
	Muscle biopsy		
Imaging			
	Brain		
	Spine		
	Periphery		
		Extremities	

2 Embryology of the Trigeminal Nerve

The origin of the word trigeminal is taken from the Latin "tri-" equaling three and "-geminal" meaning a mass connected to a common point. There are "three" significant branches arising from trigeminal nerve that have four definitive nuclei in the brain stem. They are classified as follows:

- Sensory nuclei: (1) mesencephalic trigeminal nucleus located in the midbrain, (2) principal/chief/main trigeminal nucleus located in the pons, and (3) spinal trigeminal nucleus located in the medulla and spinal cervical region
- Motor nucleus: trigeminal motor nucleus located in the pons

These types of nuclei form early during neural development and sensory afferent fibers are sent to the brain stem in the ventral medial pons. These structures form from the structures known as the first pharyngeal and/or branchial arch. The branchial arches are embryologic structures that develop into anatomic structures. The branchial arches give rise to the lower face, neck, and part of the upper thorax, while the frontonasal process gives rise to the forehead and nose. The structures formed by the branchial arches are the result of contributions from the three primary germ layers: endoderm, mesoderm, ectoderm, as well as neural crest cell derivatives.

The **endoderm** of the branchial arches develops into endocrine viscera of the neck, including the thymus, thyroid, and parathyroid glands. The **mesoderm** cell layer forms vasculature and musculature structures from endothelial cells and myoblasts, respectively, in the head, neck, and upper thorax. **Ectoderm** gives rise to nervous system derivatives, while the lateral domain of surface ectoderm gives rise to the skin. The neural ectoderm crest cells migrate to give rise to the bones of the skull, jaw, ear, as well as cartilage found in the head and neck. The peripheral nervous system itself derives from a dual origin of surface ectoderm [2].

Structures of the first branchial arch include:

- *Bones*: maxilla, zygoma, vomer, palatine, mandible, squamous portion of the temporal bone, malleus, and incus
- *Muscles*: tensor veli tympani, tensor veli palatine, anterior belly of the digastric, mylohyoid, masseter, temporalis, lateral and medial pterygoids
- *Nerves*: trigeminal and its divisions

2.1 The Trigeminal Nuclei

In understanding the trigeminal nerve, we must first have knowledge of the different trigeminal nuclei: (A) mesencephalic trigeminal nucleus: proprioceptive information from the face; (B) principal trigeminal nucleus: light touch and discriminative information from the face; (C) spinal trigeminal nucleus: pain and temperature information from the face; and (D) trigeminal motor nucleus: motor efferent fibers for somatic control of mastication (masseter and pterygoids).

The trigeminal nerve complex courses within the middle cranial fossa before it reaches the trigeminal (Gasserian) ganglion, which lies posterolateral to the cavernous sinus in an area called Meckel's cave. Fibers from the three nuclei intermingle at this point for part of the mesencephalic, principal, and spinal trigeminal nuclei, to send fibers to the three portions of the trigeminal nerve complex: ophthalmic (V1), maxillary (V2), and mandibular (V3) nerves.

2.2 Trigeminal Nerve Branches (Fig. 1)

Ophthalmic division branches: Frontal, lacrimal, nasociliary, long ciliary nerves. Supplies sensory afferents from the top of the head to the upper eyelid, including the cornea

Maxillary division branches: Middle meningeal, nasopalatine, greater and lesser palatine, zygomatic, and infraorbital. The maxillary division supplies sensory afferents from the lower eyelid to the upper lip including sensation to the gingiva and mucosa around the hard palate and maxillary dentition

Mandibular division: Branches of the main trunk (before splitting into anterior and posterior divisions) of the mandibular division include meningeal, branch to medial pterygoid, tensor tympani, and tensor veli palatini. Branches of the anterior division include masseteric, lateral pterygoid, deep temporal, and buccal. Branches of the posterior division include auriculotemporal, lingual, and inferior alveolar, which provides sensory afferents to teeth as well as motor innervation to the mylohyoid and anterior belly of the digastric muscle

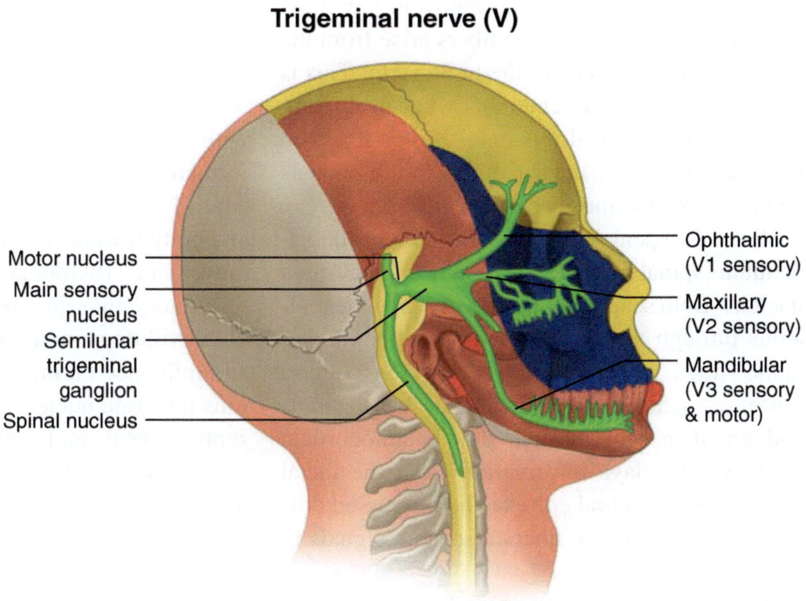

Fig. 1 Trigeminal nerve branches

3 Understanding the Trigeminal Nerve and Its Connections

The trigeminal nerve (CN 5) is the largest and most complex of 12 cranial nerves. Its vast size and influence are greatly appreciated when one attempts to diagnose and treat patients suffering from orofacial pain and temporomandibular joint disorders. Without a thorough knowledge of the trigeminal nerve, the efficacy of diagnostic and therapeutic procedures will be very disappointing. CN 5 branches into three divisions: ophthalmic, maxillary, and mandibular divisions, each of which supplies a distinct region or dermatome that carries pain, touch, temperature, and proprioception from the face, eyes, teeth, jaws, and mucosa of the nose, mouth, and anterior two-thirds of the tongue. CN 5 carries about 140,000 sensory fibers and about 8100 motor fibers.

Sensory fibers arise from the Gasserian ganglion (GG), but the sensory fibers that determine proprioception of the head come from jaw muscles and jaw position. These fibers arise from the mesencephalic nucleus in the brain stem. This is an important factor to remember when evaluating patients with cervical dystonia. Motor fibers in CN 5 originate from the trigeminal motor nucleus and innervate the muscles of mastication.

The CN 5 sensory fibers terminate in the trigeminal spinal nucleus or the principal/main nucleus. Both send secondary neurons to the thalamus through the crossed ventral trigeminothalamic tract, which terminate in the ventral posterior medial (VPM) nucleus of the thalamus and are then sent through the thalamocortical tract, which relays information from the facial region to the cerebral cortex. The uncrossed dorsal trigeminothalamic fibers also send signals to the VPM.

The CN 5 is the only cranial nerve that has direct first-order neurons that input into the reticular formation, which is another important factor in cases of movement disorders. The spinal nucleus extends caudally and merges with the substantia gelatinosa of the spinal cord and has three divisions: spinal trigeminal oralis, trigeminal spinal interpolaris, and trigeminal spinal caudalis. The trigeminal spinal nucleus is also connected to the motor nucleus along with the ocular, trigeminal, facial, vestibular, glossopharyngeal, vagal, and hypoglossal nerves in the brain stem. There are also afferent fibers to the superior colliculus, cerebellar cortex, and deep cerebellar nuclei. Nerve fibers also connect the trigeminal with cervical nerve root fibers C1, C2, and C3.

The reticular formation (RF) is the central core of the brain stem tegmentum. The RF consists of multipolar neurons with long ascending and descending axons which interact with collateral interneuron branches synaptically and form complex loops and/or circuits. It has no distinct architectural boundaries and forms the central gray matter of the midbrain, pons, and medulla. The brain stem's RF has a modulatory effect on the spinal cord, brain stem's cranial nerves, cerebrum, and cerebellar cortex. The ascending reticular pathways encompass the reticular activating system which regulates the sleep-wake cycle and moderates awareness. The descending reticular pathways moderate motor activities within the spinal cord at all levels.

The trigeminal nerve is the only cranial nerve with monosynaptic projections into the reticular formation. Other behaviors of the RF include control of body posture, orientation of the head and body towards external stimuli, control of eye movements, rhythm generator for diaphragm and respiratory muscles, blood pressure control and blood volume among organs, heart rate, reflexes, and influence on our mental states. The RF neurons integrate nuclei from the CN 5, facial, glossopharyngeal, and oculomotor that ascend and descend within the brain stem. The RF also connects to the thalamus, hypothalamus, cerebrum, and cerebellum via ascending reticular neurons. The trigeminoreticulothalamic pathway conveys pain and temperature. There are also interneuronal connections within the RF.

The CN 5 system has many branches that supply innervation to different areas of the head and facial structures (Fig. 2). One of the structures of the face that gets utilized the most is the temporomandibular joint (TMJ). It is constantly used for mastication, speaking, facial expression, swallowing, and airway maintenance. The TMJ is the

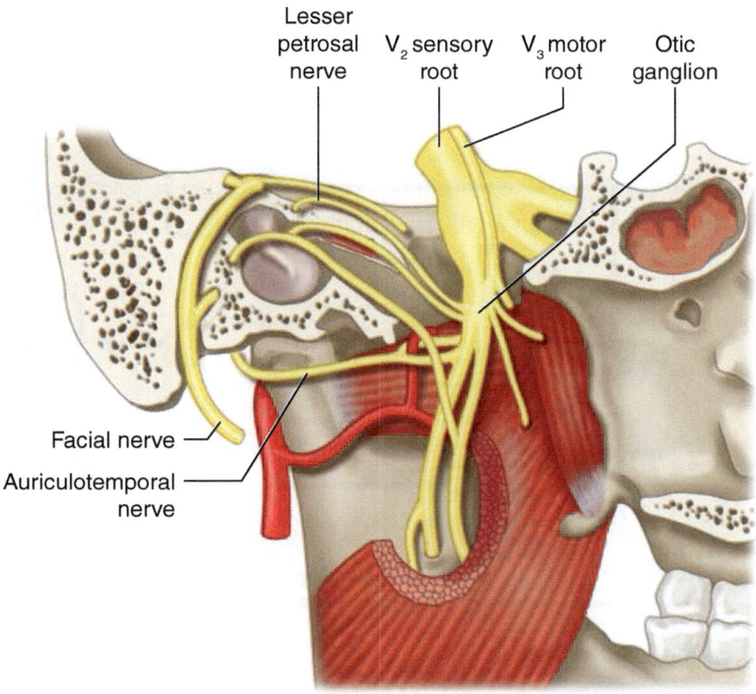

Fig. 2 https://www.muhadharaty.com/lecture/19573/%D8%AF%D9%83%D8%AA%D9%88%D8%B1-%D8%B3%D8%B9%D8%AF/mandibular-nerve-pptx

articulation between the mandible and the cranium. This articulation is a bilateral movable fulcrum. The major skeletal components of the TMJ are the mandible and the temporal bone. The sphenoid and hyoid bones play a secondary supporting role in the articulation. There are two cartilaginous components, the articular cartilage and the fibrocartilage disc, which separate the temporal bone from the mandible creating upper and lower compartments within the TMJ, which contain the stylomandibular, sphenomandibular, and Pinto's (malleomandibular) ligaments. The muscles that support the TMJ are the temporalis, the masseter, the medial and lateral pterygoids, the suprahyoids, the infrahyoids, the geniohyoid, the digastric, the mylohyoid, the styloid, and a multitude of cervical muscles. The main innervation of the TMJ is the mandibular branch (V3) of CN 5 via the auriculotemporal (AT) nerve.

The AT nerve arises typically by two roots, which encircle the middle meningeal artery. The nerve passes posteriorly deep to the lateral pterygoid and is sandwiched between the sphenomandibular ligament and the neck of the mandible condyle. The AT nerve is intimately associated with the parotid gland, and it then travels posterior to the TMJ. The terminal branches of the AT nerve go on to innervate the scalp around the temple. In addition, the AT nerve anastomoses with the facial nerve and the otic ganglion. The two branches which communicate with the facial nerve do so at the posterior aspect of the masseter muscle.

The AT nerve has five main branches. These are the anterior auricular, articular, parotid, superficial temporal, and branches to the external auditory meatus. The anterior auricular branches innervate the skin overlying the tragus as well as the adjacent part of the helix. The articular branches go on to innervate the posterior aspect of the TMJ, to which it is closely related. The parotid branches provide secretomotor innervation. Another component of this originates from cranial nerve IX, the glossopharyngeal nerve, via its tympanic branch and transverses to the otic ganglion. The fibers then pass with the AT nerve and innervate the parotid gland. The superficial temporal branches run with the superficial temporal artery. These branches innervate the tissue over the temple and coalesce with the facial nerves. The branches to the external auditory meatus run between the cartilaginous and bony

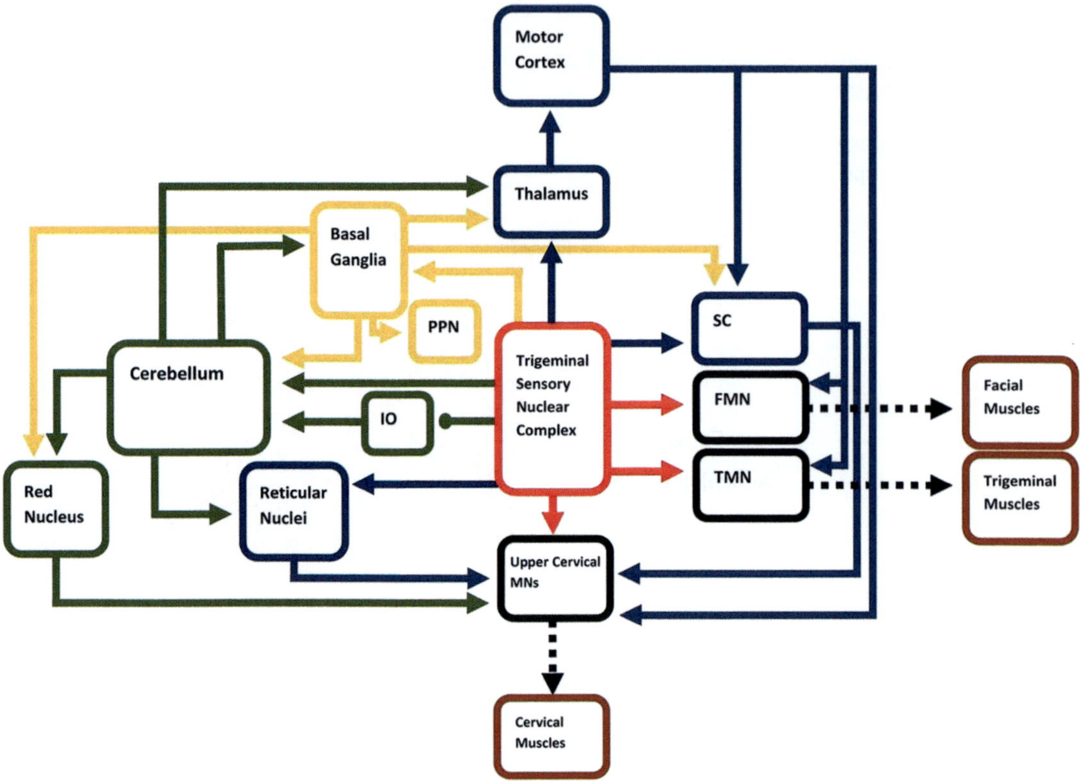

Fig. 3 Schematic of an integrated network model including the trigeminal sensory nuclear complex (TSNC) neurons in the facial motor neurons (FMNs), trigeminal motor neurons (TMNs), and upper cervical motor neurons. Projections to muscles most affected by dystonia are indicated by the hatched arrows. Ascending projections from the TSNC to the motor cortex via the thalamus, and to the superior colliculus (SC) and the reticular nuclei, also modulate excitability via descending tracts to motor nuclei (blue). Excitatory inputs to the cerebellum and inhibitory inputs via the inferior olive (IO; green) contribute to cortical and bulbar descending modulation of motor neurons innervating muscles affected by dystonia via cerebellar outputs to the red nucleus, reticular nuclei, basal ganglia, and motor cortex via the thalamus. TSNC projections to the basal ganglia (yellow) modulate excitability of descending projections to motor neurons by outputs to the motor cortex (via the thalamus), superior colliculus, red nucleus, and pedunculopontine nucleus (PPN). Connections from pedunculopontine nucleus to spinal cord are not shown in the simplified figure. [From Bradnam L, Barry C. The role of the trigeminal sensory nuclear complex in the pathophysiology of craniocervical dystonia. J Neurosci. 2013 Nov 20;33(47):18358–67]

ear canals and innervate the skin of the meatus and also provide innervation to the tympanic membrane (Fig. 3).

4 Temporomandibular Joint (TMJ)

The temporomandibular joint (TMJ) is a diarthrosis, better defined as a ginglymoarthrodial joint, which means a composite anatomical joint of which one element has an axial or hinge motion and the other a simple gliding motion. The TMJ is composed of a synovial cavity, articular cartilage, and a capsule that covers the same joint. The TMJ through its complex movements, in different orthogonal planes and multiple rotation axes, works in synergy with all the structures just listed. The TMJ must also work in coordination with the contralateral TMJ to coordinate tandem dynamic function with the head's cranial system, the neck musculature, the dental occlusion, the facial structures, and the nervous system components within these structures.

There may be developments within the TMJ system that may cause various disorders to occur. These include growth, disease, arthritis, dysfunction, and microtraumas or macrotrauma disorders. Whenever there is a mal-relation between any of these structures, a dysfunction may result within the trigeminal afferent nervous system, which in turn may cause the various central nervous systems, as discussed above, to be a factor that produces movement disorders.

4.1 Growth Disorders

Disorders of the facial structure and the TMJ are due to several factors in their development. There may be maxillary or mandibular overgrowth or undergrowth, which can be a result of (1) airway obstruction (poor swallowing habits), (2) parafunctional habits (bruxism, thumb/finger sucking), (3) allergies (enlarged tonsils and/or adenoids), (4) misaligned teeth (maxillary and mandibular teeth do not occlude properly), and (5) family genetics (familial growth patterns). Growth disorders such as condylar hypoplasia or hyperplasia and neoplasms may need to be treated to harmonize the facial structures in certain cases.

4.2 Arthritic Disease

Osteoarthritis (OA) is a disease that causes degeneration of the articular cartilage sometimes known as degenerative joint disease of the condyle or the articular eminence of the temporal bone. The cartilage within the joint begins to break down, and the underlying bone changes. These changes develop slowly and worsen over time. OA can cause pain, stiffness, and swelling. Crepitus sensation of sound could be the result of disk degeneration or perforation, causing bone-on-bone contact and erosion. Joint involvement is usually bilateral. X-rays or cone beam CT may show degeneration and/or flattening of the condylar head.

4.3 Infectious Arthritis

Infection of the TMJ may result from an infection of blood-borne organisms. The joint becomes inflamed, and jaw movement is painful with decreased motion. X-rays are usually negative early but may show bony degeneration in the later stages. Diagnosis should be made early to prevent permanent joint dysfunction.

4.4 Traumatic Arthritis

Acute injury (e.g., from difficult tooth extraction or endotracheal intubation) is a consistent factor that leads to arthritis of the TMJ. Pain, tenderness, and limitation of mandibular motion may occur. Diagnostic history is the most important element when X-ray results are negative or when intra-articular edema or hemorrhagic widening of the joint space is not present.

4.5 Rheumatoid Arthritis

Rheumatoid arthritis of the TMJ affects approximately 17% of adults and children. Limited movement, pain, and swelling are the most common symptoms. Children display destruction of the condyle which results in mandibular growth disturbance and facial deformity, and ankylosis may develop in which surgery for correction may be necessary. X-rays of the TMJ are usually negative in early stages but often show late-stage bone destruction, which may result in an anterior open-bite malocclusion.

5 Dysfunction of the TMJ

Research from the National Institutes of Health in the United States purports that the prevalence of temporomandibular joint dysfunction in the current population is between 5 and 12%. TMJ disorders are at least twice as prevalent in women as men. The most frequent sign for this dysfunction was a clicking sound in the TMJ, which was reported in all age groups. Clicking is the main distinctive sign of an "internal derangement" or dysfunction of the TMJ. Internal derangements of the TMJ can be classified as:

1. Reciprocal clicking (dislocation with reduction)
2. Intermittent clicking (dislocation with reduction)
3. Closed lock (dislocation without reduction)

Internal derangements of the TMJ involve a temporary, semipermanent, or permanent destruction of the normal relationship between the condyle, the disc, and the articular eminence. The etiologies of internal derangements are categorized as:

1. Acute macrotrauma possibly due to mandibular whiplash, a blow to the mandible, and/or mandibular hyperextension (intubation)
2. Chronic microtraumas possibly due to bruxism and/or clenching, excessive joint overload causing joint degeneration, and loss of posterior teeth which support the dental arches
3. Occlusal interferences, possibly causing stressful bruxism and/or malocclusion
4. Development from mandibular hyper- or hypoplasia with/without facial asymmetry

Whenever clinicians speak about dysfunction of the TMJ and neurological aspects of the joint, the main complaint is pain. There are many levels of pain from light touch or slight irritation to severe pain. Pain during mechanical stimulation of the joint and spontaneous pain are major symptoms of degeneration. An important neuronal process of mechanical hypersensitivity of the joint is the sensitization of thin myelinated A-delta fibers and nonmyelinated C fibers innervating the joint.

Pain is a human primate instinct and can be defined as a distressing sensation, as well as an emotional experience that is linked to actual or potential tissue damage, with the sole purpose of notifying the body's defense mechanism to react towards a stimulus in order to avoid further tissue damage. Both nociceptors remain silent during homeostasis in the absence of pain and are activated when there is a potential of noxious stimulus. Both these nociceptors have specialized free nerve endings that are widely located in the skin, muscle, joint capsule, bone, and some major internal organs.

There are three major roles for the receptors in the primary afferent neurons which are excitatory, sensitizing, and inhibitory responses. Once these receptors are being stimulated and have reached the pain threshold, the resulting impulses are propagated along the afferent fibers towards the dorsal horn (peripheral nervous system) and medulla (cranial). The auriculotemporal nerve, a branch of the mandibular portion (V3) of the trigeminal nerve, was found to innervate the lateral capsule of the TMJ. In 75% of the specimens, the masseteric nerve, a branch of the maxillary portion (V2) of the trigeminal nerve, was also found to innervate the anteromedial capsule of the TMJ.

5.1 Relationship to Cervical Spine

The cervical spine plays a major role in the stabilization of the cranium and balancing of the masticatory musculature through specific joint articulations and muscle attachments. Postural abnormalities that affect the static relationship between the head and neck can possibly lead to temporomandibular dysfunction, and the reverse is also true. Abnormal posture can result in compression of the suboccipital muscles, produce referred pain to the TMJ area, and alter the normal resting position of the mandible through compression forces of the musculature or compression of the nerves that supply the TMJ. Some patients progress to the point of chronic pain and are given a diagnosis of myofascial pain dysfunction syndrome (MFPDS).

The upper quadrant of the cervical spine consists of the suboccipital muscles, cervical spine from C1 to C7, mandible, TMJ, cranium, maxillary and mandibular dentition, cervicothoracic area, first and second ribs, hyoid bone, sternum, clavicle, shoulder girdle, sternocleidomastoid muscle (SCM), and upper extremities. A dysfunction from one area of the quadrant or any combination can elicit pain and/or a dysfunction of other portions of the quadrant. The quadrant acts as one unit to convey proper movement and position of the rest. These muscles and bones are innervated by cranial nerves C1–C4, facial, glossopharyngeal (IX), vagus (X), and trigeminal nerve (V). The interface between these nerves is called the trigeminocervical complex, and sometimes differentiation between them is difficult to discern.

The subnucleus caudalis of the trigeminal nerve contains a portion of the substantia gelatinosa that is continuous with the dorsal horn of the spinal cord. The spinal accessory nerve (XI) connects with the superior ganglion of the vagus, anastomoses with neurons from C2 to C4 spinal segments, and is an efferent portion of the pharyngeal plexus and vagus. A large portion of the spinal accessory nerve crosses the midline, which may cause referred pain or dysfunction from the SCM. The inferior ganglion of the vagus receives transmission from the hypoglossal nerve, which also joins with the pharyngeal plexus and spinal C1 nerves to form the ansa cervicalis. Therefore, the trigeminocervical complex involves cranial nerves 5, 7, 9, 10, 11, and 12 and spinal nerves C1–C4 and must include the reticular formation.

5.2 Trigeminal Nerve and Posture

Posture refers to the position of the human body when standing and its orientation accounting for its effects from gravity (Fig. 4). Through mechanisms of feedback and feed-forward, postural adjustments play a critical role in orthostatic and dynamic postural control. Afferent inputs that control posture are exteroceptive (skin sensitiveness of feet), proprioceptive (especially from the cervical, hip, ankle, and knee joints), vestibular (utriculus, sacculus, and semicircular canals), and visual (movement of the surrounding environment).

The neurons for **proprioception** are exceptional. Their unipolar cell bodies constitute the **mesencephalic trigeminal nucleus**, which is lateral to the periaqueductal gray matter and extends rostrally to the level of the superior colliculus. The axons of these neurons form the **mesencephalic trigeminal tract** and are then distributed with the maxillary and mandibular divisions of V. They go to muscle spindles, receptors in the temporomandibular joint, and pressure receptors around the roots of the teeth. This pressure sense is related to proprioception; reflex connections to the motor trigeminal nucleus regulate biting and chewing.

The stomatognathic system (SS) also plays an important role in postural control. The SS is a functional unit characterized by several structures: skeletal components (maxilla and mandible), dental arches, soft tissues (salivary glands, nervous and vascular supplies), and TMJ and masticatory muscles (MM). When the occlusal relationship is lost either unilaterally or bilaterally, the body posture may take on an unusual position, causing neck or shoulder pain. In patients with TMJ disc dysfunction, there can be hyperlordosis of the thoracic spine (rectification) and head (deviation to the right or left).

The muscle combinations of the SS are a part of the cervical muscular chain, and the musculoskeletal system is composed of several muscular chain groups. They are all integrated together. Any disorder of one body segment will result in a reorganization or adaptation of other muscular segmental group [3]. For example, studies have shown that the simulation of a flatfoot increased muscular stimulation of the temporal and masseter musculature.

The cerebellum regulates the cognitive and automatic processes of posture-gait control by acting on the cerebral cortex via the thalamocortical projection and brain stem, respectively. The basal ganglia may also contribute to the modulation of each process through projections to the cerebral cortex and brain stem. It is also generally agreed that the reticulospinal tract (RST) contributes to regulation of the level of muscle tone. There may exist functional organization in the reticular formation in relation to the control of postural muscle tone. Muscle tone related to RST participates in the execution of locomotion so that locomotor rhythm and muscle tone can be simultaneously regulated by the reticulospinal system during locomotion.

The trigeminal spinal nucleus has extensive projections to motor neurons in the spinal cord, the brain stem's reticular formation, the cerebellum, and the basal ganglia, and via the thalamus to the motor cortex. Aberrant cerebellar circuitry is linked to many forms of spinocerebellar ataxias

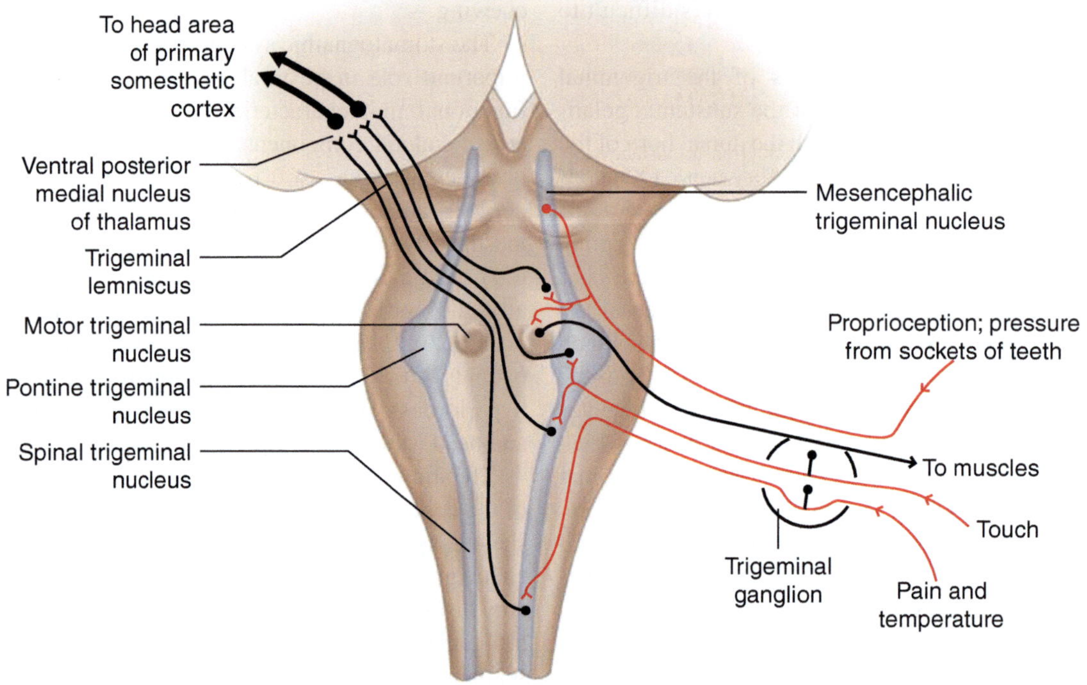

Fig. 4 The pathway of trigeminal pain. The spinal trigeminal tract connects the pons to the cervicomedullary junction, where trigeminal pain impulses are sent to the deeper second-order nucleus caudalis. Signals to the contralateral thalamus are sent by the ventral trigeminothalamic tract

including impaired balance and motor coordination. In order to achieve smooth and balanced muscle movement, the cerebellum receives input from the sensory systems which includes the trigeminal nerves, the spinal cord, the reticular formation, and other parts of the brain. The trigeminal nerve is the only cranial nerve that carries primary afferent neurons to the reticular formation, thus having primary influence on the reticulospinal system through which the nervous system can facilitate or inhibit motor movement and posture.

6 Movement Disorders

Movement disorders can be *defined* as neurological syndromes in which there is either an excess of movement (hyperkinesia) or a paucity of voluntary and automatic movements, unrelated to weakness or spasticity (hypokinesia). The abnormal movement in these disorders is in a conscious patient. Some movement disorders are known to be associated with hereditary changes, environmental exposures, and pathological changes. Some have a well-known origin (i.e., Parkinson's disease) where others are not totally clear and thought to be idiopathic (i.e., Tourette syndrome, tremor).

6.1 Hyperkinetic Movement Disorders

Hyperkinetic movements are unwanted or excess movements that are frequently seen in children with neurologic disorders. Dystonia is a movement disorder in which involuntary sustained or intermittent muscle contractions cause twisting and repetitive movements, abnormal postures, or both. Chorea is an ongoing random-appearing sequence of one or more discrete involuntary movements or movement fragments. Athetosis is a slow, continuous, involuntary writhing movement that prevents maintenance of a stable posture. Myoclonus is a sequence of repeated, often nonrhythmic, brief shock-like jerks due to sudden involuntary contraction or relaxation of one or more muscles. The previous three movement disorders will not be addressed in this chapter. Tremor is a rhythmic back-and-forth or oscillating involuntary movement about a joint axis. Tics are repeated, individually recognizable, intermittent movements or movement fragments that are almost always briefly suppressible and are usually associated with awareness of an urge to perform the movement. Stereotypes are repetitive, simple movements that can be voluntarily suppressed.

6.2 Hypokinetic Movement Disorders

Hypokinetic movement is the term used concerning slow or reduced movement regarding speed and amplitude. Hypokinetic movement disorders are often referred to as Parkinsonism because they display clinical features of idiopathic Parkinson's disease (IPD) such as rigidity and/or bradykinesia. Tremor and postural and gait instability are usual signs and symptoms. Parkinson's disease is under the umbrella of Parkinsonism. Though the assemblage of symptoms for Parkinson's disease may include the former, Parkinsonism may have other causes or origins.

7 Dystonia

Dystonia is an abnormal movement depicted by sustained muscle contractions that frequently produce involuntary twisting and repetitive movements, abnormal postures, and/or any combination of these. Dystonia often involves various body parts and according to the site determines its classification. Classifications are (1) focal: usually involving a specific part; (2) segmental: usually involving two or more contiguous body parts; (3) multifocal: involving two or more body parts that are not contiguous; (4) hemidystonia: usually involving one half of the body; and (5) generalized: usually involving the legs.

The disease course can be either static or progressive. The variability can have four different patterns: (1) persistent: dystonia that persists to approximately the same extent throughout the day; (2) action specific: dystonia that occurs only during a particular activity or task; (3) diurnal fluctuations: dystonia fluctuates during the day, with recognizable circadian variations in occurrence and severity; and (4) paroxysmal: sudden self-limited episodes of dystonia usually induced by a trigger with return to preexisting neurological state.

The etiology of the disorder is thought to be either (A) inherited, (B) acquired, or (C) idiopathic. The classification "primary dystonia" indicates that there are no obvious neurological degenerative changes or other structural defects. They are either generalized or focal dystonia. Dystonia has been associated with injury to the basal ganglia, in particular the putamen and globus pallidus. However, recent research has demonstrated that no basal ganglia injury can be identified, and recent evidence from both human disease and animal models suggests that other brain areas including cerebellum, brain stem, or sensory cortex can be causes of dystonia.

7.1 Types of Dystonia

7.1.1 Cervical Dystonia

This is the most common form of primary focal dystonia. It was once thought to have a psychogenic etiology. It usually begins between 30 and 50 years of age and is more prominent in women than men. Cervical dystonia is also known as spasmodic torticollis and is a rare neurological disorder that is believed to originate in the brain. It is classified by involuntary muscle contractions in the neck that cause abnormal movements and postures of the head and neck. These contractions may be unremitting or unabating; they may also present as spasms that can resemble tremor. The severity of cervical dystonia can vary, but the disorder can cause significant pain and discomfort as well as difficulties due to abnormal postures.

Abnormal head postures encompass combinations of rotation (torticollis), extended head posture (retrocollis), forward flexion (anterocollis), and lateral tilt (laterocollis). Dystonia tends to increase with fatigue, stress, and upset emotions and is relieved with rest and sleep. One factor that is interesting about dystonia is the temporary relief a patient may get utilizing what is called a "sensory trick" or geste antagoniste. It was recently renamed as "alleviating maneuver" by Patel et al.

The phenomenology is varied, and the exact mechanism remains elusive. These tricks are usually tactile or from proprioceptive stimuli. For cervical dystonia, the patient places their hand on the chin or side of the face to relieve their symptoms. There is no single strategy for the treatment of cervical dystonia. Most therapies are to relieve symptoms of pain, disturbed postures, functions, and/or spasms.

The three treatment options, which may be used alone or combined, are (1) botulinum toxin injections, which is the first-choice treatment; (2) oral medications, of which there is no current FDA-approved medication, levodopa, baclofen, and clonazepam; and (3) deep brain stimulation surgery, which involves placement of electrodes into the brain and to reset brain wave patterns. The precise mechanism action for this is not clear. Currently, a combination of DBS and botulinum toxin injections is being utilized as treatment.

Blepharospasm is an abnormal contraction of the eyelid muscles. It often refers to benign essential blepharospasm (BEB), which is a bilateral condition and a form of focal dystonia leading to episodic closure of the eyelids. Symptoms usually begin as mild and infrequent spasms that progress over time to forceful and frequent contractions of the eyelids, in advanced cases causing functional blindness from inability to temporarily open the eyes. The first-line treatment for BEB is periodic injection of botulinum toxin into the eyelid muscles. Meige's syndrome is a combination of eyes, jaw, and facial dystonias.

Blepharospasm is an increased frequency of blinking and/or forceful eyelid closure with difficulty or inability in opening the eyes. Eyelid closure may last for seconds to minutes. This may result in difficulty in reading, driving, or watching television. These symptoms can become severe enough to cause the patient to have a "functional blindness." Patients often complain of sensitivity to bright light (photophobia). There are alleviating maneuvers such as humming, singing, talking, and even chewing gum. Treatment for blepharospasm is the same as with other dystonias: oral medications, botulism toxin injections into the upper eyelids, and orbicularis oculi myectomy surgery (removing part of the eyelid muscle) (Fig. 5).

7.1.2 Oromandibular Dystonia (OMD)

Patients experience spasms of the face, mouth, tongue, and lower jaw. The masticatory muscles upon opening or closing produce lateral torsion, protrusion, spasms, and/or a combination of these symptoms of the jaw. Dystonic spasms may be seen as nasal contractions, facial grimacing, lip pursing or sucking, bruxism, tongue dyskinesia, mouth corner retractions, and platysma spasms. Breathing difficulties have also been reported. Dysfunctions include impaired mastication, dysphagia, speech alterations (dysarthria and dysphonia), unconscious opening and closing of the mandible, pulling and twisting of the mandible forward or laterally, and temporomandibular disorders (TMDs). Lingual dystonia is produced by lateral deviation of the tongue and/or protrusion of the tongue.

Trismus, bruxism, and forceful involuntary jaw closure or temporomandibular joint (TMJ) dislocation can lead to trauma and damage of the oral cavity structures, dental restorations, dentures, excessive dental wear, dental fractures, and trauma of the lips, gums, and tongue, while jaw-opening dystonia may be associated with TMJ overload. Alleviating maneuvers of OMD are touching the chin, talking, chewing gum, and biting on a toothpick. Some common predisposing factors associated with OMD movement disorder include tooth loss, loss of vertical dimension, ill-fitting full dentures, an edentulous state, trauma, and long dental procedures. Treatment of choice for OMD is botulism toxin. OMD rarely improves with medication, whereas there are no surgical options. Even botulism toxin has its difficulties because it can be complicated by postinjection swallowing difficulties, which could render the procedure life-threatening.

Fig. 5 Blink reflex. Diagram shows presumed location of the bulbar interneurons serving the two components of the blink reflex: (*1*) interneurons serving the ipsilateral early components; (*2*) interneurons serving the bilateral late component. (*Vm* indicates trigeminal motor nucleus, *Sp V co* spinal trigeminal complex, *Sp V tr* spinal trigeminal tract, *VI* abducens nucleus, *VII* facial nucleus, *VII* facial nerve, *VN* trigeminal sensory root, *XII* hypoglossal nucleus, *Lat tegm field* lateral tegmental field, *Med tegm field* medial tegmental field.) (Modified and used with permission)

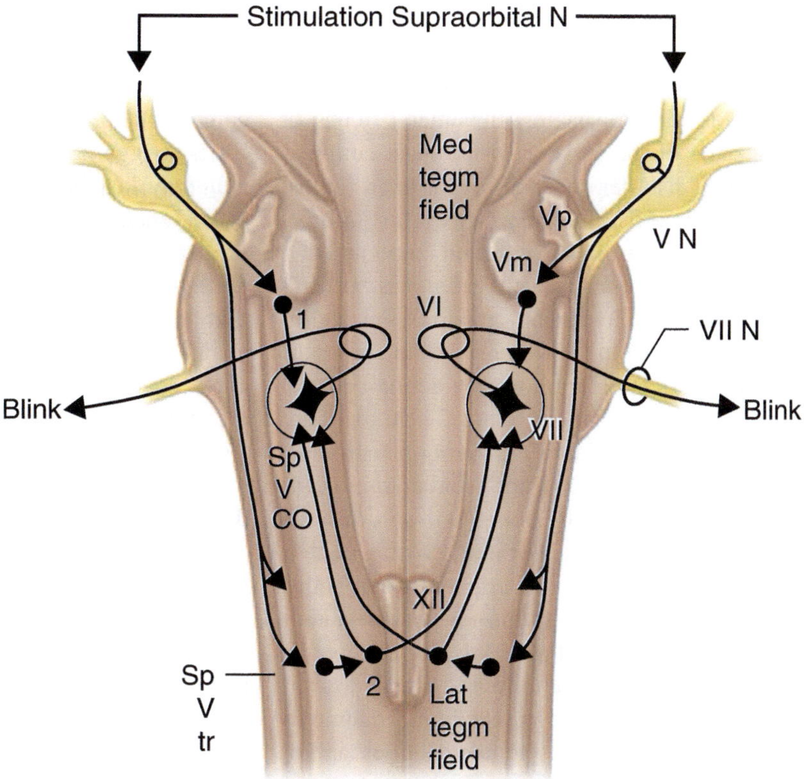

7.1.3 Limb Dystonia (LD)

This is a focal dystonia which produces involuntary twisting and other repetitive movements and/or postures of the arms, legs, and toes. LD can produce a flexion or extension of the hands or fingers and an inversion or eversion flexion of the foot. LD patients usually participate in highly skilled motor tasks such as writing, instrument playing, and golfing. These are sometimes referred to as cramping disorders. Writer's cramp is the most common. Treatment option for focal dystonia is injections of botulinum toxin. Simple orthopedic intervention with braces can help manage the patient's condition.

7.1.4 Restless Leg Syndrome (RLS)

RLS is an overwhelming urge to move your legs. It is an unpleasant limb sensation that occurs when a patient is at rest or during times of inactivity or while lying down. Patients mention the feeling of crawling or creeping sensation in the feet, calves, or thighs. Restless leg syndrome is also associated with involuntary jerking of the arms and legs during the first two stages of sleep, which is known as periodic limb movements of sleep (PLMS).

The median age for RLS is between 30 and 50 years. One etiology for RLS may be iron deficiency anemia or kidney failure though there may be many other factors associated with it (i.e., pregnancy, peripheral nerve abnormalities, multiple sclerosis).

When sensory RLS symptoms co-occur with periodic limb movements of sleep (PLMS), there is additional activation in the red nuclei and brain stem close to the reticular formation. PLMS are often associated with cortical arousal, previously thought to occur because of movement, a product of the reticular activating system. The first line of treatment is a dopamine agonist, but other medications have been used such as benzodiazepines, clonidine, and opioids.

8 Tremor

Tremor is an involuntary, rhythmic muscle contraction leading to shaking movements in one or more parts of the body. It is the most common movement disorder. It can affect the hands, arms, head, vocal cords, trunk, and legs. Most tremors get worse with stress, anxiety, and emotional distress but lessen during sleep. Tremor is not life-threatening, but it can be embarrassing and/or disabling. There are different classifications of tremor: (a) resting tremor, (b) action-postural tremor, and (c) intention tremor. Then, there are specific tremor disorders: (1) tremor from toxins, (2) essential tremor, (3) Parkinsonian tremor, (4) cerebellar tremor, (5) tremor of Wilson's disease, (6) orthostatic tremor, (7) primary writing tremor, (8) tremor associated with peripheral neuropathy, and (9) palatal tremor. In this chapter, the author will address only one type of tremor, cerebellar. Tremor following brain trauma is usually associated with lesions of the cerebellum. Treatments consist of various types of medications and/or DBS surgery.

8.1 Paroxysmal Kinesigenic Dyskinesia (PKD)

PKD is a rare condition characterized by abnormal involuntary movements that are precipitated by a sudden movement or startle. Patients might present with dystonic, ballismus, chorea, hyperkinesias, or combinations of the abnormal movements, and they may be unilateral or bilateral. Patients experience attacks without loss of consciousness. The prevalence of PKD is unknown, as epidemiologic data are not available owing to the rarity of paroxysmal dyskinesias. Paroxysmal dyskinesias are classified according to their triggers, duration and frequency of attacks, effectiveness of medication, and associated syndromes.

There are four subtypes of PKD recognized: (1) paroxysmal kinesigenic dyskinesia (PKD), which is induced by sudden movement; (2) paroxysmal non-kinesigenic dyskinesia (PNKD) precipitated by, for instance, alcohol or caffeine; they can also be triggered by excitement, stress, or fatigue or can be spontaneous, and attacks last minutes to hours; (3) paroxysmal exercise-induced dyskinesia (PED) triggered by longer lasting activity and that may last between 5 and 30 min; and (4) paroxysmal hypnogenic dyskinesia, which is a rare clinical entity characterized by intermittent dystonia and choreoathetoid movements that begin exclusively during sleep. The paroxysmal dyskinesia may be associated with ataxia, a cerebellar disorder. Treatment is with haloperidol or benzodiazepines.

8.2 Parkinsonism

Parkinsonism is used to describe neurologic disorders characterized by the existence of tremor, rigidity, and bradykinesia in addition to unstable and/or loss of postural reflexes and a freezing gait. Parkinsonism is characteristically present in Parkinson's disease (PD) and is the most common cause of Parkinsonism. These symptoms can also result from other neurodegenerative disorders, as well as specific brain lesions, head trauma, medications, metabolic conditions, and toxin exposure. In this chapter, the author will only discuss post-traumatic Parkinsonism.

Patients usually state that they had some significant head injury or trauma prior to the onset of the symptoms (i.e., car accident, whiplash). This is thought to have caused damage to the basal ganglia or the brain stem. Symptoms may occur shortly after the incident and may be unilateral. As time continues, the full symptoms of bradykinesia, tremor, dystonia, rigidity, and gait disorder may follow. Severe traumatic brain injury (TBI) has been reported to have Parkinsonian symptoms. Some authors believe that severe TBI and post-traumatic Parkinsonism may share a common midbrain network dysfunction. Dementia pugilistica or "punch-drunk" syndrome is a condition that has resulted from constant head blows. Ataxia, resting tremor, dysarthria, and dementia along with Parkinsonism may develop.

8.3 Tourette Syndrome and/or Tic Disorder

Tourette syndrome is a disorder characterized by tics. Tics are not constantly present but wax and wane. It typically begins in childhood and often improves in adult life. Tics are best described as involuntary movements made automatically so that volition is not ordinarily appreciated. The disorder can be very severe for short periods and then lessen and even transiently disappear. Exacerbation of the tic activity can occur when the patient is anxious, excited, or sleep deprived.

Tics can affect any body part including the eyes, face, and neck, which are the areas that are most commonly involved. Motor or vocal tics can be simple or complex. Simple motor tics are sudden, brief, and restricted to a single body part such as blinking or neck movements. Sometimes, they manifest as dystonic movements for a short period of time. Complex tics involve multiple body parts such as jumping, twirling, clapping, or obscene gestures (copropraxia). Complex vocal tics may be demonstrated by repeating words or phrases (echolalia) or using obscene words (coprolalia).

There is frequently an urge or premonitory phenomenon, sometimes in the form of a specific sensory feeling (sensory tic) that precedes the tic. Tourette syndrome affects boys more than girls and is associated with attention deficit hyperactivity disorder (ADHD) and obsessive-compulsive disorder (OCD). Tics are "sudden, rapid, recurrent, nonrhythmic motor movements or vocalizations, generally preceded by urge." Vocal tics present at some time with the disorder beginning before age 18 and lasting more than 1 year. Tics are not secondary to a physiological substance or other neurological disorders. A genetic etiology is assumed, but finding relevant mutations has been unsuccessful.

Treatment is symptomatic, and some patients have only mild tics; hence, treatment might be worse than the disease. Experts recommend the use of alpha-adrenergic agonists as the first line. These include clonidine and guanfacine. The next step would be the second-generation drugs or atypical antipsychotics, of which the best evidence is for risperidone and weaker evidence is for aripiprazole. Another consideration, perhaps preceding the atypical ones, would be tetrabenazine. If a patient has very severe symptoms, particularly if already an adult, then deep brain stimulation (DBS) can be considered.

8.4 PANS

PANS is an acronym for pediatric acute-onset neuropsychiatric syndrome. It is a clinical diagnosis given to children who have a dramatic onset of neuropsychiatric symptoms including obsessive-compulsive disorder (OCD) or food restriction and at least two concurrent cognitive, behavioral, or neurological symptoms such as depression, irritability, anxiety, and/or difficulty with schoolwork. It is thought to be triggered by infections, metabolic disturbances, neurological issues, psychosocial stress, and other inflammatory reactions, but no definitive cause has been established. Studies have failed to show children satisfying PANDAS/PANS criteria to have a clear immune basis. Strong evidence for treatment with antimicrobials or immunotherapy is lacking.

8.5 PANDAS

This is a subset of PANS and stands for pediatric autoimmune neuropsychiatric disorders associated with *Streptococcus*, specifically Group A Strep (GAS) infections, and has a recent positive test such as strep throat, perianal strep, or scarlet fever. The onset of symptoms, specifically OCD or tics, can occur within days of contracting GAS, or within several months of the infection. PANDAS symptoms may start during or right after an active infection, but they can start a month or two after the GAS infection has resolved.

Researchers are working to understand how GAS and other triggers result in neuropsychiatric disorders. PANDAS is the only known subset of PANS. Definitive proof of the autoimmune hypothesis of PANDAS is lacking. The interventions required to alleviate symptoms in PANS/PANDAS are different from the strategies used to manage Tourette syndrome.

9 Integration of the Trigeminal Nerve with Movement Disorders

The trigeminal or fifth cranial nerve (CN V) is the largest and most complex of the cranial nerves. It is sensory for the first two divisions (ophthalmic and maxillary) and sensory and motor for the third division (mandibular). Each division innervates specific dermatomes of the face, oral cavity, and dura mater within the cranium. These convey first-order neurons to the spinal trigeminal nucleus, which is divided into three parts and receives proprioceptive neurons from the mandible and extraocular muscles.

The spinal trigeminal nucleus also receives primary fibers from cranial nerves 7 (facial), 9 (glossopharyngeal), and 10 (vagus). It also has influence on cranial nerves 11 (accessory) and 12 (hypoglossal) and cervical nerves C1, C2, and C3 encompassing the trigemino-cervical complex. The trigeminal is the only cranial nerve that has primary fibers directly into the reticular formation, which modulates various systems of the body. It also has fibers to the thalamus, cerebellum, and vestibular regions. The lower motor neuron fibers come from the mandibular division innervating the muscles of mastication. Therefore, the trigeminal nerve can be said to potentially affect all regions and systems of the body if there is an aberrant input from CN V.

The most constantly used joint of the body is the temporomandibular joint (TMJ), and it is innervated by the auriculotemporal nerve, a branch of the third division of the mandibular division of the trigeminal nerve. This joint/nerve complex can sustain the most damage due to trauma, whiplash, constant wear, changes in vertical dimension from loss of teeth and/or tooth structure (age related), insufficient growth (from either a maxillary or a mandibular insufficiency), bruxism, and even stress.

Most evaluations of the trigeminal nerve are for pain (nociception) but are not evaluated for temperature (thermal receptors), proprioception, mechanoreceptors (pressure, vibration, or touch), balance (equilibrioceptors), and chemoreceptors (salts, ammonia, CO_2). Therefore, if the trigeminal nerve has any undetected damage to any of these receptors which interact with other cranial or cervical nerves or portions of the central nervous system, then an aberrant input can be sent to these other systems.

9.1 Trigeminal Nerve and Dystonia

Focal dystonias are rare disorders affecting muscles of the cervical (head and neck), blepharospasm (eyelid blinking or eye closure), oromandibular (facial), Meige's syndrome (blepharospasm and oromandibular), laryngeal, lingual, cranial, hand, or leg. One mechanism for increased muscle activity in craniocervical dystonia is loss of inhibition involving the trigeminal sensory nuclear complex (TSNC).

The TSNC is integrated into the functionally connected neurons under sensorimotor control of the neck and face. It mediates both excitability and inhibitory reflexes of the jaw, face, and neck. These reflexes may be aberrant in craniocervical dystonias, leading to the hypothesis that the TSNC may play a central role in certain focal dystonias. The principal sensory trigeminal nucleus receives input from fibers that have discriminative sensation in the face and intraoral structures, along with proprioceptive input from the TMJ. The spinal trigeminal nucleus processes mechanical, thermal, and nociceptive input from the TMJ, facial, and cervical neck regions, oral and laryngeal tissues, jaw and tongue, dura mater, and cerebral arteries.

The TSNC may become hyper-excitable due to loss of tonic inhibition by functionally connected motor nuclei such as the motor cortex, basal ganglia, and cerebellum. Disordered sensory input from trigeminal nerve afferents, such as aberrant feedback from dystonic muscles, may continue to potentiate brain stem circuits serving craniocervical muscle control. The TSNC has multiple connections to the primary motor cortex and brain stem motor regions, allowing it to indirectly control spinal motor neuron excitability, and is consistent with decreased inhibitory modulation through multiple descending neural pathways. Clinical studies show that the trigeminal reflexes impact the regulation of cranial, facial, and cervical muscles and are aberrant in dystonias. Stimulation of trigeminal afferents from a dental device ameliorated dystonia symptoms for some people.

9.2 Trigeminal Nerve and Blepharospasm

The trigeminal nerve demonstrates aberrant signaling in patients with blepharospasm. The corneal blink reflex is caused by a loop between the trigeminal sensory nerves and the facial motor (VII) nerve innervation of the orbicularis oculi muscles. This reflex activates when a free nerve ending, or mechanoreceptor sensory receptor, is stimulated and connects with the epithelium of the cornea. This sensory data is transmitted to the ophthalmic portion of the trigeminal nerve and synapses in the spinal trigeminal subnucleus caudalis in the brain stem. This nerve then connects to the facial nucleus and synapses with the facial nerve. The facial nerve then activates the orbicularis oculi muscle, and upon contraction of this muscle, blinking occurs (i.e., eye closure).

There are two separate stages to the blink reflex, early and late. The facial nerves are stimulated within the late stage bilaterally so that both eyes blink. Secondary motor systems (e.g., interpositus nucleus of the cerebellum, red nucleus, and reticular activating system) can modulate this late-stage reflex. The motor production of the blink reflex can vary in non-pathological conditions. Multiple components can influence the blink reflex.

One component is the duration and intensity of the sensory input. A secondary component may include a diversity of brain stem and cortical inputs that synapse directly or indirectly with the trigeminal spinal and facial nuclei. Yet another circuit may modulate the strength of blink reflex based on conditioning. Together with the oculomotor nucleus, this pathway is used to reopen the eyelid. To activate this response, the ophthalmic nerves have secondary inputs within the trigeminal spinal nucleus onto nerves that project to the oculomotor nucleus. These spinal nucleus/oculomotor neurons activate the levator palpebrae muscles. The oculomotor pathway instituted the eyelid to reopen after it closed in the blink reflex. It works in conjunction with the facial motor pathway. Peripherally, damage to either the trigeminal nerve or the facial nerve will disrupt the corneal blink circuit.

Damage to the reticular formation or cerebellum will also control the blink response. These parts of the central nervous system influence facial nerve signals and can affect the strength or speed of the late-stage blink reflex response bilaterally [4]. The blink reflex recovery cycle measures the excitability of human brain stem interneurons and is abnormal in blepharospasm. The recovery cycle was significantly disinhibited in patients with blepharospasm. Stimulation of trigeminal afferents in blepharospasm patients demonstrates a higher excitation of the trigeminal neurons and of the blink reflex motor neurons.

Trigeminal afferent input provides the ability of some patients to momentarily suppress the dystonic symptoms using a sensory trick (alleviating maneuver) by touching the skin of the neck or face, and this maneuver has been used to temporarily discontinue activity in brain stem reflexes for those with blepharospasm. A changed proprioceptive input into the TMJ auriculotemporal nerve afferents explains the success of specifically designed oral orthotics that alter jaw position to decompress the pressure on the nerve, reducing the hyper-excitability of the nerve in people with cervical dystonia.

9.3 Trigeminal Nerve and Oromandibular Dystonia

Oromandibular dystonias (ODs) are focal dystonias that act on the motor neurons of the trigeminal, facial, and hypoglossal nerves, which then influence the facial muscles and the mandible. The symptoms are usually involuntary muscle spasms, which may be continuous or intermittent. They can be repetitive or sustained movements of the muscles of mastication, tongue, or face.

OD may be mistaken for temporomandibular joint disorder, condylar dislocation, hemifacial spasm, and psychogenic disorders. There are multiple types of ODs: jaw-opening OD, jaw-closing OD, perioral OD, lingual OD, and jaw-deviating OD. When OD and blepharospasm occur at the same time, the disorder is called Meige's syndrome. OD is affiliated with facial grimacing or contorting and lip pursing. When dystonic muscle contractions occur, they interfere with motor functions of mastication, both verbal and nonverbal communications, and swallowing. Depending on the type of OD, patients may also present with bruxism, clenching, oral ulcers, damage to dental restorations, TMJ disorders, lip sucking, chewing motions, and platysma contractions.

OD can be precipitated by mandibular activities such as talking, chewing, yawning, and swallowing, often causing social embarrassment and/or diminished quality of life. Peripheral trauma has been shown to be an etiological factor in multiple neurological movement disorders, but the exact cause of peripheral trigeminal trauma and the onset of OD is still unclear. Some studies theorize that some causative or predisposing factors for OD may be old ill-fitting dentures, root canal treatments, tooth extractions, prosthodontics, TMJ arthroscopy, and dental implants. The major point that is observed in these believed precipitating factors is that the mouth or mandible is open for a considerable length of time. The question that should then be asked is if there is an extended length of time having the patients' mouth open, could there be damage to the trigeminal or other peripheral nerve(s)?

Therapy of dystonia can be divided into the following categories: (1) physical, supportive, and ancillary therapy; (2) pharmacologic treatment; (3) chemodenervation with botulinum toxin; and (4) peripheral and central surgery (deep brain stimulation). Patients with jaw-closing OD responded better than those with jaw-opening OD to botulinum toxin. Oral appliances have been shown to decrease or ameliorate OD dystonic symptoms for certain situations.

9.4 Trigeminal Nerve and Restless Leg syndrome (RLS)

RLS is frequently associated with migraine headaches and insomnia and may be a major cause of bruxism ("restless jaw"). Bruxism is a common disorder of unknown etiology, which affects approximately 10% of the population. Bruxism can cause insomnia, TMJ, and periodontal problems. RLS may be the missing link connecting bruxism and temporomandibular disorders with headaches, and the headaches should be treated as migraines. Treatments with oral orthotics sometimes stop bruxism and/or reduce dental complications. No pharmacological treatments are currently used to discontinue the symptoms. Some researchers have suggested an association of RLS and bruxism in the population. Bruxism and periodic limb movement together are seen in about 80% of patients with RLS and occur in light, non-REM sleep.

Data supports a strong association between RLS and bruxism. About three-quarters of those with both conditions had a reduction in bruxism symptoms when they received dopamine agonist drugs for RLS. Patients reporting bruxism have been shown to have been treated for temporomandibular joint disorder by appliances and/or surgery. Data suggests an abnormally decreased inhibition in trigeminal motor neurons to the masseter muscle. An occlusal equilibration appliance (OEA) was shown to reduce bruxism by relaxing all mastication muscles. Therefore, within the triad of bruxism, migraine, and RLS· a decrease or discontinuance of RLS symptoms should be observed when utilizing an oral appliance such as the OEA.

9.5 Trigeminal Nerve and Tremor

Cerebellar tremor is typically a slow, high-amplitude (easily visible) tremor of the extremities (e.g., arm, leg) that occurs at the end of a purposeful movement. Another example of cerebellar tremor typically seen after head injury is "titubation," an oscillatory (swinging to-and-fro) movement of the head and trunk. It is caused by damage to the cerebellum and its pathways to other brain regions. The trigeminocerebellar fibers are fibers in the inferior cerebellar peduncles, which transmit proprioceptive information from the face to the cerebellum. This information originates in proprioceptors (e.g., muscle spindles) in the face/mandible. Primary cell bodies are in the mesencephalic nucleus of the trigeminal nerve. These fibers transmit information to secondary afferent cell bodies in the spinal trigeminal nucleus plus the principal nucleus. Axons from the spinal nucleus and from the principal nucleus then form the trigeminocerebellar tract and ascend to the cerebellum. The cerebellum receives sensory information of all modalities, not just proprioception. Indirect pathways bring auditory, visual, somatosensory, and cortical information to the cerebellum. Damage to the trigeminal nerve could potentially then cause damage to the trigeminocerebellar pathway resulting in cerebellar tremor of the arms and/or legs. Temporomandibular joint dysfunction which can damage the auriculotemporal nerve, a division of the mandibular nerve, may be one of the factors in the etiology of cerebellar tremor.

9.6 Trigeminal Nerve and Gait/Balance

Gait and balance are also a result of normal cerebellar activity. Thus, any aberrant signal to the cerebellum from the trigeminal nerve may be the etiology of a gait imbalance. In addition, the trigeminal nerve has primary afferent neurons to the reticular formation (RF). Other axons in the inferior cerebellar peduncle come from the vestibular nerve and nuclei, reticular formation, and trigeminal nuclei. The RF is another portion of the brain stem that coordinates gait and balance. The reticulospinal tracts project to spinal cord motor neurons and help to modulate tone, balance, posture, and coordination of body movements with the assistance of other sensory stimuli, such as visual, auditory, vestibular, and proprioceptive information. The inferior olive is a hub for convergent inputs from the spinal cord (spino-olivary tract), motor cortex, superior colliculus, vestibular nuclei, trigeminal nuclei, and pretectum. In this manner, the olivocerebellar system provides multimodal input that contributes to error-based motor learning and shapes subsequent motor output by modulating the activity of cerebellar nuclei. Again, if the trigeminal nerve is damaged, the pathways that modulate gait and balance may be affected.

9.7 Trigeminal Nerve and Paroxysmal Dyskinesias

Paroxysmal dyskinesias are thought to be inherited or acquired from secondary causes. Paroxysmal dyskinesias may be secondary due to multiple sclerosis, cerebral palsy, metabolic disorders, physical trauma, central nervous system or peripheral nervous system trauma, cerebrovascular disease, and miscellaneous conditions including supranuclear palsy and AIDS. PKDs have also been associated with encephalitis and injury to the brain.

There are three types of peripheral nerves in the peripheral nervous system. They are motor, sensory, and autonomic nerves of which the trigeminal nerve is a principal example. The peripheral nervous system is a network of 43 pairs of motor and sensory nerves that connect the brain and spinal cord (the central nervous system) to the entire human body. These nerves control the functions of sensation, movement, and motor coordination. They are fragile and can be damaged easily.

The spinal accessory nerve is a peripheral nerve (CN 11) which originates in the brain stem. It allows two sets of muscles in the neck to function: the sternocleidomastoid (SCM) muscles, which allow the head to tilt and rotate, and the trapezius muscles, which allow for several motions such as shrugging the shoulder or moving the shoulder blades. It is connected to the trigeminal nerve through the trigeminocervical complex (C1–C2), which also innervates the

SCM and a majority of the neck muscles. C1 and C2 must coordinate with the spinal accessory nerve for smooth movement of the head and neck. Aberrant input from C1–C2 may cause improper/uncoordinated movement of the SCM.

The reticular formation connects the brain stem and spinal cord to modulate movement, contribute to posture, and regulate muscle tone from the peripheral nervous system. The trigeminal nerve is the only cranial nerve that has primary afferents to the RF. Therefore, aberrant impulses from the trigeminal nerve can influence and/or affect the peripheral nervous system through its RF connections.

9.8 Trigeminal Nerve and Parkinsonism

Severe traumatic brain injuries have been reported to have Parkinsonian symptoms. Post-traumatic Parkinsonism symptoms include bradykinesia, tremor, dystonia, rigidity, and gait disorder. Severe traumatic injuries and post-traumatic Parkinsonism may share a common midbrain network dysfunction. In Parkinson's disease, MRI shows atrophy of the midbrain with enlargement of the third ventricle, tegmental atrophy and an abnormal superior profile of the midbrain, signal increase in the midbrain and in the inferior olives, as well as frontal and temporal lobe atrophy. In Parkinsonism, the MRI shows normal anatomy and activity, but both have the same symptoms. Therefore, the symptoms must have two differing etiologies. The possible etiologies for tremor, dystonia, and gait disorder have been discussed previously, which may be from the brain stem and/or cerebellum.

9.9 Trigeminal Nerve and Tourette Syndrome (TS)

Tourette syndrome is a hyperkinetic movement disorder characterized by tics. Tics are categorized as either simple or complex. Please refer to a chart of some symptoms (Fig. 6).

Certain qualities of tics are the same qualities of a sternutation (sneeze). A sneeze is an autonomic protective involuntary response mechanism caused by the irritation of the nasal mucosa, which

Simple Motor Tics	Complex Motor Tics
• Winking, blinking, eye-rolling, wide eye-opening (without moving the eyebrows) • Eyebrow-raising • Wrinkling or turning up the nose • Puffing up the cheeks • Mouth opening, pulling the corners of the mouth • Lip movements • Sticking out the tongue • Jaw movements • Frowning • Grimacing • Tooth-chattering • Head-shaking, throwing, turning, twitching, or twitching, or nodding • Shoulder-shrugging • Arm and hand movements • Abdominal movements	• Seemingly intentional movements, facial expressions, gesticulations with the head, hands, arms, trunk, legs, feet • Picking at clothes • Hopping, jumping • Clapping, finger-tapping • Spinning • Bending and bowing the trunk • Wide arm movements • Foot-stamping • Dystonic tics (rare) with slow turning movements • Writing tics • Echopraxia: non-purposeful imitation of other other p ersons' observed movements • Copropraxia: making obscene gestures such such as showing the middle finger, indecent indecent movements of the trunk and pelvis, pelvis, crotch-holding

Fig. 6 Tourette syndrome is a hyperkinetic movement disorder characterized by tics. Tics are categorized as either simple or complex

is innervated by the trigeminal nerve. Sternutation can also be triggered by a sudden exposure to bright light, known as a photic sneeze from a trigeminal response. The neural regions involved in the sneeze reflex are located in the brain stem along the ventromedial part of the spinal trigeminal nucleus and the adjacent pontine-medullary lateral reticular formation. Characteristics of a sneeze are head shaking, turning, nodding, winking, blinking, eye-rolling, mouth opening, jaw movements, lip and tongue movements, abdominal movements, arm and hand movements, frowning, premonitory urge, and vocal sounds. These are the same listed as simple motor tics, which are usually the first signs seen in those with TS. Therefore, it is a good possibility that there is an irritation of the trigeminal nerve as an etiology of these symptoms.

The spinal trigeminal nucleus is a sensory tract located in the lateral medulla of the brain stem. It is responsible for relaying various sensory modalities including temperature, deep or crude touch, and pain from the ipsilateral portion of the face. The spinal trigeminal nucleus incorporates sensory information from different cranial nerves including the trigeminal nerve/ branches, ophthalmic (CN V1), maxillary (CN V2), and mandibular (CN V 3), as well as the facial (CN VII), glossopharyngeal (CN IX), and vagus nerves (CN X). The facial nerve is responsible for facial movements, the glossopharyngeal nerve is responsible for coughing, and the vagus nerve is responsible for vocal sounds and abdominal movements. When the trigeminal nerve is activated and/or irritated, it can also activate these nerves.

The trigeminal nerve is the only cranial nerve that has direct input into the reticular formation (RF). The RF is responsible for arm and leg movements. The trigeminal also has secondary neurons to the cerebellum, which is responsible for head movement, head shaking, and head nodding. It also has proprioceptive properties for the head's position in space along with the proprioceptive neurons from the mandibular division of the trigeminal as discussed earlier. The most utilized joint in the body is the temporomandibular joint (TMJ).

It is common for malpositioning of the maxilla and mandible to occur as in orthodontic cases or a genetic malocclusion. The auriculotemporal (AT) nerve may be more susceptible to trauma in these cases and in whiplash, falls, and/or through iatrogenic means such as in extraction of teeth. This leads to diminished verticality between the maxilla and mandible, which may lead to TMJ injury or incoordination within the joint. The possibility of the auriculotemporal (AT) nerve becoming injured thus increases.

The AT nerve runs medial to lateral behind the mandibular condyle. If the AT nerve is more rostral within the joint, the condylar head would irritate the nerve more than it would below the condylar head due to the morphology and shape of the condyle. In such a case, the AT nerve branch of the mandibular trigeminal division would transmit more aberrant impulses into the trigeminal nucleus and into its neuronal connections. The possibility of movement disorders then increases knowing and understanding the multiple connections of the trigeminal nerve as previously stated.

This hypothesis was tested by utilizing MR imaging to determine condylar spacing within the TMJ and determine if the symptoms decreased or ameliorated when there was increased spacing within the joint to stop the irritation or compression of the AT nerve (Fig. 7a–c). An intermittent irritation of the trigeminal nerve would be a factor for those with Tourette syndrome as it is for those with a sneeze. A constant irritation or compression on the AT nerve may be the etiology for the many dystonias or Parkinsonism.

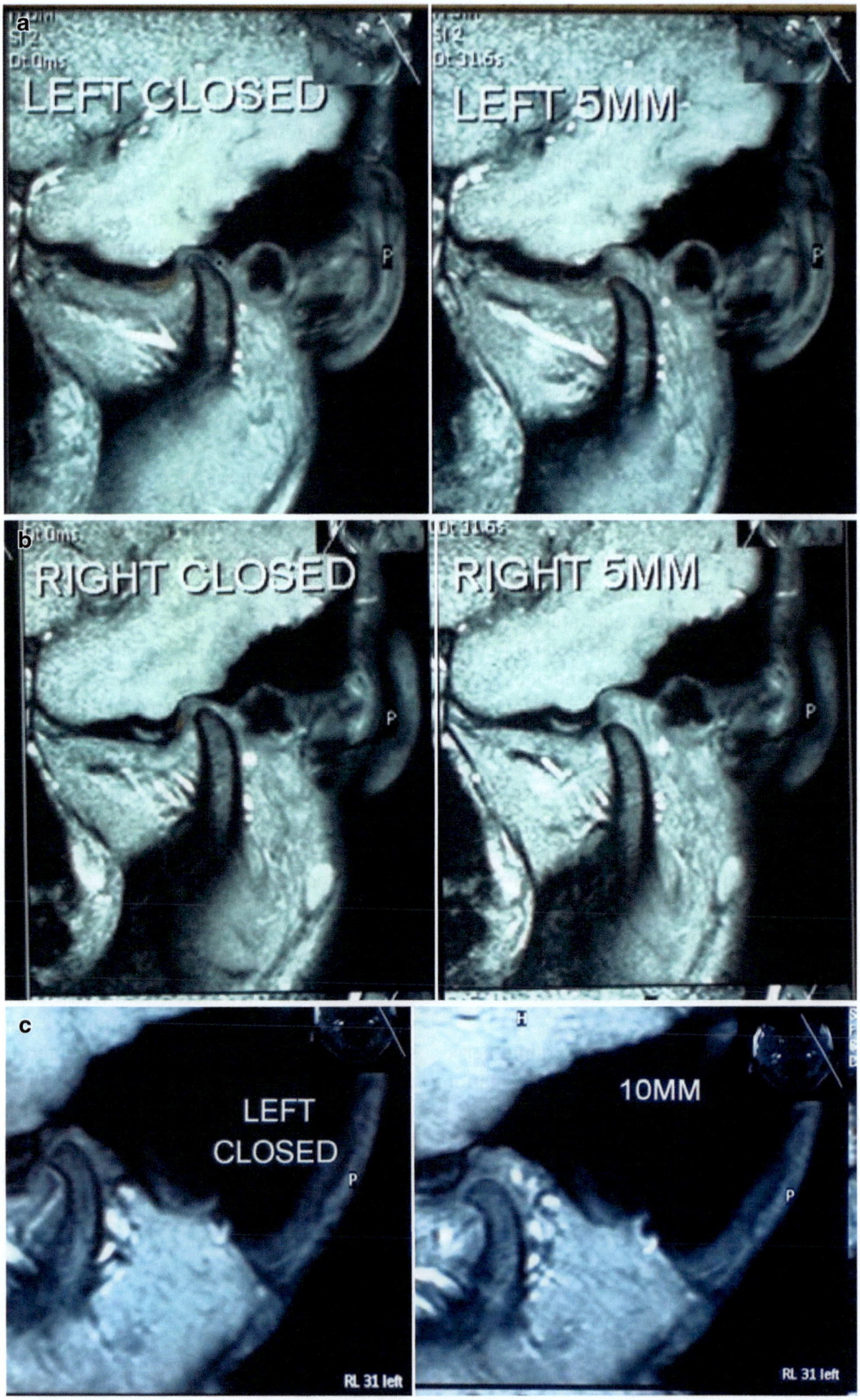
a
LEFT CLOSED
P
LEFT 5MM
P
b
RIGHT CLOSED
P
RIGHT 5MM
P
c
LEFT
CLOSED
P
RL 31 left
10MM
P
RL 31 left

Fig. 7 MRI of TMJ in patients with Tourette syndrome. (**a**) Patient JG went from 105 tics/3 min to 4 tics/3 min after increasing volumetric spacing within the TM joint. Courtesy *Dr. Anthony Sims*. (**b**) Patient BH went from 15 tics/3 min to 2 tics/3 min after increasing volumetric spacing within the TM joint. Courtesy *Dr. Anthony Sims*. (**c**) Patient HL went from 60 tic/3 min to 2 tics/3 min after increasing volumetric spacing within the TM joint. (Courtesy *Dr. Anthony Sims*)

10 Summary

As has been described meticulously above, there are many neurologic connections between the trigeminal nerve nucleus and other elements of the central nervous system in the brain stem and spine. These connections set the stage for the possible mechanisms of temporomandibular joint dysfunction and related movement disorders. An understanding of this neuroanatomy, combined with clinical observation, can assist in the diagnosis and treatment of those movement disorders which may benefit from the treatment of TMDs.

Suggested Reading

1. Rosenberg RN, Pascual JM, editors. Rosenberg's molecular and genetic basis of neurological and psychiatric disease. 5th ed; 2015.
2. Casale J, Giwa AO. Embryology, branchial arches. In: StatPearls [Internet]. Treasure Island (FL): StatPearls Publishing; 2022. https://www.ncbi.nlm.nih.gov/books/NBK538487/.
3. Lee WY, Okeson JP, Lindroth J. The relationship between forward head posture and temporomandibular disorders. J Orofac Pain. 1995;9(2):161–7.
4. Manning KA, Evinger C. Different forms of blinks and their two-stage control. Exp Brain Res. 1986;64(3):579–88. https://doi.org/10.1007/BF00340495.

A Journey to Understanding and Treating TMD/Craniofacial Pain: Rediscovering the Structure Often Overlooked in Orthodontics and Facial Orthopedics: The TMJ

Lidia Yavich

1 Introduction

As a specialist in orthodontics and facial orthopedics and a specialist in temporomandibular disorder (TMD) and orofacial pain, I work primarily with patients seeking pain relief. As our clinic deals with TMJ pathologies, the prevalence of TMD will not be discussed here. How orthodontics and facial orthopedics can cause TMD will not be discussed. The pathogenesis of TMD is far from settled, even with all the studies that cases have generated.

What is important is the discussion about what procedures can cause TMD and the importance to evaluate the situation of the temporomandibular joints in patients before beginning any therapy. When patients are evaluated, it is important to know whether they have undergone orthodontic and/or orthopedic treatments, to be aware of the signs and symptoms, and to look at patient posture and movements. A good history, clinical examination, and images help to differentiate the lesions that affect the TMJ. It is fundamental to distinguish the cases that can benefit from routine orthodontics and the cases that need to be referred to other specialists and/or need to have a multidisciplinary team.

Orthodontists and facial orthopedists are professionals who have general training in dentistry and extensive specialized education to diagnose, prevent, control, and treat anomalies in the form, position, relationship, and function of dento-maxillofac ial structures. This is an integral part of patient care, making diagnoses on the early or late detection of the disease and monitoring the response to treatment. Many patients who seek malocclusion correction present with noise and pain in the TMJs. Their TMJ images show facets and erosions, and these patients feel more pain when retrodiscal palpation is performed. Many who finish orthodontics and/or facial orthopedics treatments have clicks in the TMJ, signs of joint wear in images, and pain in the retrodiscal palpation.

In training, the temporomandibular joint, which connects the jaw with the skull, the most used of all articulations, is wholly ignored. This joint performs different functions such as chewing, swallowing, speaking, and breathing. Just like all the other synovial joints of our body, the TMJ can also suffer from different diseases. What differentiates the TMJ and makes it unique when compared to the other synovial joints of the body is that in addition to all the structures that the other synovial joints have, such as the capsule, ligaments, and others, the TMJ is also subordinated to the teeth (occlusion).

Primary pathologies of the temporomandibular joint can affect the occlusal relationship, change the spatial alignment of the joint, and affect all of its body alignment. Infections and trauma can initiate processes that sometimes cause permanent damage to TMJ ligaments, even in cases where the teeth are aesthetically aligned and in an occlusal relationship that seems healthy.

L. Yavich (✉)
SBPAT, The Brazilian Society for Diagnosis and Treatment of Temporomandibular Joint Pathologies, Attending, Clinica My, Porto Allege, RS, Brazil

B. C. Stack Jr. et al. (eds.), *Craniofacial Pain*, https://doi.org/10.1007/978-3-031-57563-1_11

Technological advances have allowed for a deeper understanding of the pathologies that affect the temporomandibular joint. The images of nuclear magnetic resonance (NMR or MRI) and bioinstrumentation have been migrated to the realm of clinicians, no longer being the exclusive domain of the investigators. These advances play a fundamental role together with the clinical examination, carefully integrated with the history and pathophysiology of the patient.

2 Pain

Controlling pain in a patient with temporomandibular dysfunction is crucial. Presently, it is also possible in certain cases to improve damaged structures as well. The evaluation of the TMJ and the diagnosis of its pathologies must be an inseparable part of all fields of dentistry. Examining the curricula of different universities of the world today, TMD is not included or, if it is, it is very abbreviated. Embryology, morphology, and neurological and proprioceptive connections are studied but there is often nothing about the pathologies and/or joint dysfunctions. In this education, TMJ is often a "ghost," and its pathologies and dysfunction are not discussed.

One frequent question encountered is: How many of our patients that present for malocclusion correction or prosthodontics, or just simple clinical procedures, have among other things, a clicking TMJ, signs of wear in any TMJ images, limitation in opening the mouth, and/or pain during retrodiscal palpation? How many patients that finish orthodontics or facial orthopedic treatments continue with or develop the signs and symptoms during or after treatment? For many practitioners, the answer would be none because they did not check for that.

3 Training

Many are trained as a dentist, an orthodontist, and a facial orthopedist as though the TMJ did not exist. Training may presume that no pathology affects the head of the mandible or its morphology. Many believe that a "good occlusion" was a guarantee of healthy joints. The famous quote of the philosopher Giacomo Leopardi, "**Ignorance is the greatest source of happiness,**" can be a painful lesson. Continuing with the analysis of my training, everything depended on my diagnosis, my ability, my knowledge to balance the occlusion, the cognizance of the most modern techniques, understanding of the latest generation of materials, and the biological response of the patient.

3.1 Where was the TMJ in this Planning? Without Considering the TMJ, There Is No Diagnosis!

Without knowing what the status of the foundation, can one effectively balance the occlusion? That is, considering occlusion like the relation of the arches, without muscles, joints, and neural innervation. Without considering the TMJ, the knowledge of the most modern techniques and the latest generation of materials is like constructing a beautiful building without having any awareness of the ground, like a project without an engineer or an architect. The temporomandibular joint was an abstract entity. The vast majority of the anatomy texts assumed that the head of the mandible has no pathology in its localization nor in its size or shape. This does not coincide with new technologies and diagnostic methods. Temporomandibular joints can be affected by local and systemic pathologies, trauma, autoimmune diseases, and occlusal problems.

A functional lesion is one which presents an alteration of the function without an anatomical change. An organic lesion however is one which presents with anatomical alterations. How can one determine anything without images? Imaging is the only method for obtaining visual information about the joint's tissues and is fundamental to differentiate the lesions that affect the TMJ. It is not uncommon to see publications in orthodontics and facial orthopedics where panoramic radiographs do not show the condyles considering that they are not an important part of a diagnosis; even in many international meetings and conferences, the panoramic radiographs do not show the condyles. Panoramic radiographs are not the ideal images for TMJ, but in many cases, they can show that a problem exists; therefore they need to be investigated deeper.

4 A New Look at Familiar Basic Images

4.1 Panoramic Radiograph

Every orthodontist requests a panoramic radiograph which, as its name indicates, gives a general scenario of odontogenic and maxilofacial alterations. Some structural alterations of the mandibular condyles can be identified as asymmetries, erosions, large osteophytes, and fractures. Comparing both images in Fig. 1a with round condyles beside image (Fig. 1b) where the condyles present asymmetries and erosions demonstrates the utility of the panorex. The panoramic radiograph alone is not adequate to treat TMJ pathologies as more accurate information is needed. The panoramic radiograph image is still a good image and one from where to begin evaluation of the TMJ.

With the use of cone beam CT, the panoramic radiograph obtained through tomography and the conventional panoramic radiograph have different image qualities because they have different acquisition principles. Conventional panoramic radiography (Fig. 2a) is an imaging technique with a specific device with a cutting zone in which the structures that are within the zone are clearly visible in the image. It has diagnostic capacity. The panoramic radiograph (Fig. 2b) obtained through tomography has no diagnostic

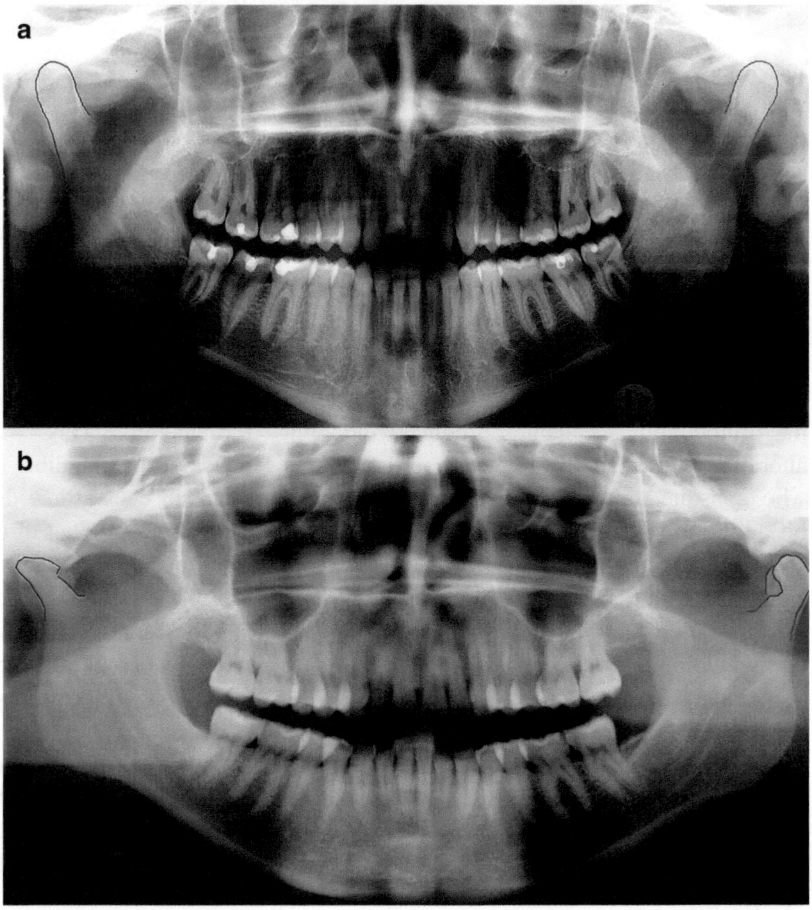

Fig. 1 Comparative example of panoramic radiographs with healthy heads of the mandible (**a**) and pathological heads of the mandible (**b**)

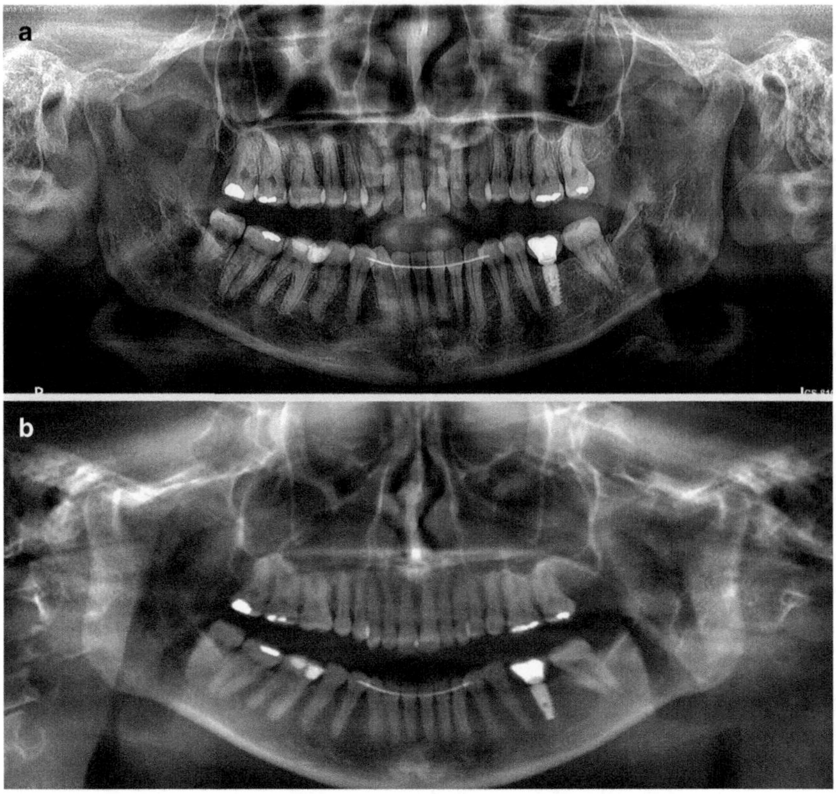

Fig. 2 Comparative example of a conventional panoramic radiograph (**a**) and a panoramic radiograph obtained through tomography (**b**)

value. It is a reconstruction of a tomographic volume.

In many publications and conference presentations, the mandibular heads are omitted from images of cases showing the before and after treatment (Fig. 3). One cannot specify whether the orthodontic mechanics produced the joint alteration shown in the image. For the patient who consulted after treatment due to an open bite, little joint pain, and significant loss of balance, everything needs to be investigated. One cannot disregard portions of images as if they were insignificant. One should consider the panoramic radiograph as a first clue of TMD looking at it in an in-depth way.

4.2 TMJ Plain Films

Plain films allow one to observe the joint's bony components: the head of the mandible, the articular fossa, and also the articular eminence. This is the basic reference in the field, and its significance may be compared to that of panoramic radiography for general dentistry or a modified panoramic radiography for TMJ. A comparative example of a plain film is with healthy heads of the mandible (Fig. 4a) and with pathological heads of the mandible Fig. 4b. Different pathologies can cause three-dimensional joint changes. They are a product of different etiologies. These "tridimensional anatomical variations" provoke morpho-functional pathologies.

One cannot call these joint changes an "adaptation" where it does not increase the system efficiency or improve health. Different cuts of mandibular condyles in the closed mouth position show severe structural alterations of the mandible heads. Image (Fig. 5a) without coloring and image (Fig. 5b) with color to mark the condylar geometry are not compatible with optimal mechanics of the temporomandibular joint.

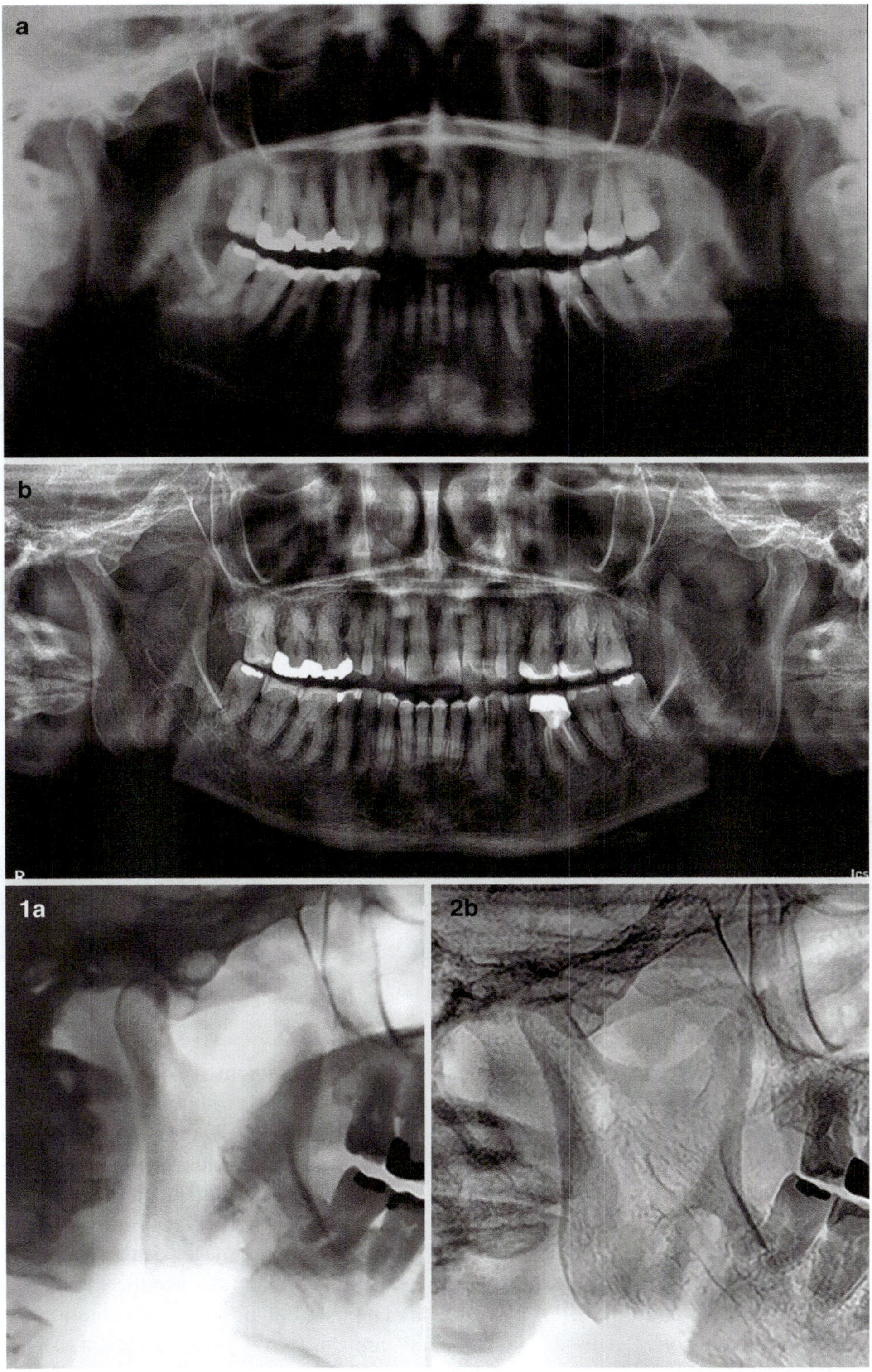

Fig. 3 Comparison of a panoramic radiograph before (**a**) and (**b**) after orthodontic treatment. Cross section of the comparative condyles with image inversion to highlight the deformation of the mandibular condyle and the articular eminence (1a) before treatment and (2b) after treatment

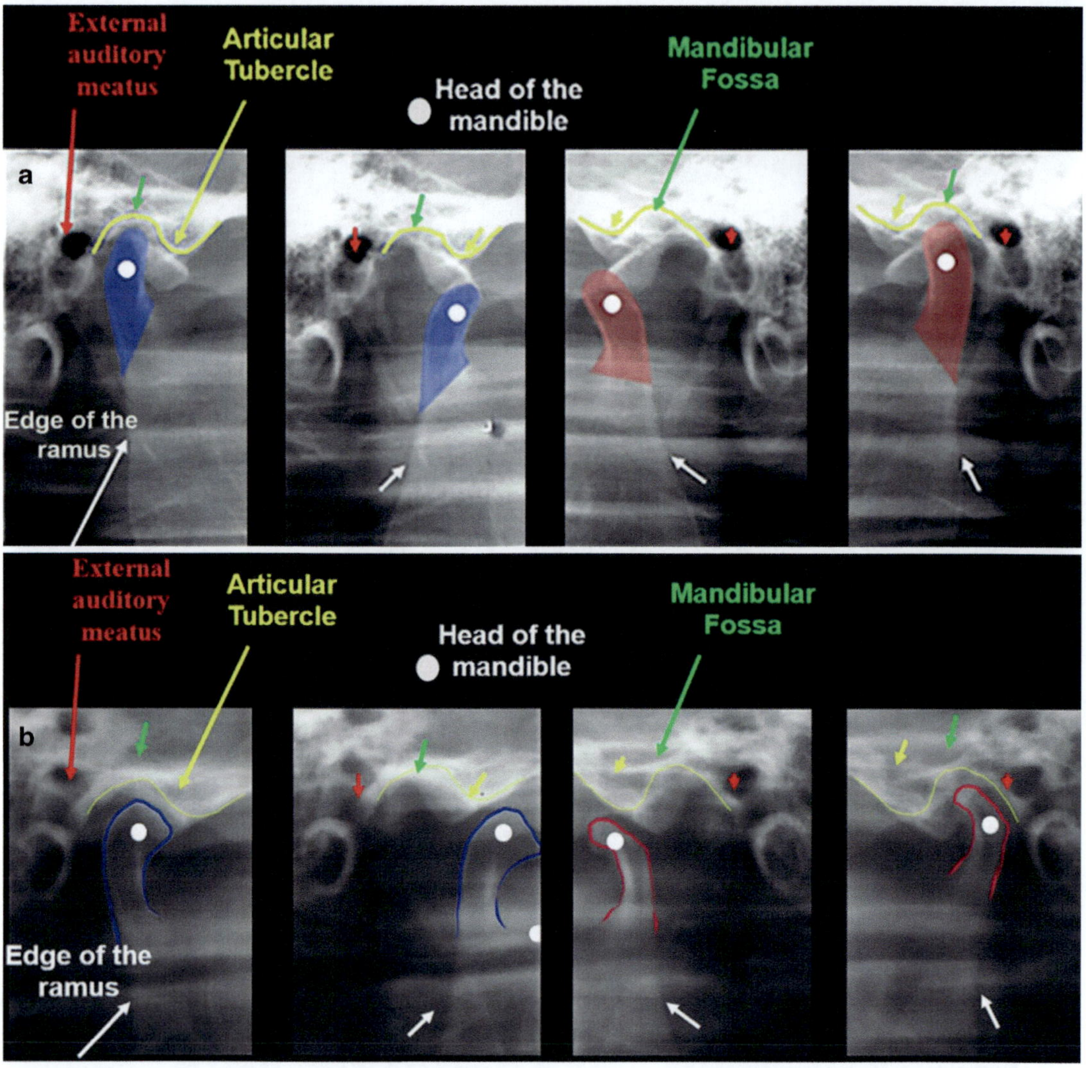

Fig. 4 TMJ plain films: right and left TMJ, open and closed mouth, color highlighted

Congruence of articular surfaces is a basic biomechanical principle of any synovial joint. Anatomy is the platform where physiology acts. Many of the lesions that are labeled as functional assessed only with a clinical exam are organic joint lesions.

It is necessary to understand that differences in structures caused by several etiological agents produce diverse effects on muscle performance, soft tissues, and sensory response, even when the patient is in occlusion. Let us consider in Fig. 6 a patient that came in the middle of the orthodontic treatment with this image of significantly deformed condyles. In this specific case, did the treating dentist know the joint situation before initiating orthodontic treatment? If the colleague was not aware of this situation, this is a problem. If the professional knew of this condition, there is a problem. In this specific case, the patient was diagnosed with lupus. Oftentimes, these images can give us a first clue that can be impactful since the sooner a disease like lupus is diagnosed, the greater the chance of its control. In a 9-year-old patient, it is easy to see only the crossbite without considering the resorption of the left condyle, which requires a thorough investigation (Fig. 7).

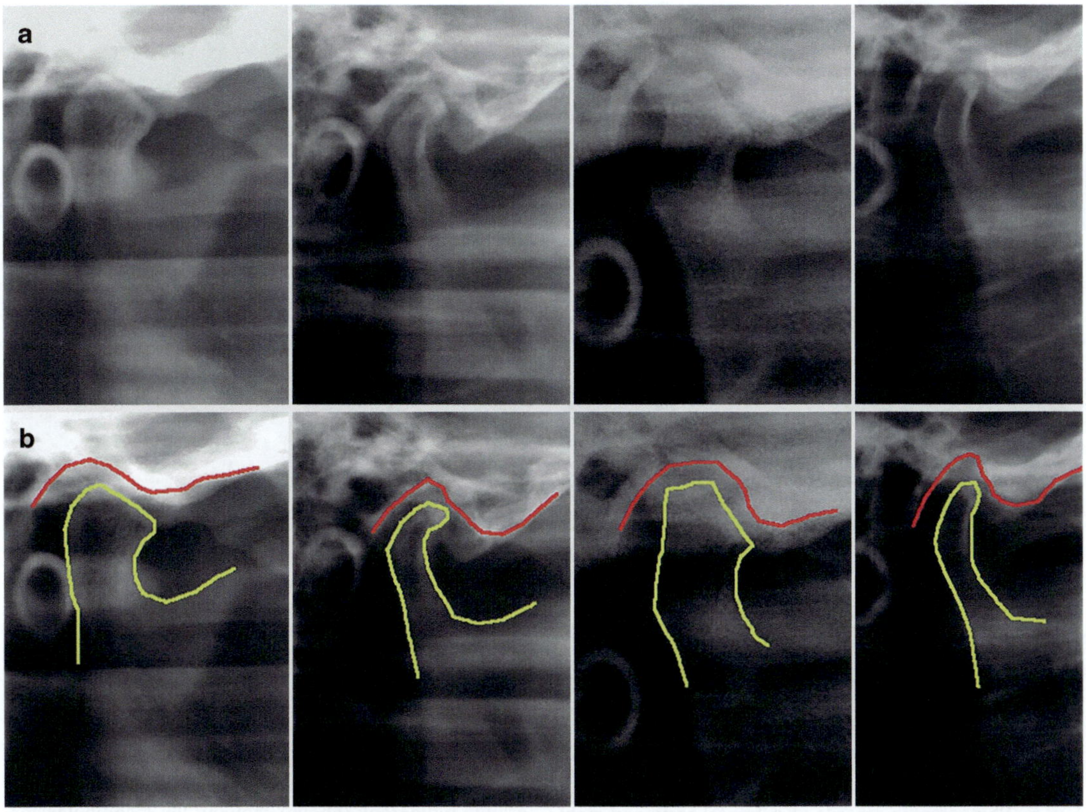

Fig. 5 TMJ plain films: different distorted shapes of mandible heads

There are a number of local and systemic factors or diseases that can cause mandibular condylar resorption. This condition can create occlusal and skeletal instability, dentofacial deformities, TMJ dysfunction, and pain. In Fig. 8, the ideal structural shape of the condyles is shown. However, the patient's TMJ plain films show a very different shape in that both condyles are deformed. This first image cannot be considered a normal finding as the corresponding plain films belong to a patient in profound pain. When joint structures undergo anatomical changes, an imbalanced system is inevitable.

4.3 Clinical Documentation

Documentation in the study of patients can change many times in a career based on professional growth and introduction of new technologies, but also noticing new data that was not previously considered. One of the fundamental things to be changed in documentation is the request for photos of the patient's entire body: front, back, right, and left profiles, and not exclusively photos of the patient's head (Fig. 9). Do not forget that the head is joined to the rest of the body! It is very important to evaluate posture.

Orthodontists and facial orthopedists do not treat posture like other professionals, but it is fundamental to have the insight to assess the postural problems that can be observed in TMD patients. Many of these problems may have descending triggers from the oromandibular complex, and, with this awareness, patients can be directed to trained professionals to make precise diagnoses and to improve posture. Posture is bidirectional from ascended and descendent pathways. As for the descendent pathway, craniomandibular intervention is decisive.

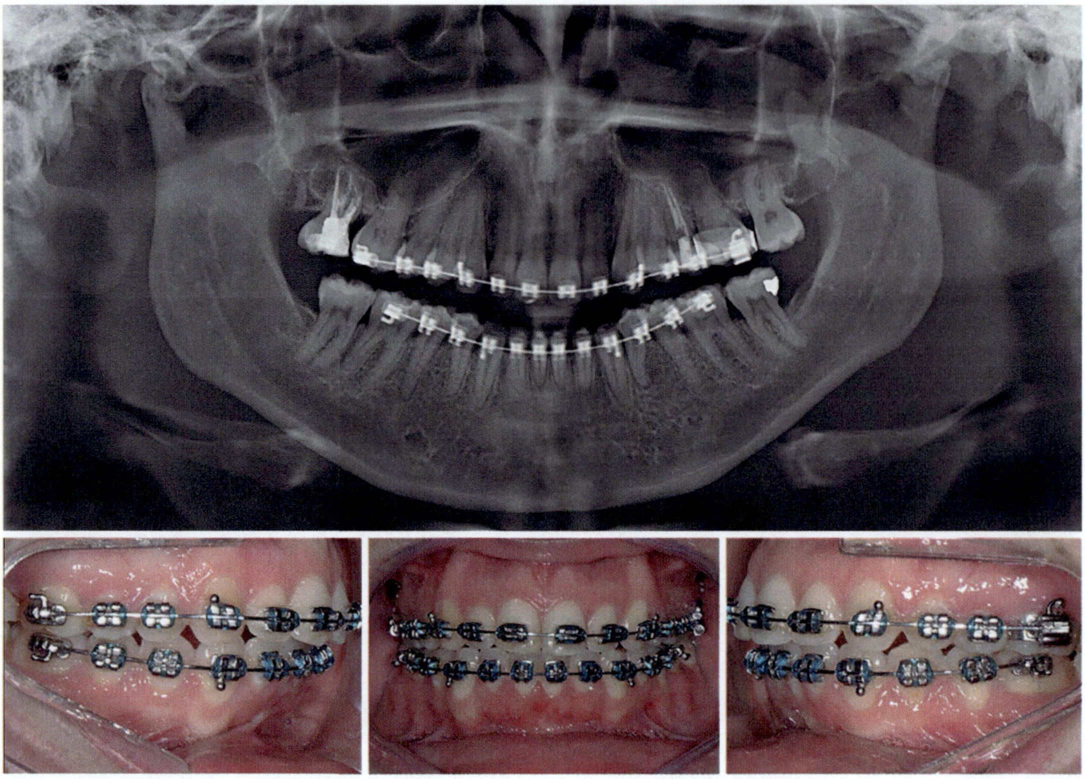

Fig. 6 Photographic records of a frontal view and right and left lateral views in maximum intercuspation in the middle of orthodontic treatment, together with a panoramic radiograph (above) showing the mandibular condyles with significant erosions

Observable postural images:

- Uneven shoulder height
- Lateral tilt and cervical rotation to the right
- Cervical straightening
- Cervical anteriorization
- Gluteal line parallel to the scapular line
- Uneven anterior superior iliac spines
- Dorsal curve rectification

Physiotherapists like to assess the patient's posture in a natural stance and not with aligned feet, but, for dentists, it is very difficult to compare the natural posture from day to day.

4.4 Structural Misalignment Related to Temporomandibular Joint Pathology

4.4.1 Intraoral photographs

This patient underwent orthodontic treatment, and one can observe a beautiful alignment of the teeth, class 1 molar and canine, and aligned dental midlines. Despite the aesthetic result, she had difficulty in opening her mouth; severe headaches; pain in the back of the neck, in the forehead, in both shoulders, and in both temporomandibular joints; as well as vertigo. In a quick analysis of the patient's teeth, in Fig. 10, some questions arise:

- Does the wear on the lower incisors stand out?
- Did this wear exist before the treatment?
- Can the wear represent a misplaced incisor guide?

The colleague who treated the patient placed her in permanent retainers on the worn lower and upper incisors. This is also appreciated in the lower dental photographs and also in the panoramic radiograph (Fig. 11a). Why would upper incisors need retaining if they do not have periodontal problems, and why would they open? Does the habitual closing trajectory coincide with the closing neuromuscular trajectory? These

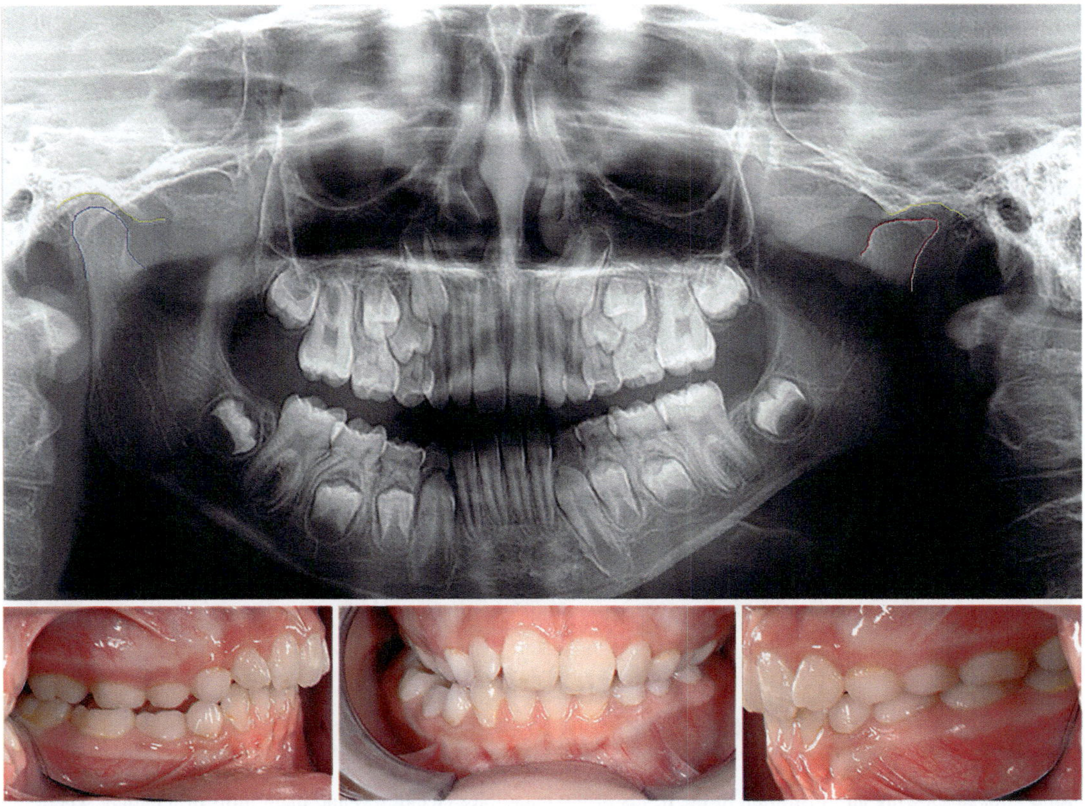

Fig. 7 Photographic records of a frontal, right, and left lateral views in maximum intercuspation in a patient in mixed dentition. The panoramic radiograph (below) shows the left mandibular condyle with significant resorption

are some of the questions that should be asked. "When we believed that we had all the answers, all of a sudden, all the questions changed," **Mario Benedetti**.

Significant distortions cannot be seen in the mandible heads in the panoramic X-ray (Fig. 11a). It is important to understand that the panoramic radiograph can sometimes show distortions but not always. In this case, it is noticeable only in the laminography. In the TMJ panoramic radiography of the same patient, the posterior displacement of the right and left mandibular condyles in the joint cavity with consequent reduction of the joint space is clearly visible. One can also notice the alteration of the growth axis in both mandibular condyles (greenstick fracture), more evident in the left condyle (highlighted in red); greenstick fractures will be explained further in a following section.

Pain can occur due to the posteriorizing of the condyle and anteriorization of the disc when compression of the retrodiscal tissue occurs. Mandibular retrusion, whether caused by iatrogenesis, trauma, or malocclusion, often results in otalgia (ear pain) due to excessive compression of the retrodiscal tissues. Mandibular retrusion invades the retrodiscal tissue, impairs TMJ metabolism, reduces the blood supply of the TMJ, wears down the posterior band of the articular disc, and stretches TMJ ligaments.

Fundamental questions:

- Was the mandibular retrusion present before the orthodontic treatment?
- Was the mandibular retrusion a result of the orthodontic treatment?
- How and in what tridimensional location were the temporomandibular joints before the treatment?

These are important questions not only because of legal issues but also for the health of patients. It is important to highlight that in these images, the structural alterations do not appear in

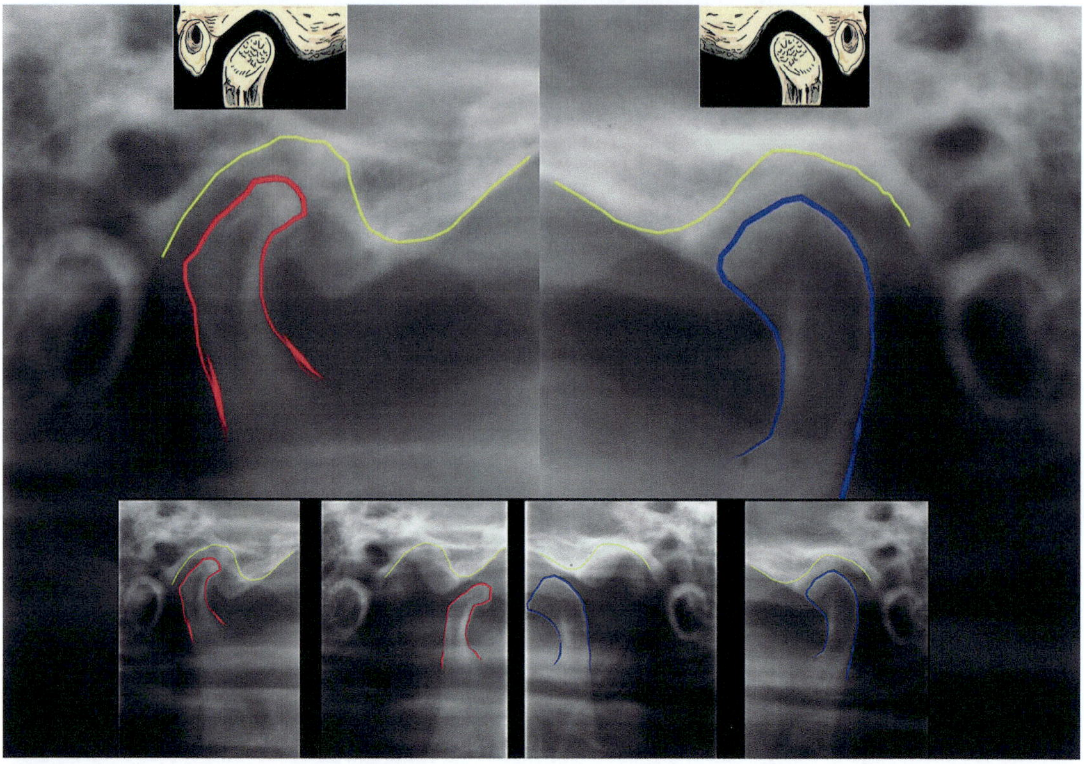

Fig. 8 Image showing an illustration of the heads of the mandibles (windows) and plain films of a patient where the structures bear no resemblance to the healthy physical structure of the illustration

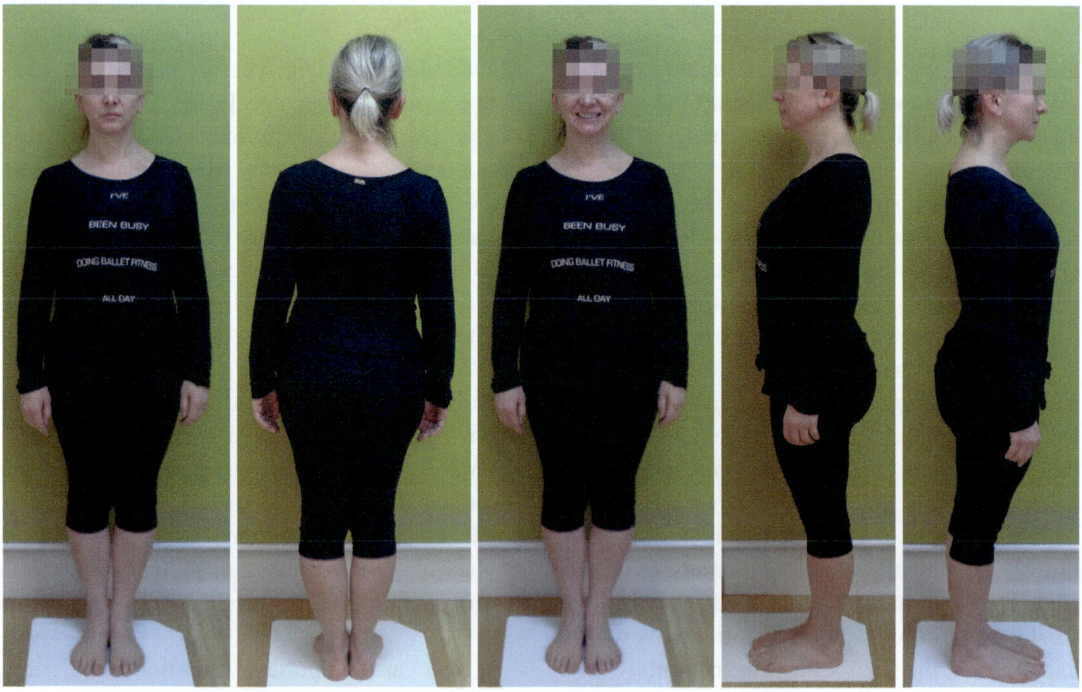

Fig. 9 **Whole-body** postural photos: front, back, right, and left profile and front smiling

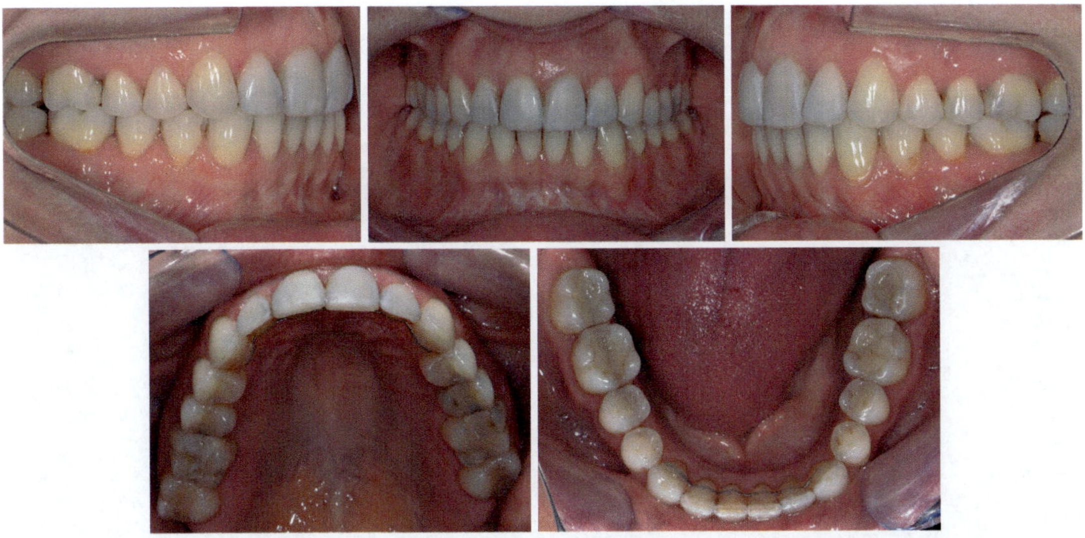

Fig. 10 Photographic records of a frontal view, right and left lateral views in maximum intercuspation (above), and superior and inferior occlusal views

the panoramic view but in the plain films. In previous examples of Figs. 6 and 7, the structural deformities already appeared in the panoramic view. This is not describing cephalometric analysis but rather pointing out the lack of parallelism of the frontal planes in the frontal radiograph.

The head is balanced over the cervical spine and is in equilibrium with the bi-pupillary and occlusal planes. An important third plane is the transverse mandibular, which must be parallel to the nasal, auricle, and pupillary planes.

When the head loses its optimal gravitational relationship with respect to the surface of the earth, the patient's balance is disturbed, which can cause vertigo, nausea, and frequent myalgias in postural muscles. The neuromuscular system is in a state of constant activity in order to keep those planes in an optimal physiological relationship with each other both while sitting and standing.

A healthy cervical spine should not be straight as seen in Fig. 12b, but concaved posteriorly, described as cervical lordosis. A change in head posture can be devastating to the neuromuscular system. Notice an important loss of space between the fifth and sixth cervical vertebrae and also osteophytes in the same vertebrae. Symptomatically, the cervical region overlaps with the craniofacial region. The superior cervical nerves, discs, facets, and muscles are a potential source of referred pain, and the second and third cervical nerves innervate the angle of the mandible, lower region of the TMJ, and parts of the ear, mastoid, and nape of the neck. Any irritation or dysfunction of these nerves can be associated with cervicofacial pain.

In this patient, there was an anterior displacement of the joint disc in closed mouth with recapture in open mouth in both temporomandibular joints. MRI of the cervical spine showed the reduction of the intervertebral discs between C6 and C7 where a disc-osteophytic complex is observed, normally associated with a bulging (protrusion) of the intervertebral disc in the cervical spine. With the loss of intervertebral space and the retro-positioned condyles on the plain films together with the clinical data, it is strongly suspected that an anterior displacement of the articular disc as well as protrusions in the cervical spine, both confirmed by MRI (Fig. 13), are related. This is why it is fundamental to look at all our patient's data as a puzzle to be solved. It seems logical to look at the patient as a whole.

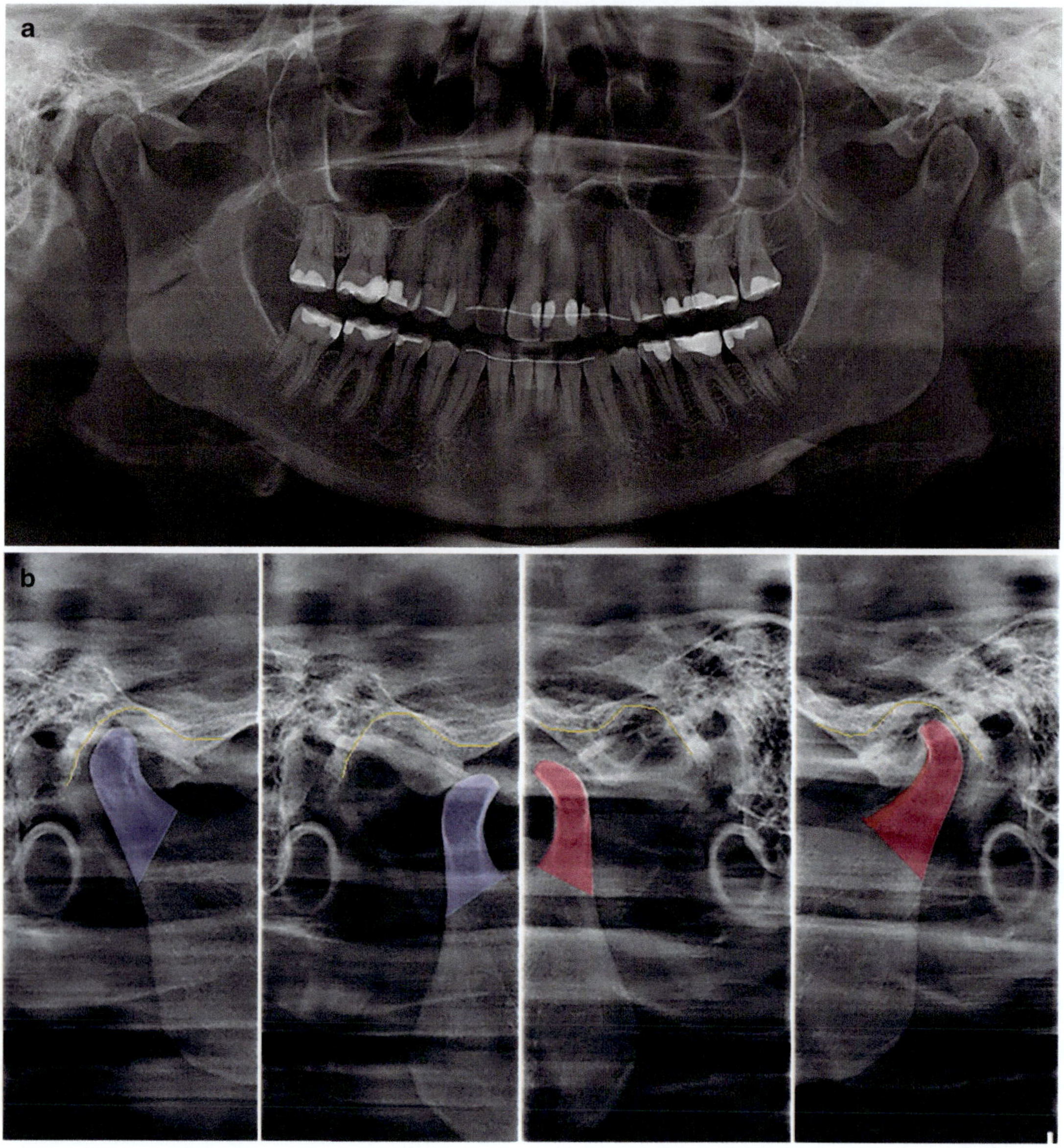

Fig. 11 (a) Panoramic and (b) TMJ plain films of the patient with condyle color highlights

4.5 Structural Misalignment Related to Temporomandibular Joint Pathology

A 17-year-old patient who had already been treated orthodontically returned to the clinic complaining of headache, ear pain, shoulder pain, and bilateral joint clicks. She had pain in her TMJs and a stronger ache when retrodiscal palpation was performed, an indication of condyle retro-position. The patient showed an "ideal occlusion" without relapses from the orthodontic treatment, which was finished 5 years previously (Fig. 14). She exhibited no interference in jaw protrusion nor lateral translation. A surface electromyography was performed to measure the right and left anterior temporalis muscle and right and left masseter muscle activity in maximum intercuspation and clenching. The masseter muscles, the most powerful of the

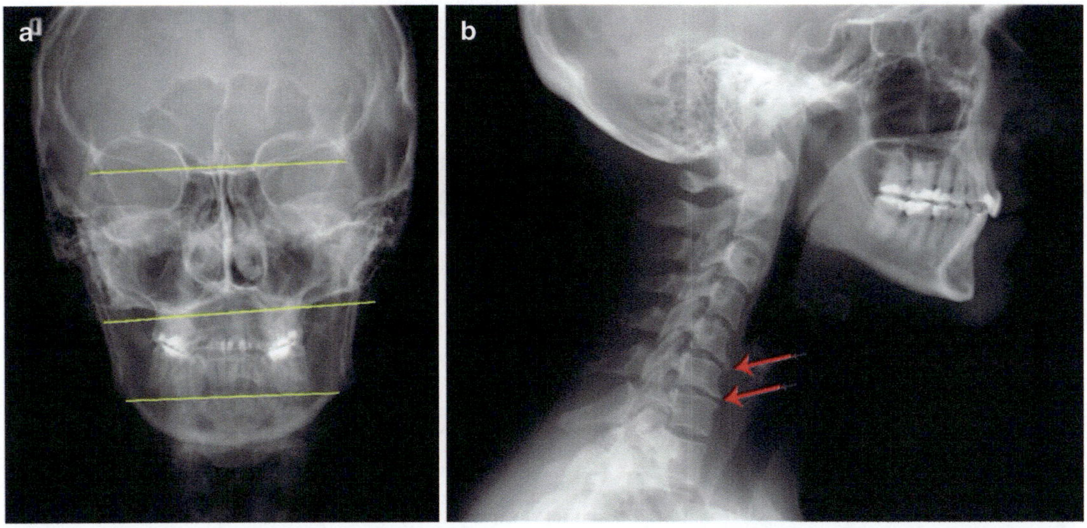

Fig. 12 Frontal and lateral radiographs including C7. (**a**) Notice that planes are not parallel to the horizon. (**b**) Arrows highlight the loss of space between the fifth and sixth cervical vertebrae and also osteophytes in the same vertebrae

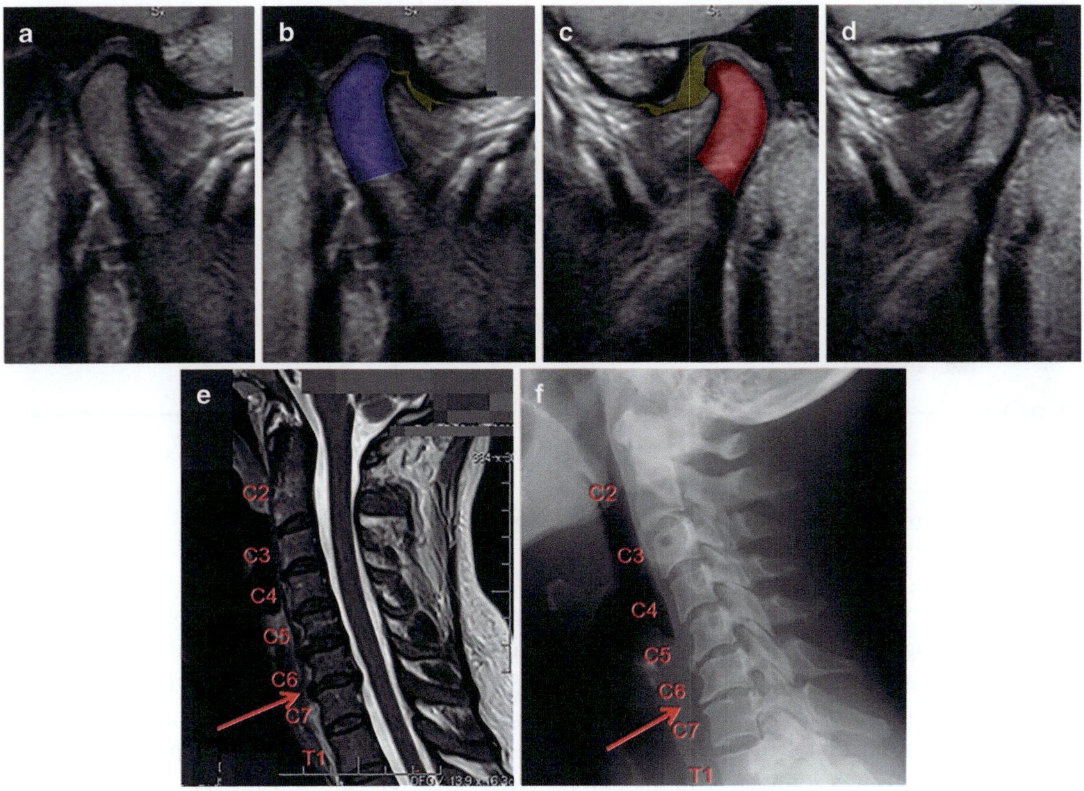

Fig. 13 Top, TMJ MRI. (**a** and **d**) Original color and (**b**, **c**) colored to make the dislocated articular disc easier to visualize. Bottom, (**e**) cervical spine MRI, and (**f**) cervical spine X-ray

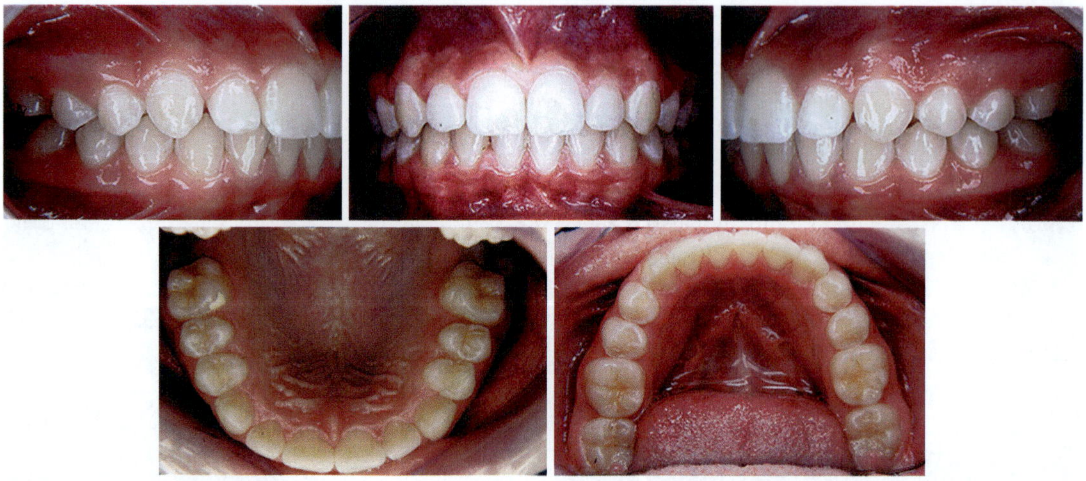

Fig. 14 Patient's habitual occlusion; frontal, right, and left lateral photograph (above); and upper and lower occlusal view

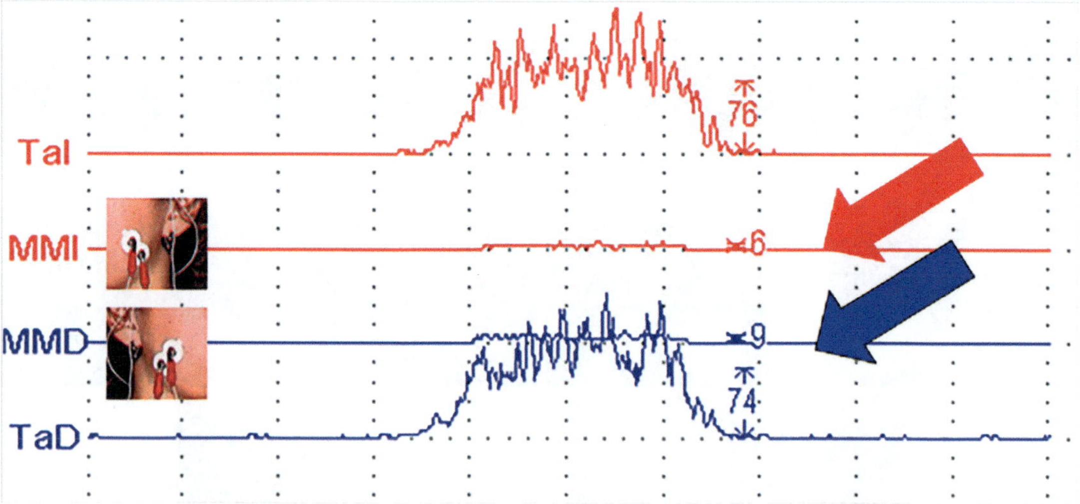

Fig. 15 Electromyographic record of the patient in habitual occlusion

stomatognathic system, were unable to contract during clenching (Fig. 15). Masseter muscles are unable to contract, and the patient had an ideal occlusion. The initial reaction was to think that there was a malfunction with the electromyograph or that there was some error in the placement of the electrodes. Plain films and a TMJ MRI were requested.

Laminography in habitual occlusion, the retro-position of the mandibular heads, especially on the left side (Fig. 16) (red arrow), was clearly visible. This retro-position provokes a significant retrodiscal compression. A modification of the growth axis (greenstick fracture) bilaterally caused by a trauma in infancy is also visible. The MRI shows an anterior disc displacement in the right and left TMJs with reduction (Fig. 17) (open-mouth MRI not included). The patient's masticatory muscles were electronically deprogrammed to check the differences between the neuromuscular and dental trajectories. The closing path is that which is taken during the dis-

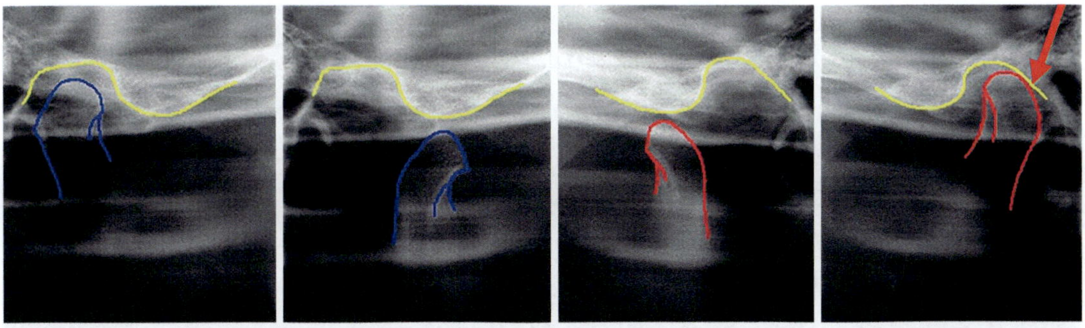

Fig. 16 Patient's laminography in open and closed mouth in habitual occlusion

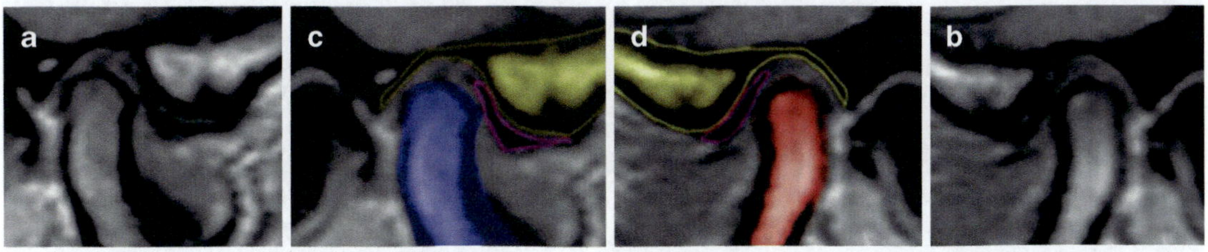

Fig. 17 (**a**, **b**) Patient's MRI in habitual occlusion in closed mouth. (**c**, **d**) Same image with color highlight

placement of the mandible when it passes from its position of rest (MRP) to the position of usual occlusion. This trajectory is the result of the various muscular contraction vectors. These vectors determine a line of mandibular displacement, which brings the mandible into contact with its antagonist (maxilla).

The neuromuscular trajectory (Fig. 18) measured after deprogramming with transcutaneous electrical neural stimulation (TENS) does not match the usual trajectory, having a discrepancy in the sagittal, frontal, and vertical directions. The patient's habitual dental path is posterior to the neuromuscular pathway. The graphic makes perfect sense coinciding with the images and the clinical tests. The patient presented a pathological freeway space of 6.2 mm and a retromandibular position of 2.5 mm. The ultimate goal in orthodontic and facial orthopedic treatments is to treat all three components of the stomatognathic system and create an environment for the synergistic function of the teeth, temporomandibular joints, and neuromuscular system.

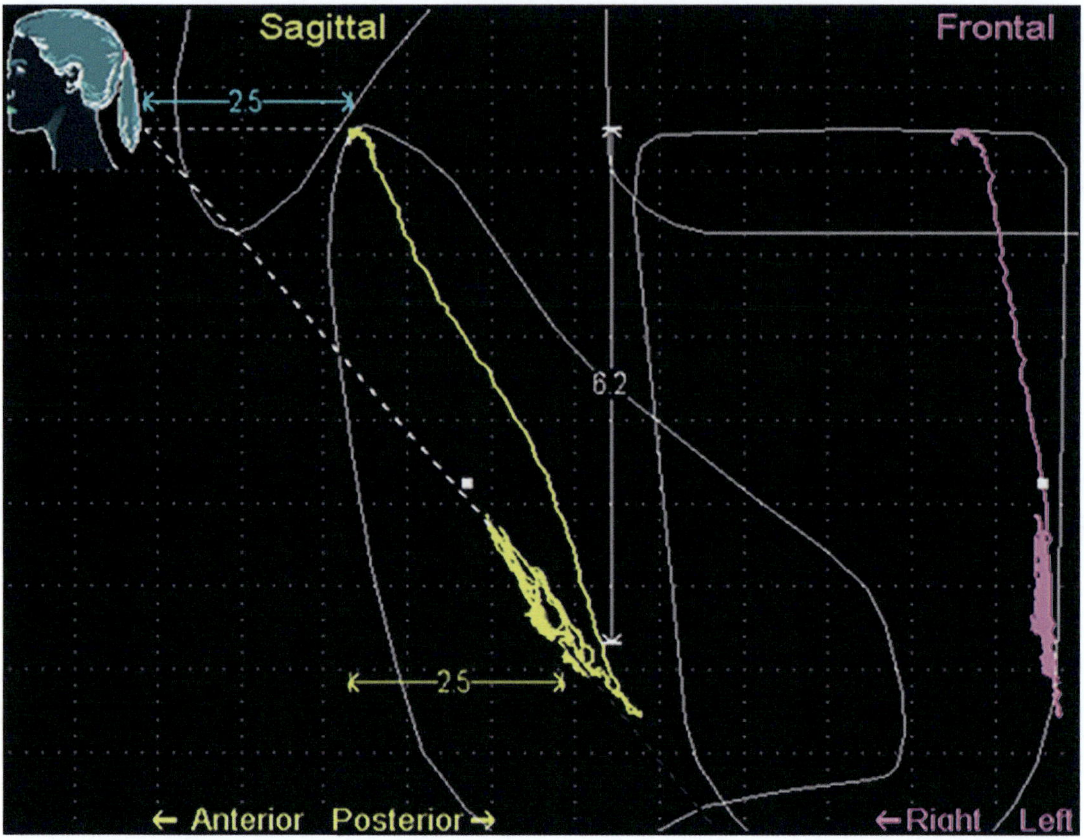

Fig. 18 Jaw tracker data after electronic deprogramming

5 Summary

A static image of beautiful occlusion does not speak of muscular harmony, does not show if there is coordination between the systems, and does not show if the patient has either local or remote pain. Occlusion needs a definition where all systems are represented. The stomatognathic system is linked primarily with the trigeminal nerve and the cervical spine and consequently with the whole body. If one does not understand that teeth are the ending point of this joint, that the temporomandibular joint can be affected by systemic and local pathologies, and that muscles move the mandible, treatment failure may not be understood, especially in cases where TMJ pathologies are present.

Understanding the complex interrelationship of craniomandibular disorders requires a broad understanding, not only of the anatomy and physiology of the head and neck, but also of the spine. Nociceptive reflexes originating from the temporomandibular joint lead to adaptive postural responses (craniomandibular, head and neck, trunk, and limbs). These will be addressed in the following chapter: ***Structural Misalignment: Postural Changes Related to Temporomandibular Joint Pathology.***

Suggested Readings

1. Abbas AK, Lichtman AH, Pillai S. Basic immunology: functions and disorders of the immune system. 6th ed; 2019.
2. Stevens A, Lowe JS. Pathology. Mosby; 2000.
3. Moses AJ. Controversy in temporomandibular disorders: clinicians' guide to critical thinking. Futa Book Publishers; 1997.
4. Arabshahi B, Baskin KM, Cron RQ. Reactive arthritis of the temporomandibular joints and cervical spine in a child. Pediatr Rheumatol Online J. 2007;5:4. https://

doi.org/10.1186/1546-0096-5-4. PMID: 17550629; PMCID: PMC1869027.

5. Bag AK, Gaddikeri S, Singhal A, Hardin S, Tran BD, Medina JA, Curé JK. Imaging of the temporomandibular joint: an update. World J Radiol. 2014;6(8):567–82. https://doi.org/10.4329/wjr.v6.i8.567. PMID: 25170394; PMCID: PMC4147437.
6. Basmajian JV, De Luca Carlo J. Muscles alive: their functions revealed by electromyography. Williams & Wilkins; 1985.
7. Bayar N, Kara SA, Keles I, Koç MC, Altinok D, Orkun S. Temporomandibular joint involvement in rheumatoid arthritis: a radiological and clinical study. Cranio. 2002;20(2):105–10. https://doi.org/10.1080/08869634.2002.11746198.
8. Cedströmer AL, Andlin-Sobocki A, Abbu N, Hedenberg-Magnusson B, Dahlström L, Berntson L. Condylar alterations and facial growth in children with juvenile idiopathic arthritis. J Orofac Orthop. 2020;81(3):163–71. https://doi.org/10.1007/s00056-020-00216-8. Epub 2020 Feb 20. PMID: 32077980; PMCID: PMC7186245.
9. Cevidanes LH, Alhadidi A, Paniagua B, Styner M, Ludlow J, Mol A, Turvey T, Proffit WR, Rossouw PE. Three-dimensional quantification of mandibular asymmetry through cone-beam computerized tomography. Oral Surg Oral Med Oral Pathol Oral Radiol Endod. 2011;111(6):757–70. https://doi.org/10.1016/j.tripleo.2011.02.002. Epub 2011 Apr 16. PMID: 21497527; PMCID: PMC3095695.
10. Conti AC, Oltramari PV, Navarro Rde L, de Almeida MR. Examination of temporomandibular disorders in the orthodontic patient: a clinical guide. J Appl Oral Sci. 2007;15(1):77–82. https://doi.org/10.1590/s1678-77572007000100016. PMID: 19089105; PMCID: PMC4327217.
11. Costen JB. A syndrome of ear sinus symptoms dependent upon disturbed functions of TMJ. Ann Otol. 1934;43(1):1–15.
12. Costen JB. Neuralgias and ear symptoms associated with disturbed function of the TMJ. JAMA J Am Med Assoc. 1936;107:252–4.
13. Cram JR, Kasman GS. Introduction to surface electromyography. Gaithersburg: Aspen Publishers; 1998. p. 408.
14. Wilson-Pauwels L, Akesson EJ, Stewart PA, Spacey SD. Cranial nerves in health and disease. BC Decker Inc.; 2002.
15. Simmons HC, American Academy of Craniofacial Pain. Craniofacial pain: a handbook for assessment, diagnosis and management. 3rd ed. Chroma, Incorporated; 2009.
16. Rozencweig D, Gerdolle D, Delgoffe C, Stricker M. Imagerie de l'ATM: aide au diagnostic des troubles cranio-mandibulaires. Editora Cahiers de prothèses éditions; 1995.
17. Defabianis P. Post-traumatic TMJ internal derangement: impact on facial growth (findings in a pediatric age group). J Clin Pediatr Dent. 2003;27(4):297–303. https://doi.org/10.17796/jcpd.27.4.2782236161p3p467.
18. Defabianis P. TMJ fractures in children and adolescents: treatment guidelines. J Clin Pediatr Dent. 2003;27(3):191–9.
19. Ortu E, Pietropaoli D, Adib F, Masci C, Giannoni M, Monaco A. Electromyographic evaluation in children orthodontically treated for skeletal class II malocclusion: comparison of two treatment techniques. CRANIO®. 2017;37:129. https://doi.org/10.1080/08869634.2017.1393916.
20. Emshoff R, Brandlmaier I, Bösch R, Gerhard S, Rudisch A, Bertram S. Validation of the clinical diagnostic criteria for temporomandibular disorders for the diagnostic subgroup—disc derangement with reduction. J Oral Rehabil. 2002;29(12):1139–45. https://doi.org/10.1046/j.1365-2842.2002.00980.x.
21. Antonio MV, Gil JG. Enfermedades reumaticas extrarticulares. Masson; 1998.
22. Ferreira CL, Da Silva MA, de Felício CM. Orofacial myofunctional disorder in subjects with temporomandibular disorder. Cranio. 2009;27(4):268–74. https://doi.org/10.1179/crn.2009.038.
23. Gary Demerjian G, Barkhordarian A, Chiappelli F. Temporomandibular joint and airway disorders a translational perspective. Springer International Publishing AG, part of Springer Nature; 2018.
24. de Souza Pinto GN, Grossmann E, Iwaki Filho L, Groppo FC, Poluha RL, Muntean SA, Iwaki LC. Correlation between joint effusion and morphology of the articular disc within the temporomandibular joint as viewed in the sagittal plane in patients with chronic disc displacement with reduction: a retrospective analytical study from magnetic resonance imaging. CRANIO®. 2019;39:119. https://doi.org/10.1080/08869634.2019.1582166.
25. Helenius LM, Hallikainen D, Helenius I, Meurman JH, Könönen M, Leirisalo-Repo M, Lindqvist C. Clinical and radiographic findings of the temporomandibular joint in patients with various rheumatic diseases. A case-control study. Oral Surg Oral Med Oral Pathol Oral Radiol Endod. 2005;99(4):455–63. https://doi.org/10.1016/j.tripleo.2004.06.079.
26. Ide Y, Nakazawa K. Anatomical atlas of the temporomandibular joint. Quintessence Publishing Co., Ltd; 2001.
27. Isberg A, Widmalm SE, Ivarsson R. Clinical, radiographic, and electromyographic study of patients with internal derangement of the temporomandibular joint. Am J Orthod. 1985;88(6):453–60. https://doi.org/10.1016/s0002-9416(85)80044-0.
28. Jankelson B. Three-dimensional orthodontic diagnosis and treatment. A neuromuscular approach. J Clin Orthod. 1984;18(9):627–36.
29. Jankelson Robert R. Sensitivity/specificity: straw men, red herrings, and dental politics. Cranio. 2013;31(3):156–8. https://doi.org/10.1179/crn.2013.023.
30. Jaunet E, Le Guern A, Le Tacon P, Thery-Dumeix C, Deshayes MJ. Uncovering and treating asymmetry

before 6 years in our daily clinical practice: option or obligation? Orthodontics or orthopedics? Int Orthod. 2013;11(1):35–59. https://doi.org/10.1016/j.ortho.2012.12.013. Epub 2013 Feb 1.

31. Guimarães JP, Ferreira LA. Atlas de diagnóstico por imaginologia das desordens temporomandibulares. Ed. UFJF; 2012.
32. McNamara JA Jr., SD Kapila KY VanRiper. Temporomandibular disorders and orofacial pain: separating controversy from consensus. (2009)
33. Kim C-W, Han M-C. Cortes anatómicos: correlacionados con RM y TC. Espanha: Doyma; 1990.
34. Kuroda S, Tanimoto K, Izawa T, Fujihara S, Koolstra JH, Tanaka E. Biomechanical and biochemical characteristics of the mandibular condylar cartilage. Osteoarthr Cartil. 2009;17(11):1408–15. https://doi.org/10.1016/j.joca.2009.04.025. Epub 2009 May 18.
35. Learreta JA, Barrientos EE. Temporomandibular joint method to study the morphology and relationship of the hard structures. Cranio. 2010;28(4):223–31.
36. Learreta JA, Yavich LG. Of healthy and pathologic images of temporomandibular joint. São Paulo: Artes Médicas; 2008.
37. Learreta JA, Yavich LG. Structural modifications of the mandibular condylar process as one of the sequels of traumatism in infancy. J Cranio Maxill Dis. 2014;3:85–8.
38. Lopes SL, Costa AL, Cruz AD, Li LM, de Almeida SM. Clinical and MRI investigation of temporomandibular joint in major depressed patients. Dentomaxillofac Radiol. 2012;41(4):316–22. https://doi.org/10.1259/dmfr/27328352. PMID: 22517997; PMCID: PMC3729006.
39. Piancino MG, Tepedino M, Cavarra F, Bramanti E, Laganà G, Chimenti C, Cirillo S. Condylar long axis and articular eminence in MRI in patients with temporomandibular disorders. CRANIO®. 2018;38:342. https://doi.org/10.1080/08869634.2018.1532647.
40. Masi M, Lederman HM, Yamashita HK, de Arruda Aidar LA. Temporomandibular joint evaluation with magnetic resonance imaging in children with functional unilateral posterior crossbite, treated with rapid maxillary expansion. Am J Orthod Dentofacial Orthop. 2009;136(2):207–17. https://doi.org/10.1016/j.ajodo.2007.10.048.
41. Melchior MO, Mazzetto MO, Magri LV. Relation of painful TMD with the speech function: what are the possible characteristics of mandibular movements and the main symptoms reported? Codas. 2019;31(2):e20180161. https://doi.org/10.1590/2317-1782/20182018161.
42. Michelotti A, Iodice G. The role of orthodontics in temporomandibular disorders. J Oral Rehabil. 2010;37(6):411–29. https://doi.org/10.1111/j.1365--2842.2010.02087.x. Epub 2010 Apr 9.
43. Maulén-Yáñez M, Meeder-Bella W, Videla-Jiménez PJ, González-Arriagada WA. Assessment of association between muscular diagnosis in temporomandibular disorders with mandibular kinematics. CRANIO®. 2018;37:365. https://doi.org/10.1080/08869634.2018.1465513.
44. Monaco A, Cattaneo R, Marci MC, Marzo G, Gatto R, Giannoni M. Neuromuscular diagnosis in orthodontics: effects of TENS on maxillo-mandibular relationship. Eur J Paediatr Dent. 2007;8(3):143–8.
45. Moncada G, Cortés D, Millas R, Marholz C. Relationship between disk position and degenerative bone changes in temporomandibular joints of young subjects with TMD. An MRI study. J Clin Pediatr Dent. 2014;38(3):269–76. https://doi.org/10.17796/jcpd.38.3.w43m8474433n7ur2.
46. Jankelson RR. Neuromuscular dental diagnosis and treatment hardcover. Ishiyaku Euroamerica; 1990.
47. Skármeta NP, Araneda L, Araya C. Destructive psoriatic arthritis of the temporomandibular joint: a clinical case, an overview of the pathophysiology and its differential diagnoses. CRANIO®. 2018;38(3):201–7.
48. Piancino MG, Cannavale R, Dalmasso P, Tonni I, Filipello F, Perillo L, Cattalini M, Meini A. Condylar asymmetry in patients with juvenile idiopathic arthritis: could it be a sign of a possible temporomandibular joints involvement? Semin Arthritis Rheum. 2015;45(2):208–13. https://doi.org/10.1016/j.semarthrit.2015.04.012. Epub 2015 May 2.
49. Pollack B. Cases of note: Michigan jury awards $850,000 in ortho case: a tempest in a teapot. J Mich Dent Assoc. 1988;70(11–12):540–2.
50. Saldanha AD, Hilgenberg PB, Pinto LM, Conti PC. Are temporomandibular disorders and tinnitus associated? Cranio. 2012;30(3):166–71. https://doi.org/10.1179/crn.2012.026.
51. Schmitter M, Kress B, Rammelsberg P. Temporomandibular joint pathosis in patients with myofascial pain: a comparative analysis of magnetic resonance imaging and a clinical examination based on a specific set of criteria. Oral Surg Oral Med Oral Pathol Oral Radiol Endod. 2004;97(3):318–24. https://doi.org/10.1016/j.tripleo.2003.10.009.
52. Shankland WE 2nd. Anterior throat pain syndromes: causes for undiagnosed craniofacial pain. Cranio. 2010;28(1):50–9. https://doi.org/10.1179/crn.2010.007.
53. Sims A, Stack B. Tourette's syndrome: a pilot study for the discontinuance of a movement disorder. Cranio. 2009;27(1):11–8. https://doi.org/10.1179/crn.2009.003.
54. Sims AB, Stack BC, Demerjian GG. Spasmodic torticollis: the dental connection. Cranio. 2012;30(3):188–93. https://doi.org/10.1179/crn.2012.029.
55. Cortes D, et al. Association between disk position and degenerative bone changes of the temporomandibular joints: an imaging study in subjects with TMD. CRANIO. 2011;29(2):117.
56. Sano T, Yajima A, Otonari-Yamamoto M, Wakoh M, Katakura A. Interpretation of images and discrepancy between osteoarthritic findings and symptomatology in temporomandibular joint. Jpn Dent Sci Rev. 2008;44(1):83–9.

57. Varol A, Sencimen M, Gulses A, Altug HA, Dumlu A, Kurt B. Diagnostic importance of MRI and CT scans for synovial osteochondromatosis of the temporomandibular joint. Cranio. 2011;29(4):313–7. https://doi.org/10.1179/crn.2011.046.
58. Voudouris JC, Kuftinec MM. Improved clinical use of twin-block and Herbst as a result of radiating viscoelastic tissue forces on the condyle and fossa in treatment and long-term retention: growth relativity. Am J Orthod Dentofac Orthop. 2000;117(3):247–66. https://doi.org/10.1016/s0889-5406(00)70231-9.
59. Wang MQ, He JJ, Chen CS, Widmalm SE. A preliminary anatomical study on the association of condylar and occlusal asymmetry. Cranio. 2011;29(2):111–6. https://doi.org/10.1179/crn.2011.019.
60. Warhekar AM, Wanjari PV, Phulambrikar T. Unilateral trifid mandibular condyle: a case report. Cranio. 2011;29(1):80–4. https://doi.org/10.1179/crn.2011.011.
61. Yajima A, Sano T, Otonari-Yamamoto M, Otonari T, Ohkubo M, Harada T, Wakoh M. MR evidence of characteristics in symptomatic osteoarthritis of the temporomandibular joint: increased signal intensity ratio on proton density-weighted images of bone marrow in the mandibular condyle. Cranio. 2007;25(4):250–6. https://doi.org/10.1179/crn.2007.038.
62. Yavich LG. Alterações na orientação do côndilo mandibular devido a traumatismos na primeira infância. JBA. 2001;1(4):270–9.
63. Yavich LG. Eletromiografia de superfície no diagnóstico e controle do tratamento das disfunções temporomandibulares. JBA. 2001;1(3):193–8.
64. Yavich LG. Paciente com disfunção temporomandibular apresentando assimetria condilar e micro nódulos no terço anterior das pregas vocais. JBA. 2002;2(5):12–9.
65. Yavich LG. Princípios neuromusculares na Odontologia, trajetória de fechamento habitual coincidente com a trajetória de fechamento neuromuscular. JBA. 2002;2(6):101–11.
66. Yitschaky O, Yitschaky M, Zadik Y. Case report on trial: do you, doctor, swear to tell the truth, the whole truth and nothing but the truth? J Med Case Rep. 2011;5:179. https://doi.org/10.1186/1752-1947-5-179. PMID: 21569508; PMCID: PMC3113995.

Structural Misalignment: Postural Changes Related to Temporomandibular Joint Pathology

Lidia Yavich

1 Introduction

Upon patient evaluation, one must analyze not only the cranio-cervical-mandibular system but also the whole posture and gait. To correctly assess the maxillomandibular relationship, one must begin to consider the physiological rest position of the mandible. This concept is no different from the physiological rest position of the body but, concerning not only the hard tissue such as teeth and bone as is usually done in dentistry, but also muscle and nerves.

The rest position of the mandible is also a result of a combination of the posterior cervical muscles and the muscles that are anterior to the cervical spine. Therefore, one can appreciate the connection from the cranium to the mandible, from the shoulder girdle to the mandible, and from the cervical spine to the mandible through a muscular chain. The hyoid is the prevertebral bone which distributes tensional forces below the mandible and in front of the cervical spine.

The important role of the tongue during swallowing also determines the mandibular posture as does the level of contraction of the genioglossus. The mandible articulates with the cranium through the temporomandibular joint. Nociceptive reflexes originating from the temporomandibular joint lead to adaptive postural responses (craniomandibular, head and neck, trunk, and limbs). Although not considered a part of the joint itself, muscles are closely related to joints. In orthopedic disorders, muscle spasms are secondary and are the result, not the cause, of pain. Skeletal asymmetries are a common source of mechanical stress. Postural stress is often a consequence of structural stress.

The vertical dimension of occlusion (VDO) is also determined by the TMJ and its state of health. Head and neck posture influences the resting position of the mandible, which subsequently alters its closure pathway for tooth–tooth contact. As mentioned in Chap. 11, one of the fundamental things to consider in a patient's documentation are photos of the patient's entire body, front, back, right, and left profile, not only photos of the patient's head and neck. In the same way as panoramic radiographs in conferences and publications are often displayed without mandibular condyles, one often sees patients' photographs focused on the face only.

Analysis of photographs of the face and part of the neck, as shown in Fig. 1a–c, has a limited view of the patient. It is important to understand that the patient's entire posture has to be analyzed, taking into account that interventions can produce postural changes that may or may not be beneficial (Fig. 1d): in this frontal view image, one can observe right and left shoulder protrusion, abdominal protrusion, forward head position, higher right nipple, and higher right shoulder. Figure 1g, h, left (g) and right (h): in these lateral images, one can observe knee flex-

L. Yavich (✉)
SBPAT, The Brazilian Society for Diagnosis and Treatment of Temporomandibular Joint Pathologies, Attending, Clinica My, Porto Allege, RS, Brazil

B. C. Stack Jr. et al. (eds.), *Craniofacial Pain*, https://doi.org/10.1007/978-3-031-57563-1_12

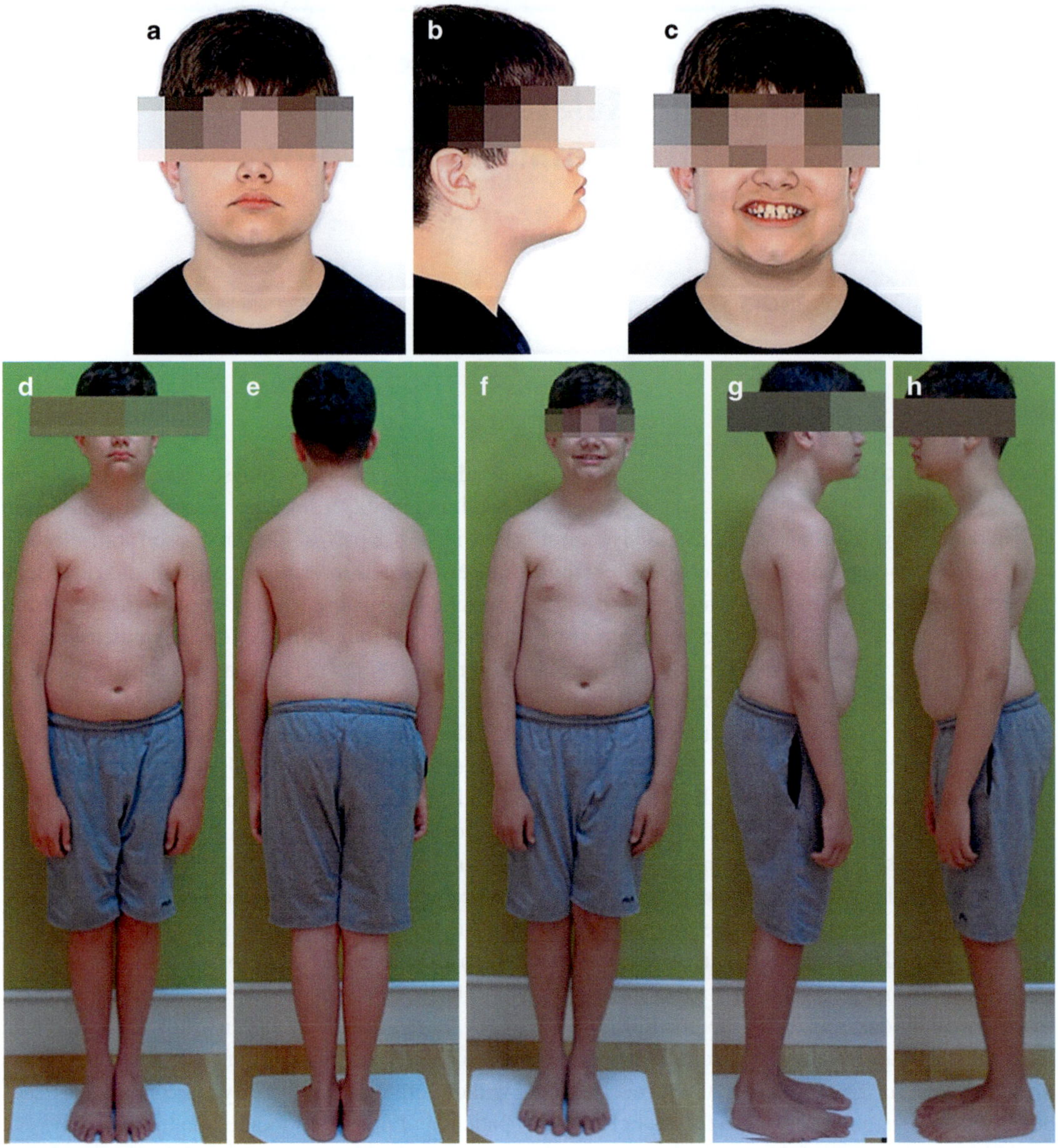

Fig. 1 Above: patient's face in frontal, profile, and smile views. Below: patient's posture, frontal, back, smiling, right, and left profile

ion, pelvic anteversion, increase in spinal curvatures (lumbar hyperlordosis and dorsal hyperkyphosis), right shoulder more protruding than the left, cervical rectification, and forward head position.

A photograph is only an image in time. It is a method that allows one to see body posture alignments and misalignments. Dentists need to detect these signs even though they are not qualified to directly treat these conditions. Such patients should be referred to specialists who will make an adequate description and diagnosis of postural problems. Dentists treat mandible tridimensional posture, which has a fundamental relation to body posture.

This patient suffered headaches, neck pain, difficulty swallowing liquids and solids, and nocturnal and daytime choking episodes. In this specific example, postural comparisons will be highlighted, as well as the patient's profile and vertical dimension with the orthotic (Fig. 2b) and the patient's profile and vertical dimension at the beginning of the treatment in habitual occlusion (Fig. 2a).

An orthotic is not a simple piece of acrylic; it represents the position where the muscles are at their best performance, with the limitations of each differential diagnosis. Teeth habitual trajectory must coincide with the neuromuscular trajectory, considering mandible posture with all its components. An improvement in cervical rectification can be observed by comparing Fig. 2a with b. Patients' evaluation should consist of complete records including conventional images, CT, and MRI of the temporomandibular joints. To make the orthotics, bioinstrumentation is utilized such as surface electromyography and a computerized jaw tracker. Patients may also be referred to a physiotherapist and speech therapist during treatment.

Comparing Fig. 3a with b: in these frontal images, note the improved shoulder positioning, right shoulder, and right iliac crest more aligned and improved knee alignment. Comparing Fig. 3 (c, e) with (d, f): in these lateral images, note the improved head and shoulder positioning, decreased abdominal protrusion, improved spine curvature alignment, knee bending no longer apparent, and pelvic anteversion correction.

It may be easier to understand what a three-dimensionally misaligned mandible can cause if one considers the mandible as the first girdle of the body (Fig. 4). The mandible is connected to the vertebral spine. TMJ pathologies not only

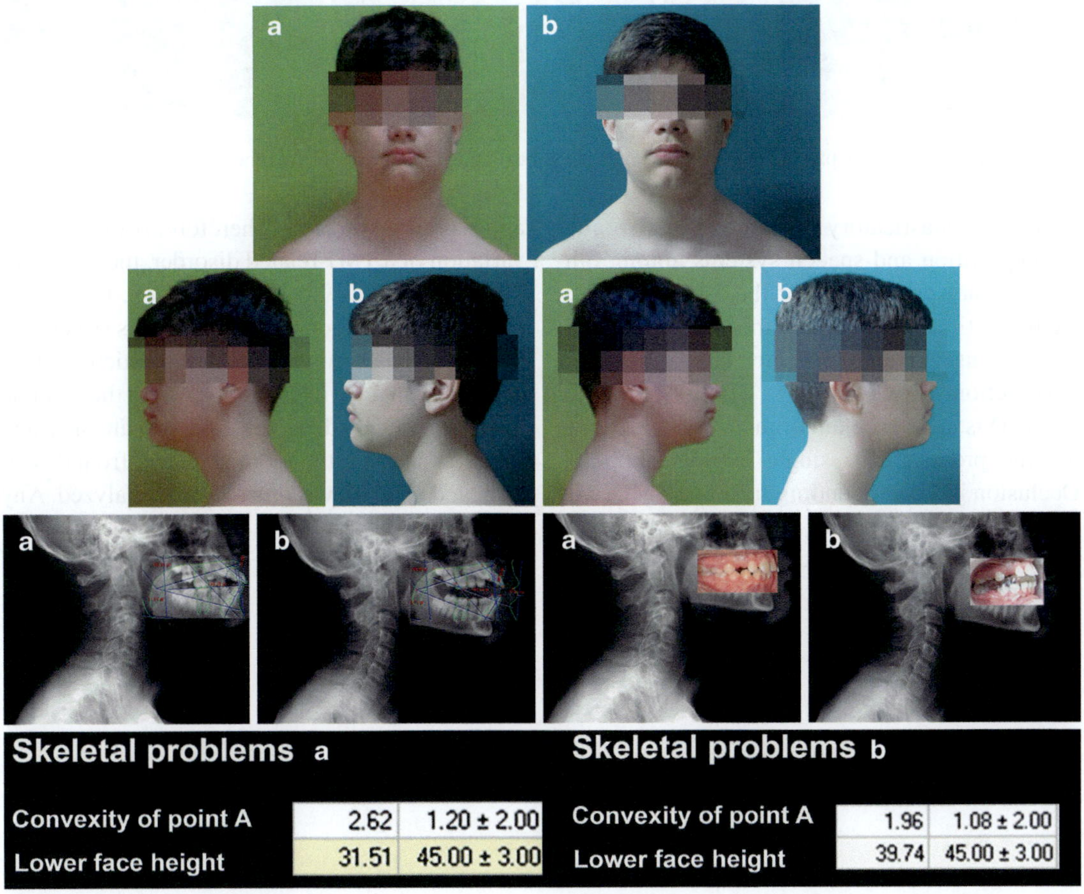

Fig. 2 Photographs and lateral radiographs including C7 of the patient with and without an orthotic appliance

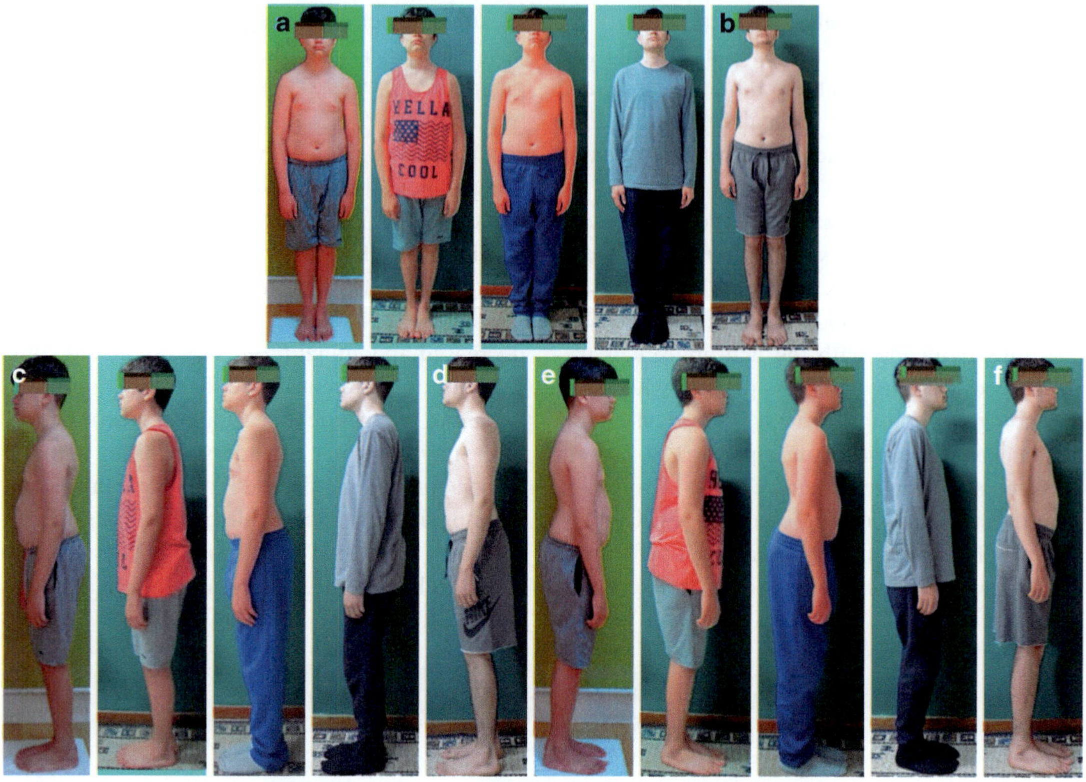

Fig. 3 Comparison of the patient's postural changes at the beginning and during the treatment

disturb the masticatory apparatus but also alter the deglutition and speech systems among others. Primary pathologies of the TMJ can affect teeth positions; sometimes, this wrong position is a consequence and not the cause of dysfunction.

TMD is not a problem of modern society; it is not the product of a single etiological factor. Occlusion is a compounding factor of TMD. The point is how occlusion is defined. A healthy occlusion requires that the TMJs are healthy and working properly and that the muscles are healthy and working correctly. Therefore, if there is any variation of a TMJ-related disorder, then, by definition, there must be a malocclusion. Upon considering the TMJ, one must analyze its structures: the mandibular condyle and the articular disc, especially in growing patients, where the condyle must be protected by the disc. Ligaments, and synovial space in three-dimensional, frontal, sagittal, and axial views, must also be analyzed. Any modification in the joint structures will cause distortions in its vertical, horizontal, and axial dimensions.

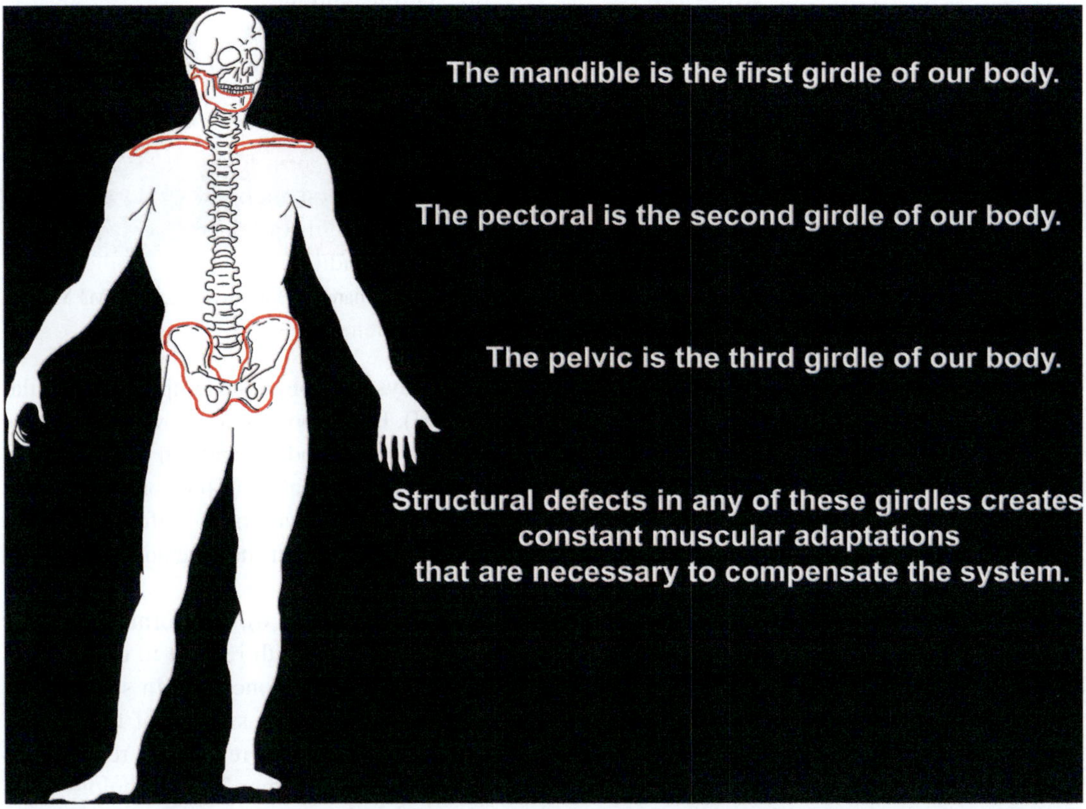

Fig. 4 Girdles on the human body, considering the mandible as the first girdle

2 Some Considerations When Dealing with TMJ Pathologies

- Can the TMJ be healed?
- Can the TMJ be improved or can TMD be prevented from worsening?
- Can TMJ articular discs be recaptured?

The first question must be: What is the problem? And only after that, the second should be: How can it be fixed? For this, a differential diagnosis must be carefully elaborated. Consider that central relation is not a dental terminology; it is a terminology that relates to the concept of stability of synovial joints. Basically, it refers to the congruency of joint surfaces. When it relates to the temporomandibular joint, it is a synovial joint. If the joint flattens, if the articular disc is displaced, the joint is no longer stable regardless of the occlusion or molar class. If there are degenerative processes affecting the mandibular condyle, if the mandibular condyle presents growth axis modification, and if the temporomandibular joint presents effusions caused by different etiologies, then there is articular pathology and resultant joint instability.

Even though there are aligned teeth and correct molar class in both patients in the top and bottom images, the articular discs shown with open mouth are dislocated and only on the right side of Fig. 5a, there is a recapture. The bottom images (c) and (d) show that the teeth are aligned and in the correct molar class, but both in the open-mouth MRI have irreducible articular disc dislocations; furthermore, the left side has an anatomic distortion. This condition can happen at any age without pain and is frequently undiagnosed. It implies that the system is compromised. Joint stability presupposes the correct functioning of ligaments, tendons, and muscular structures for the proper mechanics

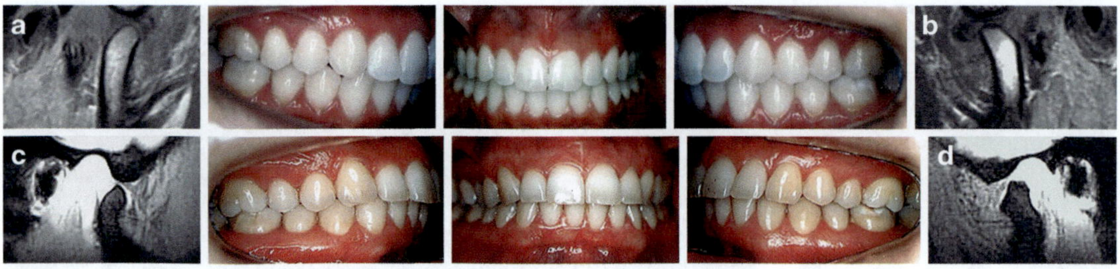

Fig. 5 Top: a slice of TMJ MRI (**a**, **b**) with intraoral photographs of the same patient. Bottom: a slice of TMJ MRI (**c**, **d**) with intraoral photographs of another patient

of the joint. Images of beautiful occlusions as shown in image Fig. 5 are not a guarantee of TMJ health.

Analyzing the TMJ in sequence, the first piece of information about the mandibular condyle can be obtained from the panoramic radiograph, but pathology may or may not be visible. The next comes from the TMJ plain film, and the third and most accurate for hard tissues can only be seen in the CT where shape, positioning, and bone alterations are evident. To be able to observe discs, soft tissues, bone edema, and effusions, among other changes, one must obtain an MRI of the TMJs. What is important when requesting a magnetic resonance image of the TMJs, apart from the knowledge to interpret the image, is the question of what can be done with that information. This is an exam that should be requested by colleagues who can apply this information to the treatment of the patient's TMJ pathology.

3 Greenstick Fractures

Mandible and condylar process fractures are well and plentifully described in the bibliography except for greenstick fractures of the condylar process which are rarely described. The name is by analogy with green (i.e., immature) wood, which similarly breaks on the outside when bent. These fractures provoke deformation of the mandibular condyle, which in turn creates a morphofunctional dysfunction of the temporomandibular joint (TMJ). It is important to know that this type of fracture can produce growth disturbances. Changes in the orientation of the condyle axis are common in patients who have suffered blows to the chin region, whether they are anteroposterior, vertical, or lateral.

In these cases (Fig. 6), a deformation of the head of the condyle with respect to curvature is seen with an anterior concavity. In some cases, the deformity can be so significant that it produces compression of the retrodiscal region, producing severe symptoms. This pathology may even be present with an apparently healthy condyle-disc relationship in those patients in whom the articular disc structures have not been obviously affected by the trauma.

Traumas are classified as direct and indirect. Direct traumas are those that have their impact upon different sectors of the mandible. Indirect traumas are those that are a result of sudden and strong dislocation of the mandible. We were taught that occlussion is guided in harmonic order, determined by the axis of rotation of the joint, and joint position in so-called centric relationship. Perhaps this is the case in ideal patients without joint pathologies. The condyle should not be a reference in patients with assymmetries, modification in the growth axis, degenerative processes, autoimmune diseases, inflammatory processes, metabolic diseases, and other conditions that affect the head of the mandible/TMJ.

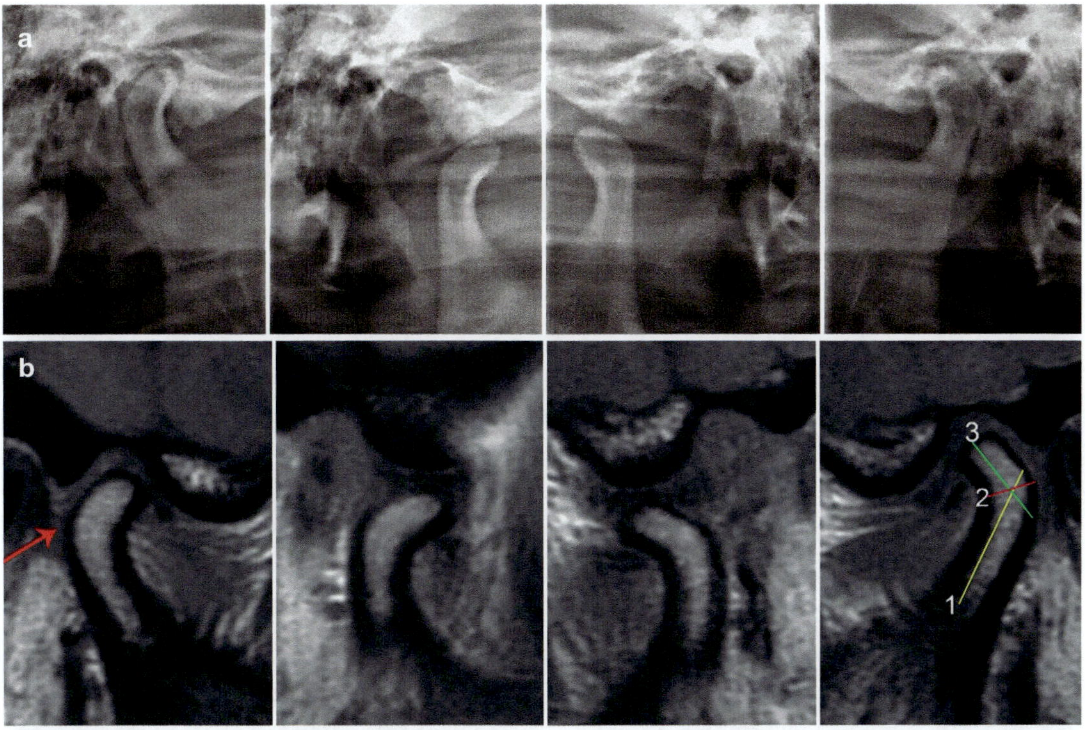

Fig. 6 Laminography (**a**) and MRI (**b**) of right and left TMJ in open and closed mouth. Pathologic mandible head. Deformity caused by traumatism in childhood. Normal growth axis (1), fracture location (2), and pathological growth axis (3). The arrow marks the compression site

4 Which TMJ Side Has a Centric Relationship?

Which side is chosen to determine the centric relationship in any one of the patients in Fig. 7, **all of them with different arthropathies?** The right condyle and the right glenoid fossa or the left condyle and left glenoid fossa? When guided only by cephalometry, there is an assumption that the mandibular heads are in a physiologic position and that the patients do not present any pathology within the temporomandibular joint. Cephalometry is traced on craniometric points in a maximal intercuspation position ignoring muscles or presupposing that they are in balance.

How can muscles be in balance when they are twisted because of structural failures? The patient's existing habitual occlusion is often a relation of the mandible to the skull, which is very far from optimal. Therefore, the diagnosis made in intercuspal models, or simply in a radiographic cephalometry in this position, reflects the pathological accommodation of the patient's muscles. Imaging is not an isolated tool and should be requested after a thorough history and a meticulous clinical examination.

Figure 8a: 3D reconstruction of a condyle in the closed mouth of a patient with a history of trauma and *Staphylococcus aureus* infection; Fig. 8b: MRI of close mouth of a patient with anterior disc displacement and a history of sudden trauma; Fig. 8c: CT patient with the change of growth axis of the condyle, history of trauma in infancy, and a retro-position of the condyle after orthodontic treatment; Fig. 8d: patient with psoriatic arthritis, change of growth axis condyle, and retro-position of the condyle after orthodontic treatment; Fig. 8e: patient with a history of rheumatic fever; Fig. 8f: patient with rheumatoid arthritis. These images help uncover etiological agents that cause the pathology that affects patients. The patient may present one of these conditions or several concom-

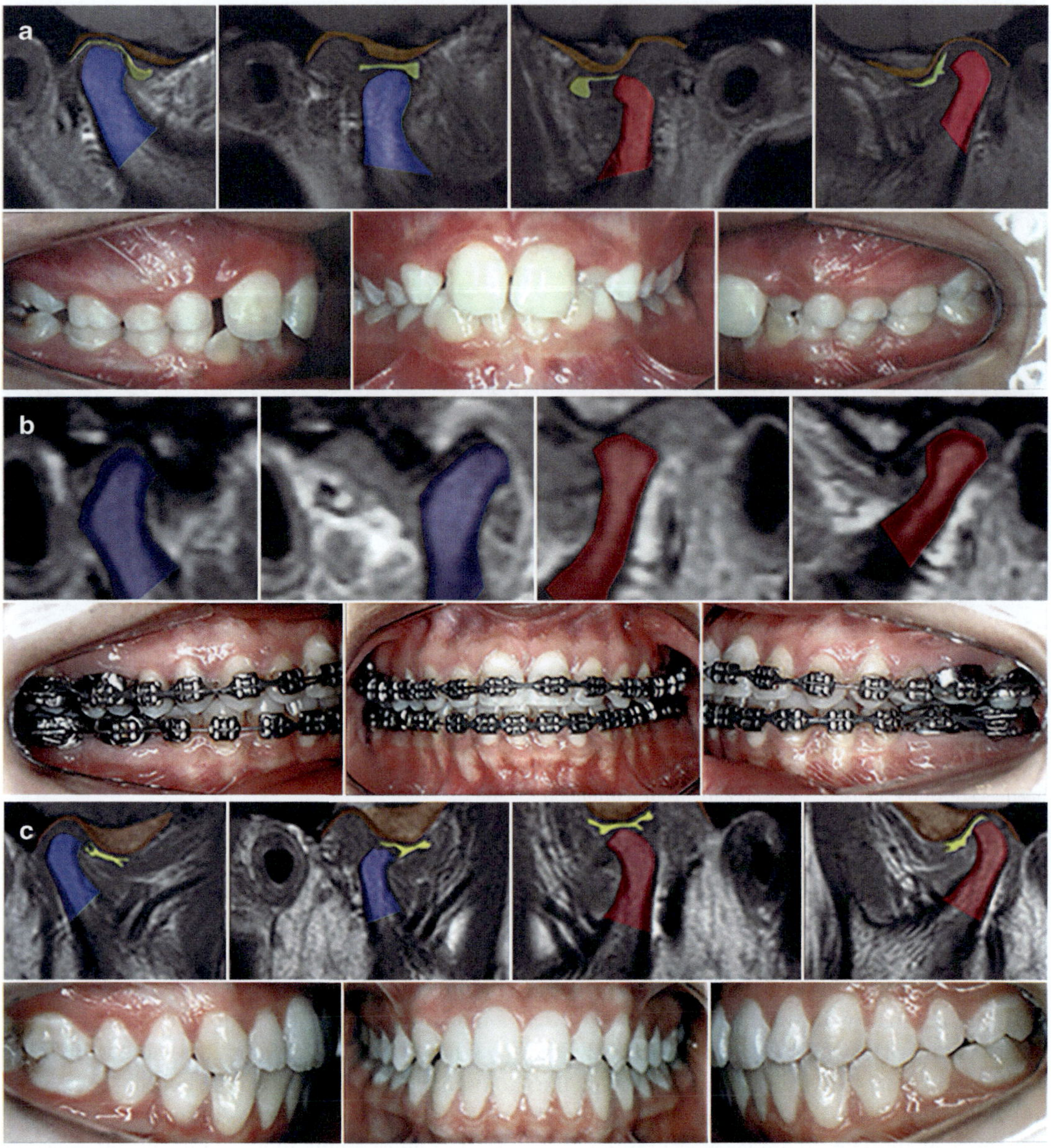

Fig. 7 Different images of occlusions of patients with the respective MRI images in closed and open mouth with color highlights

itant ones, which modifies the degree of complexity of the disease.

How is a better relationship between muscles, jaws, teeth, and temporomandibular joints achieved when several components of the stomatognathic system may be injured with different types and degrees of lesions? In the section, ***TMJ Pathology Treatment (Chap. 13)***, four clinical cases are presented with the therapeutic resources utilized. Even though the importance of full-body photographs has been emphasized heretofore, for brevity and convenience, they are not included. The focus in the third section is TMJ structural and functional changes.

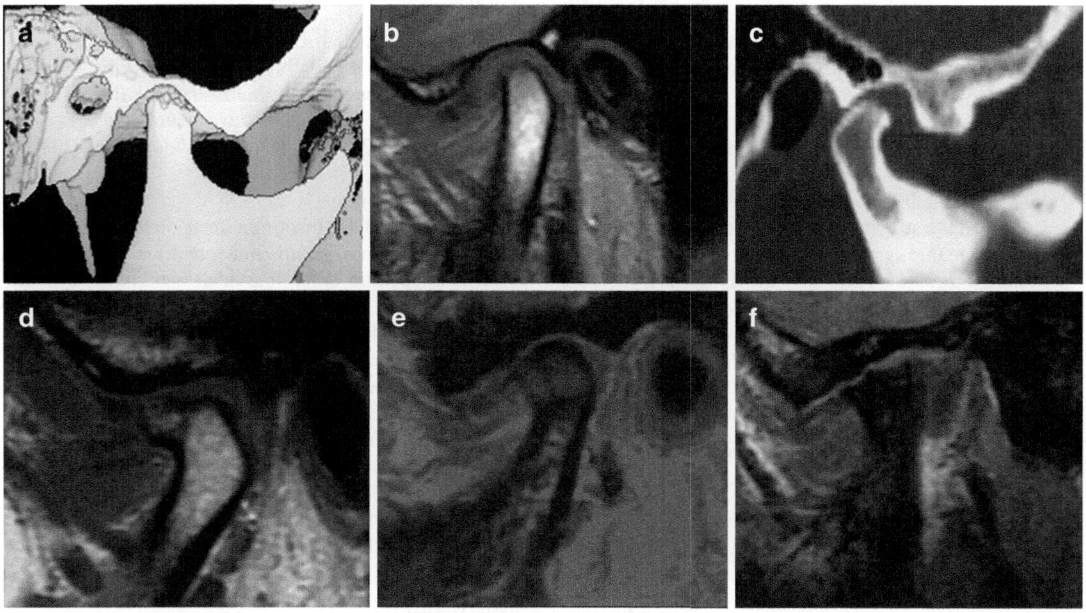

Fig. 8 Images of different patients with diverse pathologies

5 Summary

Can the TMJ be healed? Yes, in many cases, as soon as the problem is diagnosed and the structures have not undergone permanent and extensive alterations.

Can the TMJ be improved or prevented from worsening? Yes, in many cases, when positioning problems are treated and compressive mandible postures are avoided.

Can dislocated articular discs be recaptured? Yes, in many cases, the physiological relationship of the head of the mandible with the articular disc can be recovered.

Suggested Readings

1. Abdallah EF, Mehta NR, Forgione AG, Clark RE. Affecting upper extremity strength by changing maxillo-mandibular vertical dimension in deep bite subjects. Cranio. 2004;22(4):268–75. https://doi.org/10.1179/crn.2004.033.
2. Abduljabbar T, Mehta NR, Forgione AG, Clark RE, Kronman JH, Munsat TL, George P. Effect of increased maxillo-mandibular relationship on isometric strength in TMD patients with loss of vertical dimension of occlusion. Cranio. 1997;15(1):57–67. https://doi.org/10.1080/08869634.1997.11745993.
3. Alghadir AH, Zafar H, Iqbal ZA. Effect of three different jaw positions on postural stability during standing. Funct Neurol. 2015;30(1):53–7. PMID: 26329542; PMCID: PMC4520673.
4. Le Breton A. Occlusion et posture. Sciences du Vivant; 2017.
5. Ayub E, Glasheen-Way M, Kraus S. Head posture: a case study of the effects on the rest position of the mandible*. J Orthop Sports Phys Ther. 1984;5(4):179–83. https://doi.org/10.2519/jospt.1984.5.4.179.
6. Bag AK, Gaddikeri S, Singhal A, Hardin S, Tran BD, Medina JA, Curé JK. Imaging of the temporomandibular joint: an update. World J Radiol. 2014;6(8):567–82. https://doi.org/10.4329/wjr.v6.i8.567. PMID: 25170394; PMCID: PMC4147437.
7. Bergamini M, Pierleoni F, Gizdulich A, Bergamini C. Dental occlusion and body posture: a surface EMG study. Cranio. 2008;26(1):25–32. https://doi.org/10.1179/crn.2008.041.
8. Bricot B. La reprogrammation posturale globale. Sauramps Médical; 1996.
9. Bracco P, Deregibus A, Piscetta R. Effects of different jaw relations on postural stability in human subjects. Neurosci Lett. 2004;356(3):228–30. https://doi.org/10.1016/j.neulet.2003.11.055.
10. Chakfa AM, Mehta NR, Forgione AG, Al-Badawi EA, Lobo SL, Zawawi KH. The effect of stepwise increases in vertical dimension of occlusion on isometric strength of cervical flexors and deltoid muscles in nonsymptomatic females. Cranio. 2002;20(4):264–73. https://doi.org/10.1080/08869634.2002.11752122.

11. Clark RKF, Wyke BD. Contributions of temporomandibular articular mechanoreceptors to the control of mandibular posture: an experimental study. J Dent. 1974;2(3):121–9.
12. Simmons HC, American Academy of Craniofacial Pain. Craniofacial pain: a handbook for assessment, diagnosis and management. 3rd ed. Chroma, Incorporated; 2009.
13. Cuccia A, Caradonna C. The relationship between the stomatognathic system and body posture. Clinics (Sao Paulo). 2009;64(1):61–6. https://doi.org/10.1590/s1807-59322009000100011. PMID: 19142553; PMCID: PMC2671973.
14. D'Attilio M, Filippi MR, Femminella B, Festa F, Tecco S. The influence of an experimentally-induced malocclusion on vertebral alignment in rats: a controlled pilot study. Cranio. 2005;23(2):119–29. https://doi.org/10.1179/crn.2005.017.
15. Kapandji AI. Fisiología articular. Tomo 3. Tronco y Raquis. Editorial Médica Panamericana S.A.; 2002.
16. Gangloff P, Louis JP, Perrin PP. Dental occlusion modifies gaze and posture stabilization in human subjects. Neurosci Lett. 2000;293(3):203–6. https://doi.org/10.1016/s0304-3940(00)01528-7.
17. Goldstein DF, Kraus SL, Williams WB, Glasheen-Wray M. Influence of cervical posture on mandibular movement. J Prosthet Dent. 1984;52(3):421–6. https://doi.org/10.1016/0022-3913(84)90460-8.
18. De Giorgi I, Castroflorio T, Cugliari G, Deregibus A. Does occlusal splint affect posture? A randomized controlled trial. CRANIO®. 2018;38(4):264–72. https://doi.org/10.1080/08869634.2018.1511265.
19. Coskun Benlidayi I, Guzel R, Tatli U, Salimov F, Keceli O. The relationship between neck pain and cervical alignment in patients with temporomandibular disorders. CRANIO®. 2018;38(3):174–9. https://doi.org/10.1080/08869634.2018.1498181.
20. Kalia V, Singh AP. Greenstick fracture of the mandible: a case report. J Indian Soc Pedodont Prev Dent. 2008;26(1):32–5. https://doi.org/10.4103/0970-4388.40320.
21. Kibana Y, Ishijima T, Hirai T. Occlusal support and head posture. J Oral Rehabil. 2002;29(1):58–63. https://doi.org/10.1046/j.1365-2842.2002.00794.x.
22. Learreta JA, Beas J, Bono AE, Durst A. Muscular activity disorders in relation to intentional occlusal interferences. Cranio. 2007;25(3):193–9. https://doi.org/10.1179/crn.2007.030.
23. Learreta JA, Yavich LG. Structural modifications of the mandibular condylar process as one of the sequels of traumatism in infancy. J Cranio Maxill Dis. 2014;3:85–8.
24. Maeda N, Sakaguchi K, Mehta NR, Abdallah EF, Forgione AG, Yokoyama A. Effects of experimental leg length discrepancies on body posture and dental occlusion. Cranio. 2011;29(3):194–203. https://doi.org/10.1179/crn.2011.028.
25. Monaco A, Cattaneo R, Marci MC, Marzo G, Gatto R, Giannoni M. Neuromuscular diagnosis in orthodontics: effects of TENS on maxillo-mandibular relationship. Eur J Paediatr Dent. 2007;8(3):143–8.
26. Kendall HO, Kendall FP, Wadswoth GE. Muscles: testing and function. Williams and Wilkins; 1971.
27. Mehta NR. The neck–jaw interaction revisited. CRANIO®. 2019;37(1):4. https://doi.org/10.1080/08869634.2019.1546646.
28. Palazzi C, Miralles R, Soto MA, Santander H, Zuñiga C, Moya H. Body position effects on EMG activity of sternocleidomastoid and masseter muscles in patients with myogenic cranio-cervical-mandibular dysfunction. Cranio. 1996;14(3):200–9. https://doi.org/10.1080/08869634.1996.11745969.
29. Ricketts RM. Provocations and perceptions in craniofacial orthopedics. RMO; 1989.
30. Rodríguez K, Miralles R, Gutiérrez MF, Santander H, Fuentes A, Fresno MJ, Valenzuela S. Influence of jaw clenching and tooth grinding on bilateral sternocleidomastoid EMG activity. Cranio. 2011;29(1):14–22. https://doi.org/10.1179/crn.2011.004.
31. Auvenshine RC, Pettit NJ. The hyoid bone: an overview. CRANIO®. 2018; https://doi.org/10.1080/08869634.2018.1487501.
32. Rothbart BA. Vertical facial dimensions linked to abnormal foot motion. J Am Pediatr Med Assoc. 2008;98(3):189–96. https://doi.org/10.7547/0980189.
33. Saito ET, Akashi PM, Sacco IC. Global body posture evaluation in patients with temporomandibular joint disorder. Clinics (Sao Paulo). 2009;64(1):35–9. https://doi.org/10.1590/s1807-59322009000100007. PMID: 19142549; PMCID: PMC2671968.
34. Sakaguchi K, Mehta NR, Abdallah EF, Forgione AG, Hirayama H, Kawasaki T, Yokoyama A. Examination of the relationship between mandibular position and body posture. Cranio. 2007;25(4):237–49. https://doi.org/10.1179/crn.2007.037.
35. Sakar O, Calisir F, Oztas E, Marsan G. Evaluation of the effects of temporomandibular joint disk displacement and its progression on dentocraniofacial morphology in symptomatic patients using lateral cephalometric analysis. Cranio. 2011;29(3):211–8. https://doi.org/10.1179/crn.2011.030.
36. Silveira A, Gadotti IC, Armijo-Olivo S, Biasotto-Gonzalez DA, Magee D. Jaw dysfunction is associated with neck disability and muscle tenderness in subjects with and without chronic temporomandibular disorders. Biomed Res Int. 2015;2015:512792. https://doi.org/10.1155/2015/512792. Epub 2015 Mar 26. PMID: 25883963; PMCID: PMC4391655.
37. Sims AB, Stack BC, Demerjian GG. Spasmodic torticollis: the dental connection. Cranio. 2012;30(3):188–93. https://doi.org/10.1179/crn.2012.029.
38. Souza JA, Pasinato F, Corrêa EC, da Silva AM. Global body posture and plantar pressure distribution in individuals with and without temporomandibular disorder: a preliminary study. J Manipulative Physiol Ther. 2014;37(6):407–14. https://doi.org/10.1016/j.jmpt.2014.04.003. Epub 2014 Aug 6.

39. Stack B, Sims A. The relationship between posture and equilibrium and the auriculotemporal nerve in patients with disturbed gait and balance. Cranio. 2009;27(4):248–60. https://doi.org/10.1179/crn.2009.036.
40. Wiest DM, Candotti CT, Sedrez JA, Pivotto LR, da Costa LMR, Loss JF. Severidade da disfunção temporomandibular e sua relação com a postura corporal. Fisioterapia E Pesquisa. 2019;26(2):178–84. https://doi.org/10.1590/1809-2950/18037026022019.
41. Xiao CQ, Wan YD, Li YQ, Yan ZB, Cheng QY, Fan PD, Huang Y, Wang XY, Xiong X. Do temporomandibular disorder patients with joint pain exhibit forward head posture? A cephalometric study. Pain Res Manag. 2023;2023:7363412. https://doi.org/10.1155/2023/7363412. PMID: 36776487; PMCID: PMC9911253.
42. Yitschaky O, Yitschaky M, Zadik Y. Case report on trial: do you, doctor, swear to tell the truth, the whole truth and nothing but the truth? J Med Case Rep. 2011;5:179. https://doi.org/10.1186/1752-1947-5-179. PMID: 21569508; PMCID: PMC3113995.

TMJ Pathology Treatment

Lidia Yavich

1 Introduction

Four clinical cases are presented and the cases are to emphasize their respective nuances and encourage reporting and publication of complex TMD cases. Images and bioinstrumentation measurements are presented as well as highlights from the clinical histories. One case is presented in its two complete phases, and the other three clinical cases aim to point out the improvements that can be achieved.

As mentioned previously, TMJ can be affected by local and systemic pathologies, trauma, infections, autoimmune diseases, and occlusal problems among other etiologies. All these etiological factors can act separately or in concert, making the clinical case more difficult to resolve and modifying expectations of the patient and practitioner for resolution.

2 Case 1

2.1 TMJ Pathologies in Children and Teenagers: The Overlooked Diagnosis

The importance of this case report is that structural improvements were achieved in the first phase of treatment. Can treatment sometimes improve the TMJ pathological situation, or prevent it from worsening? This case report draws attention to TMJ pathologies in children and teenagers where the TMJ may be compromised.

2.2 Case Report

A 14-year-old female patient presented to the clinic complaining of pain in the lower teeth, shoulder pain, and TMJ clicking on the left side. Aesthetic correction is an important issue for the patient, but she and her mother were also concerned with the pain in the lower teeth and the origin of the clicking noise (Fig. 1). The patient's occlusion suggests a simple case. It is expected to be very easy to evaluate and diagnose the need for a superior expansion to accommodate and advance the mandible and afterward to treat the vertical deficiency (Figs. 2 and 3). With this laminography, one can see the retro-position of the left closed-mouth TMJ (highlighted in red), the change in the growth axis direction on this same side, and the loss of joint space on both sides. These images do not show the articular disc condition or the ligaments which can only be seen in an MRI. The panoramic radiograph for the temporomandibular joints cannot be compared to a CT scan of the temporomandibular joints and is a basic examination for the TMJ.

When evaluating a functional failure, one must consider all the etiologic factors involved in the dysfunction. The patient reports a trauma

L. Yavich (✉)
SBPAT, The Brazilian Society for Diagnosis and Treatment of Temporomandibular Joint Pathologies, Attending, Clinica My, Porto Allege, RS, Brazil

B. C. Stack Jr. et al. (eds.), *Craniofacial Pain*, https://doi.org/10.1007/978-3-031-57563-1_13

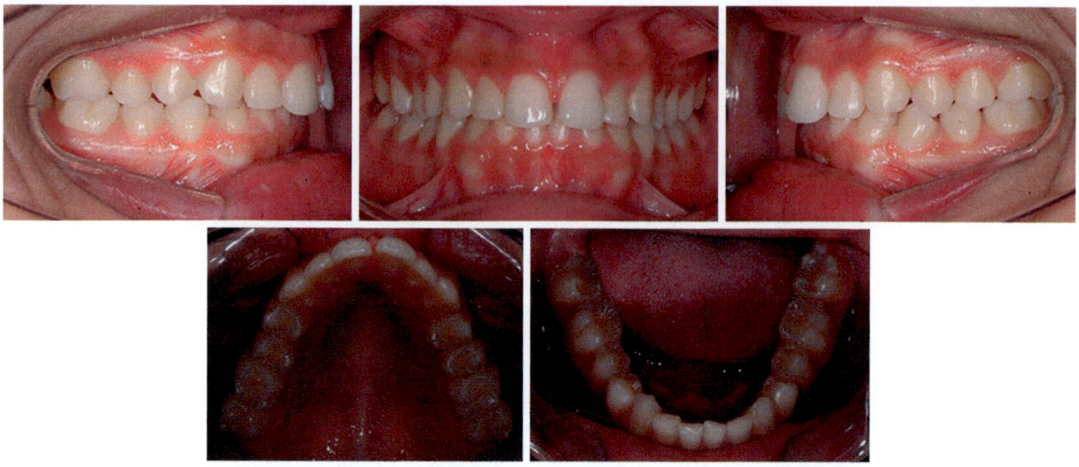

Fig. 1 Intraoral records of the patient's habitual occlusion

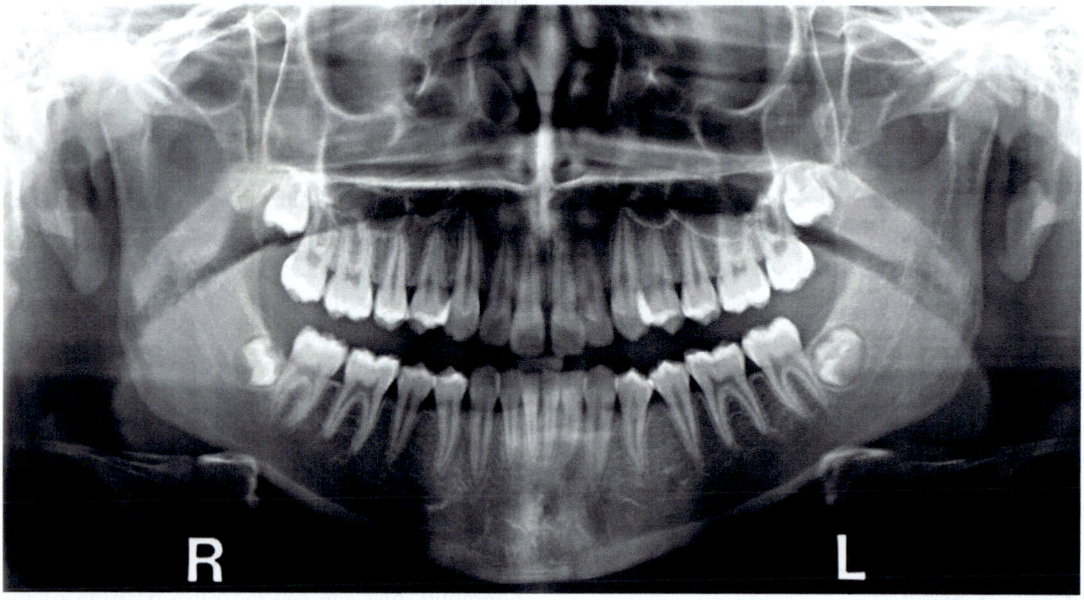

Fig. 2 Patient's initial panoramic radiograph

when she was a child, "I hit my neck, near my chin, playing on the bedside table." A change in the direction of the growth axis does not happen physiologically. It is very common for patients not to remember these childhood traumas.

Besides the rectification of the cervical spine, there is the start of an inversion of the physiological curvature from C4 (Fig. 4). Cephalometry is a very important part of the diagnosis and treatment of cases, both in orthodontics and facial orthopedics; however, it is not an exam to show the pathology of temporomandibular joints. An MRI of the temporomandibular joints was ordered (Figs. 5 and 6).

The two slices, (1) external and (2) medial, show irregularity of the bone cortex and anterior articular disc dislocation. Even though CT is the method par excellence for observing bone erosions, studies comparing bone erosion scores and quantitative measures of erosions in RA joints on CT and MR images demonstrate very high intramodality and intermodality agree-

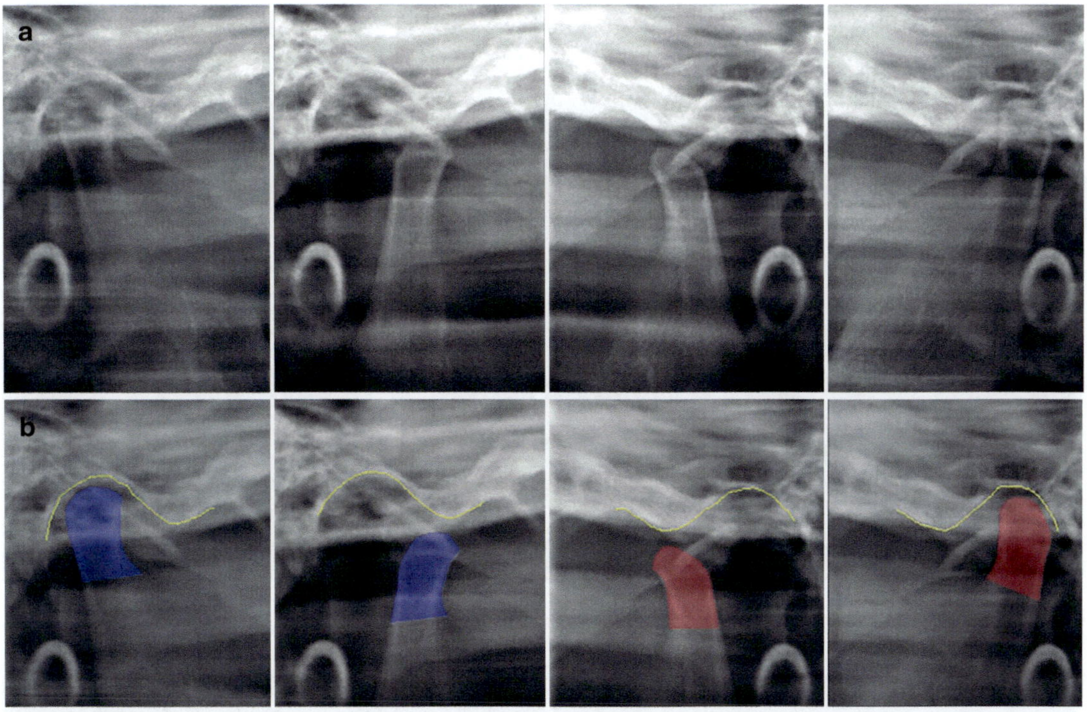

Fig. 3 Laminography of the temporomandibular joints in the closed and open mouth (**a**). (**b**) The same images with **color highlights**

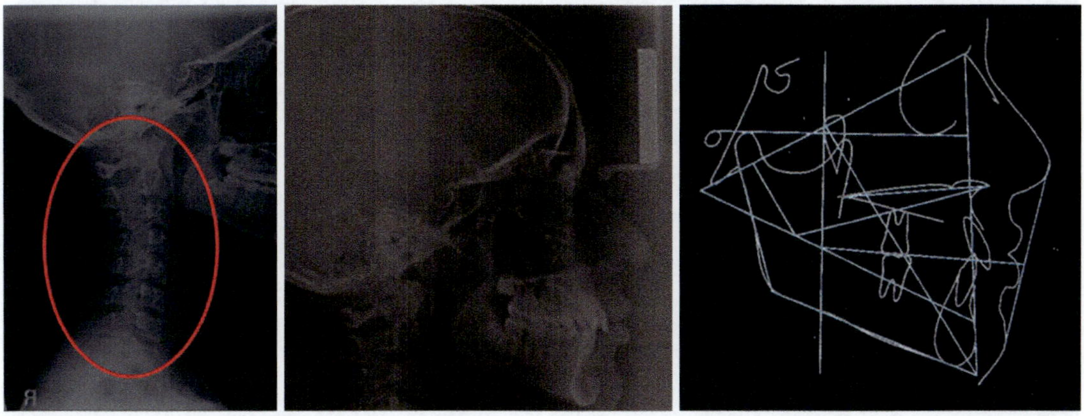

Fig. 4 Patient's initial lateral and cervical spine (left) radiograph with a cephalometric tracing (right), all before treatment

ment. Medial slice (1) shows superior flattening, an anterior marginal osteophyte, and articular disc dislocation. External slice (2) also shows superior flattening and anterior articular disc dislocation. This is the TMJ of a 14-year-old girl!

Systemic diseases, traumas, infections, damage to growth centers, and muscle balance disruption can profoundly influence the craniofacial complex during this critical growth phase. There was no crepitus, nor pain in the TMJ was present, only a click.

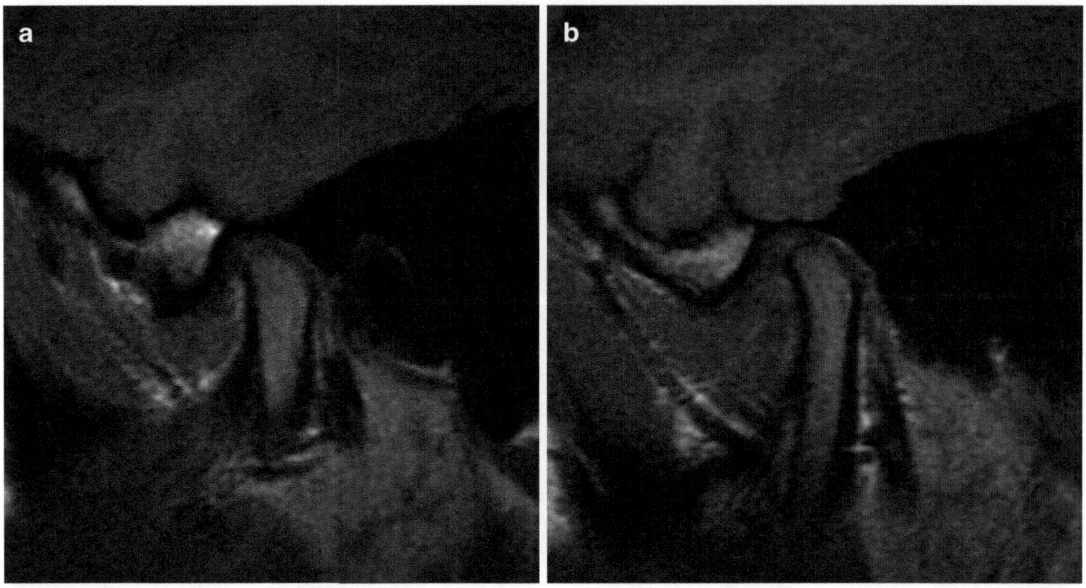

Fig. 5 MRI: two slices of the left TMJ closed mouth before treatment

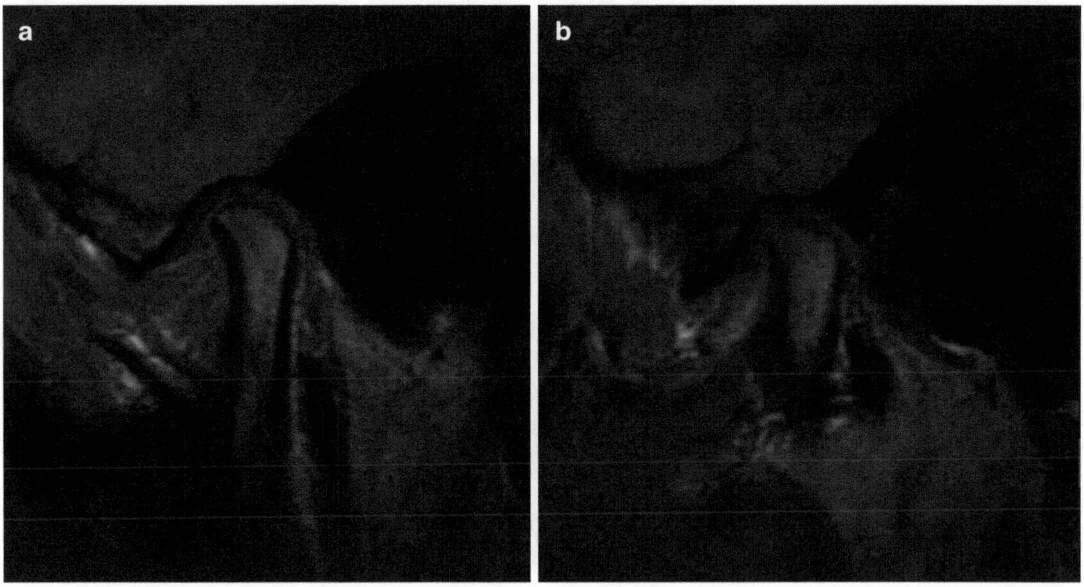

Fig. 6 MRI two slices of the right TMJ closed mouth before treatment

If one cannot improve this situation because of the sequelae of different etiologies, the next step is to analyze if one can prevent it from worsening and improve the patient's life quality. The patient should be informed about the difficulties and limitations of their cases.

For a dynamic record of SEMG (Fig. 7), the patient is asked to open her mouth, clench, and swallow. In this record, one can observe that the patient cannot maintain strength in clenching, even though she was instructed to clench her teeth and not to open for the duration of the

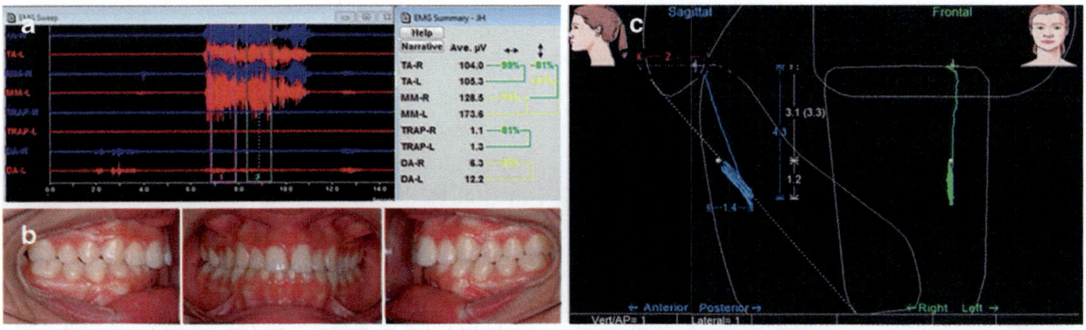

Fig. 7 Initial dynamic electromyography (**a**) in habitual occlusion (**b**) and jaw tracker data (**c**)

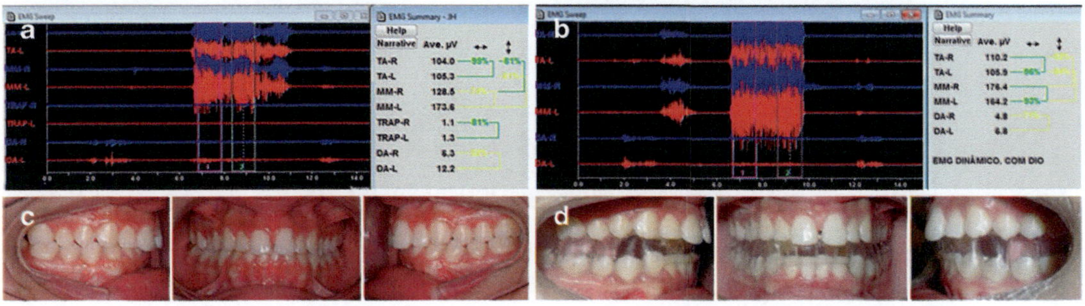

Fig. 8 Comparison of the SEMG records of the patient, (**a**, **b**) in habitual occlusion and (**c**, **d**) with orthotic in place

exam. Her masticatory muscles were electronically deprogrammed with a dental TENS unit, and a bite record in neuromuscular physiological position was registered using a jaw tracker. The information obtained from the images and the individualized objectives for each clinical case should always be considered in the bite registration. Bioinstrumentation is a useful tool but is only a part of the decision on bite registration.

The patient had a pathological free space of 4.3 mm and a retro-position of 2.1 mm. With this data, an orthotic can be fabricated. This device is electromyographically tested to represent the ideal muscle position. With dynamic electromyography (Fig. 8), and with the orthotic in a neuromuscular physiological position, the patient can maintain the strength of the bite. In fact, she increased the strength of the masseters and balanced both digastric muscles.

These images showing the joint decompression (Fig. 9) do not reveal the position of the articular disc nor the improvement of the irregularities on the cortical bone observed in the initial MRI. We can notice an improvement in the cervical spine physiological curve and an increase in the intervertebral spaces (Fig. 10). In all these images, Figs. 11, 12, 13, 14, 15 and 16, we can observe the improvement in the relationship between the mandible head and the articular disc and the positive remodeling of the cortical bone.

In this specific case, the questions that have to be asked are the following:

- Was there a pathologic condition of the patient's TMJ? If so, which structures were affected?
- Is it possible to heal or improve the damaged structures?

The goal is to bring these structures as close to a healthy function as possible. Is this always possible? When it is possible, the structures must be improved. Differential diagnosis allows us a differential prognosis: favorable or not. Not all arthropathies will have the same result as this case.

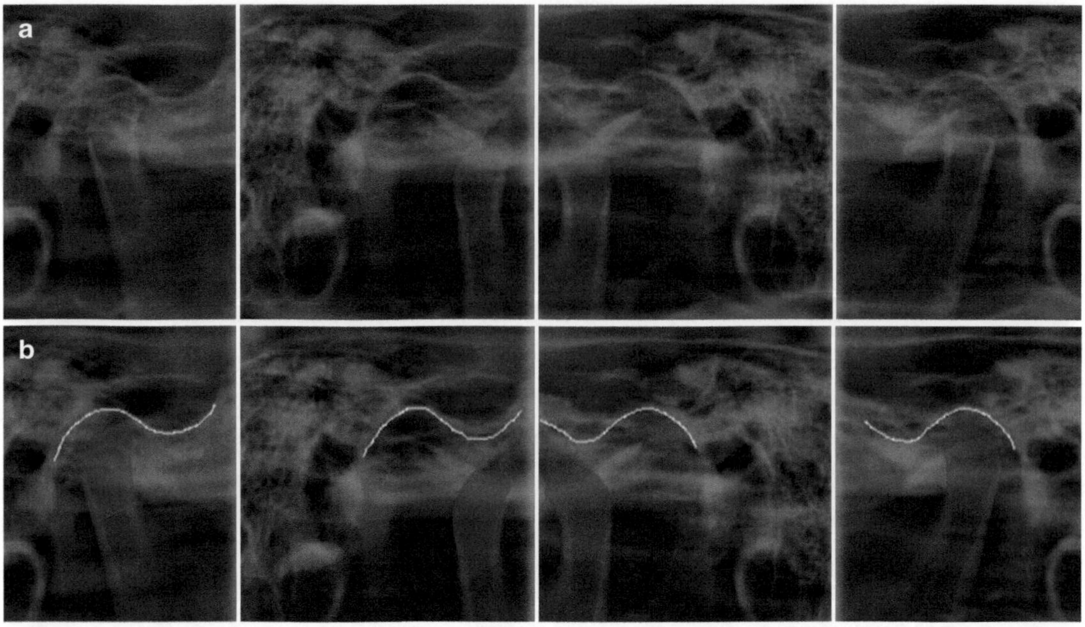

Fig. 9 (**a**) Laminography of the temporomandibular joints in the closed and open mouth with the orthotic constructed in neuromuscular physiological position; (**b**) the same image with color highlights

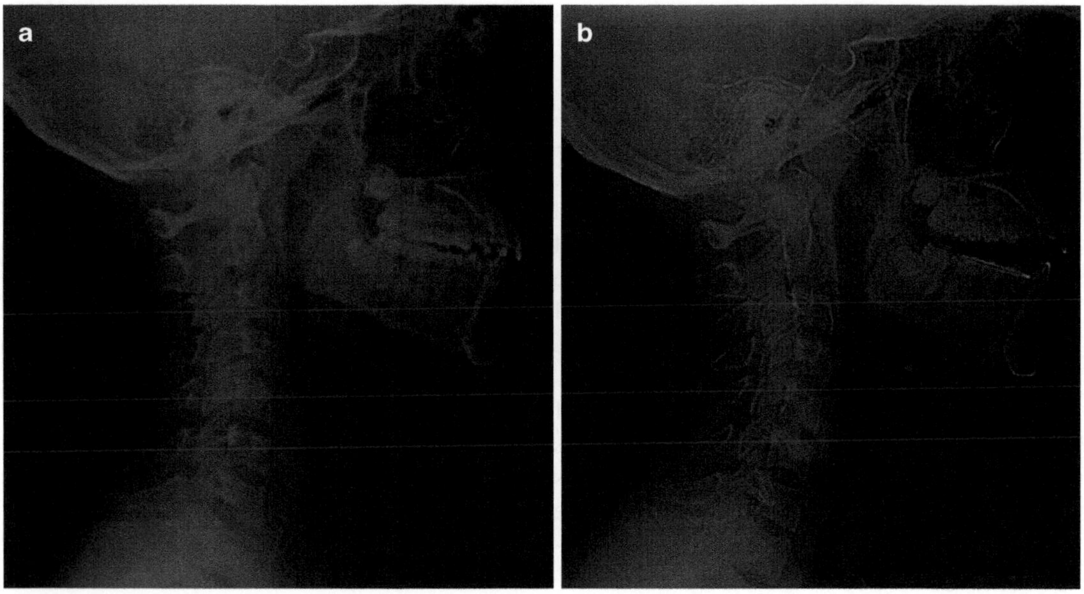

Fig. 10 Patient's lateral and cervical spine comparison: (**a**) in habitual occlusion and (**b**) with the orthotic constructed in neuromuscular physiological occlusion

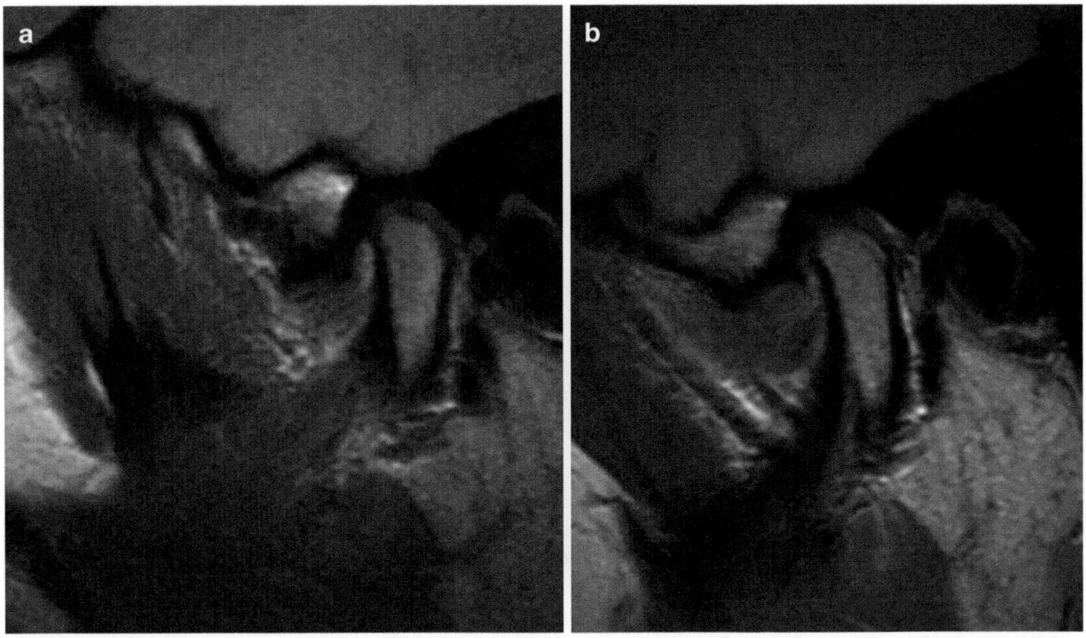

Fig. 11 Comparative MRI images of the left TMJ sagittal external slice, closed mouth position, (**a**) before treatment and (**b**) after the first phase of the treatment

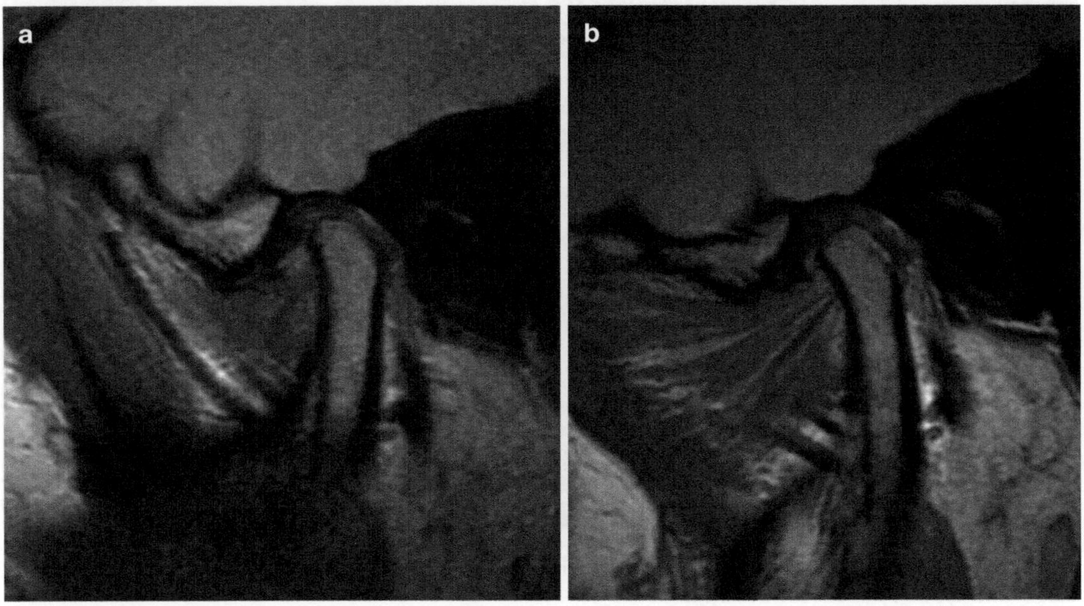

Fig. 12 Comparative MRI images of the left TMJ, sagittal medial slice, closed mouth position, (**a**) before treatment and (**b**) after the first phase of the treatment

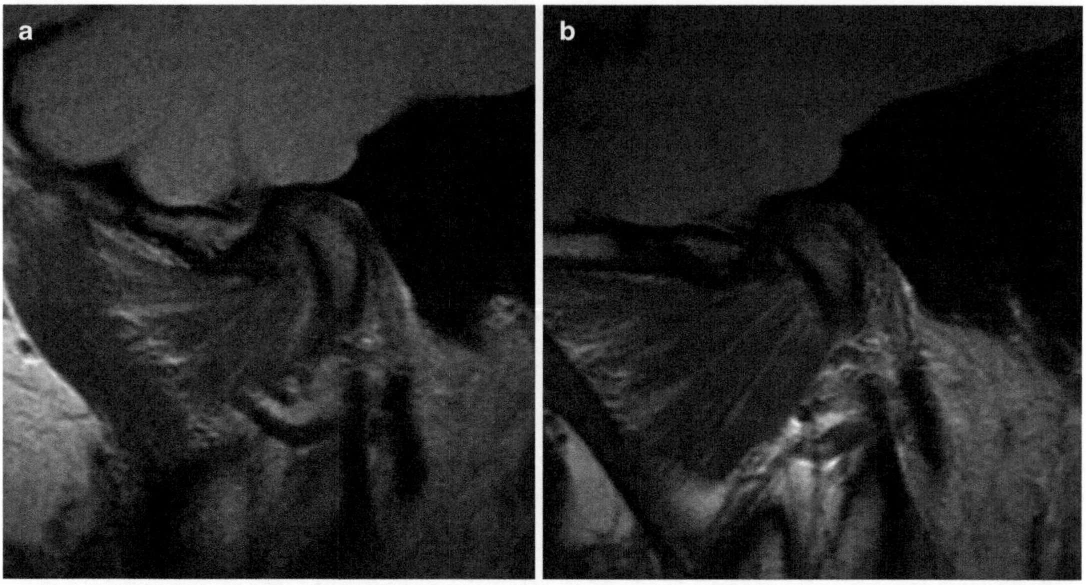

Fig. 13 Comparative MRI images of the left TMJ, sagittal internal slice, closed mouth position, (**a**) before treatment and (**b**) after the first phase of the treatment

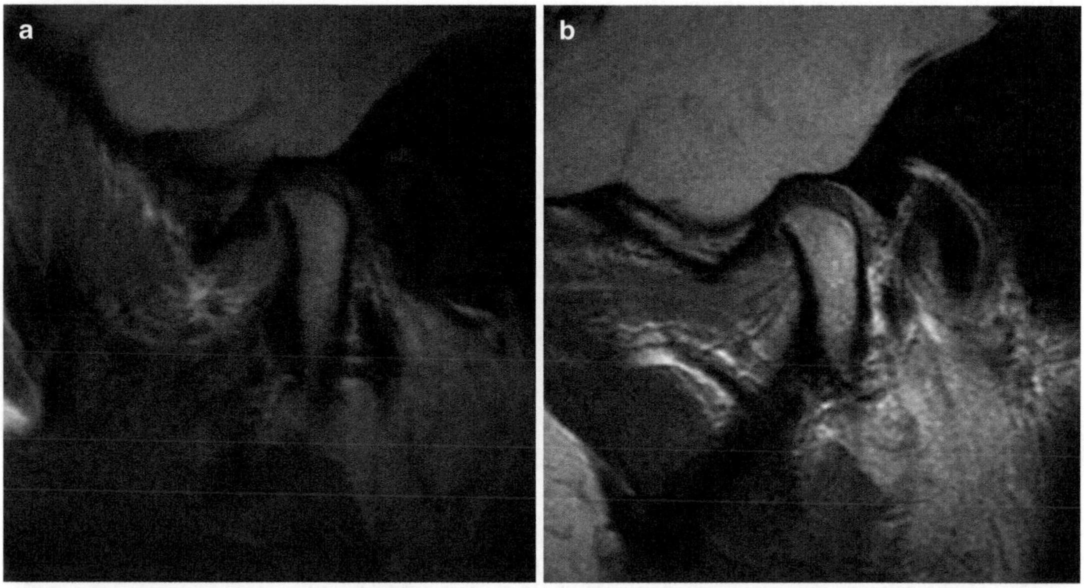

Fig. 14 Comparative MRI images of the right TMJ, sagittal external slice, closed mouth position, (**a**) before treatment and (**b**) after the first phase of the treatment

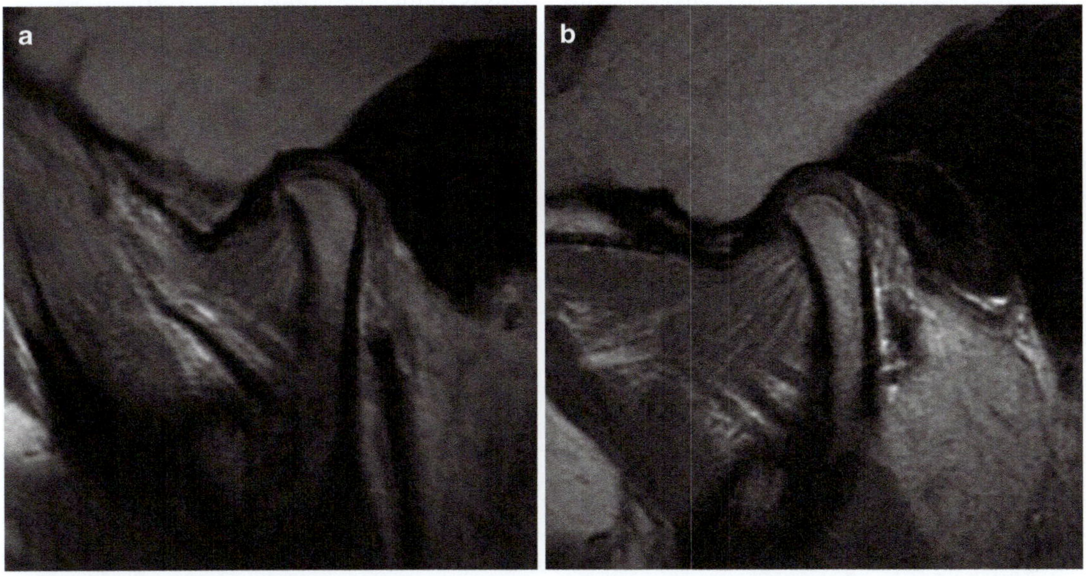

Fig. 15 Comparative MRI images of the right TMJ, sagittal medial slice, closed mouth position, (**a**) before treatment and (**b**) after the first phase of the treatment

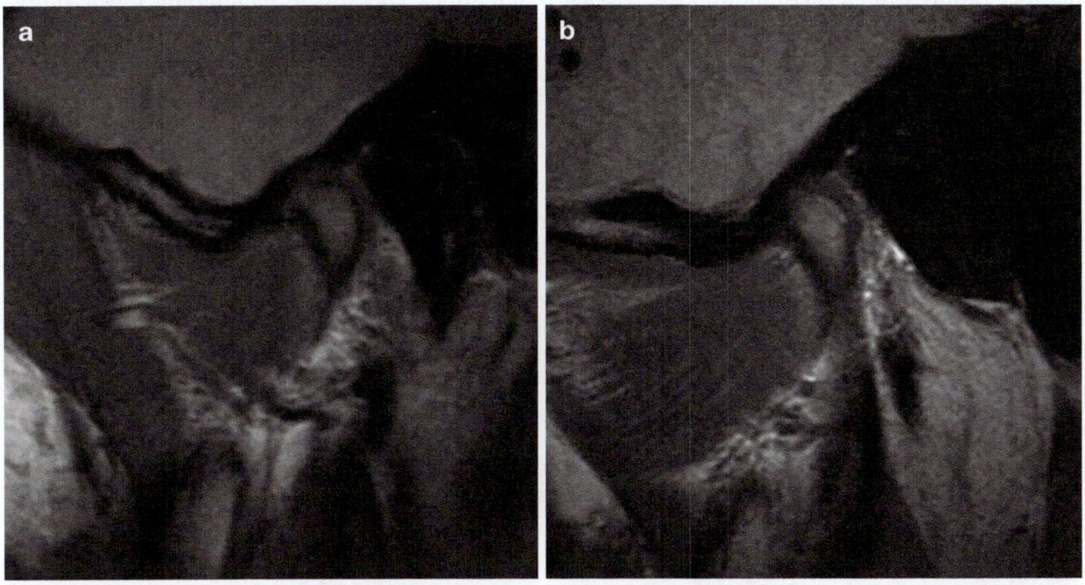

Fig. 16 Comparative MRI images of the right TMJ, sagittal internal slice, closed mouth position, (**a**) before treatment and (**b**) after the first phase of the treatment

3 Case 2

3.1 Conductive Hearing Loss Resulting from Eustachian Tube Dysfunction Initiated by TMJ Disorders. When Measuring Makes the Difference

Symptoms of mild hearing loss occurring in childhood may go unnoticed. The early detection of this disability is vital. Various physical and psychological activities of children and adolescents may be affected due to hearing impairment. The conductive hearing loss resulting from Eustachian tube dysfunction initiated by TMJ disorders is often not considered; however, it is essential to think about this etiologic origin.

There are two general types of hearing loss, conductive and sensorineural. Conductive hearing loss results from a disruption in the passage of sound from the external ear to the oval window. Anatomically, this pathway includes the ear canal, tympanic membrane, and ossicles (middle ear). Such loss may be due to cerumen impaction, tympanic membrane perforation, otitis media/middle ear effusion, otosclerosis, intra-aural muscle dysfunction, or displacement of the ossicles by the malleolar ligament.

Sensorineural hearing loss results from otologic abnormalities within the cochlea and auditory nerve (CN VIII). Such abnormalities may affect the sensory cells of the cochlea or the neural fibers of the eighth cranial nerve. Hearing loss from loud noise exposure or from advanced age (presbycusis) is an example of sensorineural hearing loss. Cerebellopontine angle tumors rarely lead to such hearing loss.

3.2 Case Report

An 11-year-old male patient arrived at the clinic for consultation complaining of headache, pain on the back of the head, shoulder pain, neck pain, hand numbness, tingling in hands, and limited mouth opening. The patient also reported pain in the left ear, a sensation of ear blockage on the left, as well as tinnitus and diminished hearing in both ears. An antecedent of trauma on the chin in early childhood is relevant to the patient's medical history. It is also important to consider a history of recurrent ear and throat infections and severe pneumonia that required hospitalization when he was 8 months old. A significant overbite and lack of space for the correct positioning of the left maxillary canine can be seen (Fig. 17). One can observe in Figs. 18 and 19 (1) the superior and posterior position of the left condylar process in the articular cavity when the jaw is in the position of maximum intercuspation. Rectification of the cervical spine is observed in this radiograph (Fig. 20).

The disc is slightly anteriorly dislocated (Fig. 21a) in the right TMJ; Fig. 21b the same

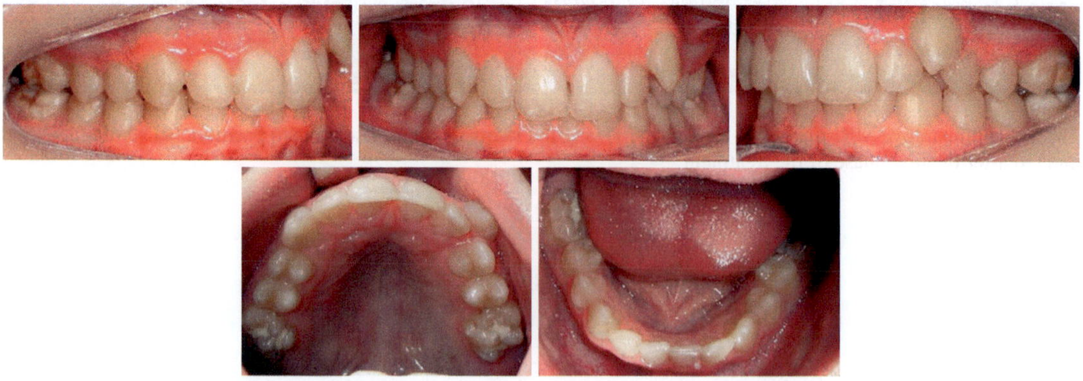

Fig. 17 Patient's habitual occlusion (above). Upper and lower occlusal view (below)

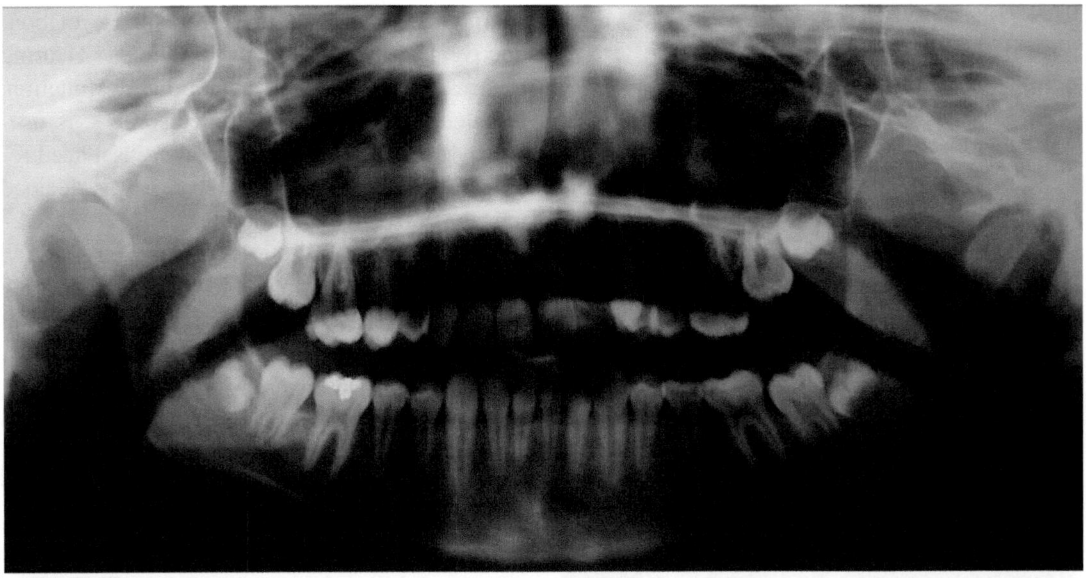

Fig. 18 Patient's panoramic radiograph

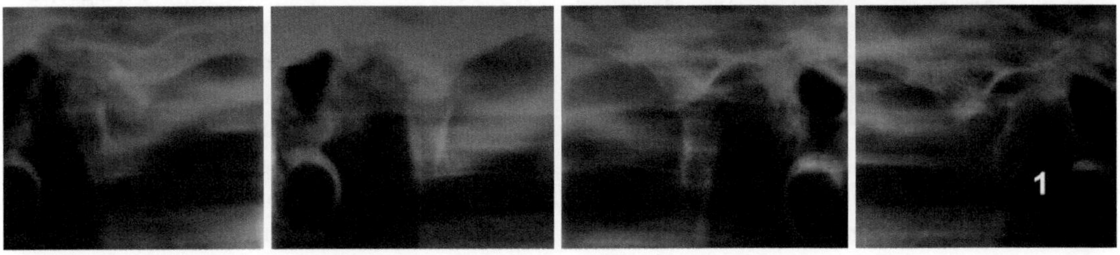

Fig. 19 Patient temporomandibular joint laminography, open and closed mouth

image is given with a color highlight. The anterior dislocation is more evident in the left TMJ Fig. 21c, where the head of the mandible is backed on the retrodiscal zone; Fig. 21d the same image is given with a color highlight. We can also observe anterior facets on both the right and left mandibular heads. Both mandibular condyles cannot translate, limiting mouth opening (Fig. 22). Anterior right and left temporalis muscles, right and left masseter muscles, right and left digastric muscles, and right and left superior trapezius muscles are recorded in dynamic surface electromyography (Fig. 23) (2) in habitual occlusion, open mouth, close mouth, bite clenching, and to swallowing in this order for this exam.

One can see the activation of the digastric muscles when the patient closes the mouth. These muscles should be active when opening but not closing. During the examination, there was an activation of the right and left upper trapezius muscles, even when the patient was instructed to lower his shoulders. He had activated both trapezii throughout the examination. Because of the patient's reported hearing symptoms, we requested an audiogram, which can be seen in Fig. 24 from the patient's otorhinolaryngologist.

An audiogram is produced by using a relative measurement of the patient's hearing as compared with an established "normal" value. It is a graphic representation of auditory threshold responses that are obtained from testing a patient's hearing with pure-tone stimuli. The parameters of the audiogram are frequency, as measured in cycles per second (Hz), and intensity, as measured in decibels (dB). The first audiometry of the patient

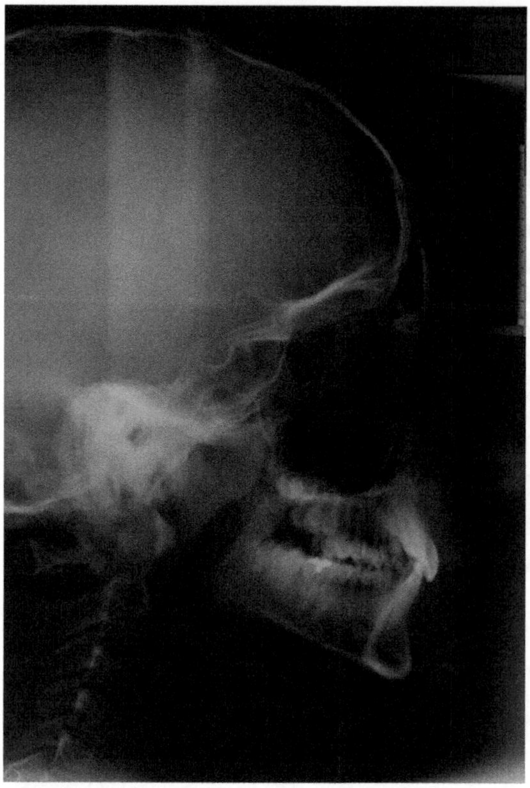

Fig. 20 Patient's lateral radiograph

revealed a mild hearing loss in his left ear and moderate hearing loss in his right ear. Hearing loss is classified as mild when the ear is unable to detect sounds below 40 dB, which makes it difficult to understand human speech. In the moderate loss, sounds below 70 dB are not heard.

The mandibular rest position was recorded after electronic deprogramming, together with the information from the MRI to orient decisions regarding bite registration, for the three-dimensional construction of the orthotic (Figs. 25 and 26). The patient had a pathological free space of 8.6 mm and 8 mm of mandibular retro-position. The retrusion of the mandible, whether iatrogenically induced or because of malocclusion, often results in otalgia due to excessive compression of the neurovascular retrodiscal tissues. The patient can feel ear pain. The degree of compression determines the degree of pain for the patient.

The parents of the patient were informed that the priority at this stage was the patient's health, focusing on improving function, controlling symptoms, and observing the response of conductive hearing loss to the treatment. Hearing loss resulting from Eustachian tube dysfunction, initiated by craniomandibular disorders, is usually subjective; for this reason, there is a need for objective control by audiometry. It was decided to stage corrective orthodontics.

The installed orthotic is controlled through surface electromyography (SEMG) to evaluate its function (Fig. 27). A significant reduction in digastric muscle activity was realized, the trapezius muscles were not activated during clenching, and the masseter muscles increased their activity. Controlling the orthotic with SEMG is important to check the improvement of motor unit recruitment and the requirement for recalibration or orthotic substitution. It takes time and effort to stabilize the muscles and the TMJ, when possible, during treatment; this time and effort vary with different patients, different ages, and different pathologies. Even a decompressed joint takes time to recover. Some structural lesions can be recovered, while others cannot.

The patient's third audiogram shows normal thresholds in the left and in the right ear (Fig. 28). With the normalization of the conductive hearing loss, the remission of symptoms, and the improvement of images from the exams, second phase of the TMJ treatment commenced. This includes three-dimensional orthodontics, neuromuscular physiological rehabilitation, or a combination of both, to remove the orthotic used during the first phase of the treatment (Fig. 29). In the second phase, the use of the orthotic during the active eruption of the teeth must be continued, and the mandible should maintain the best position possible to that which was achieved with the first orthotic. This means equilibrium with the muscular planes and the temporomandibular joint.

In tridimensional orthodontics, during the active eruption of the teeth in the second phase of TMJ treatment, the orthotic is changed and/or recalibrated, as required (Fig. 30). Not every case will allow the implementation of a second phase of treatment. There are cases where the TMJ is severely damaged and/or patients with active autoimmune diseases will have an affected joint (Fig. 31). There was no recovery of the physio-

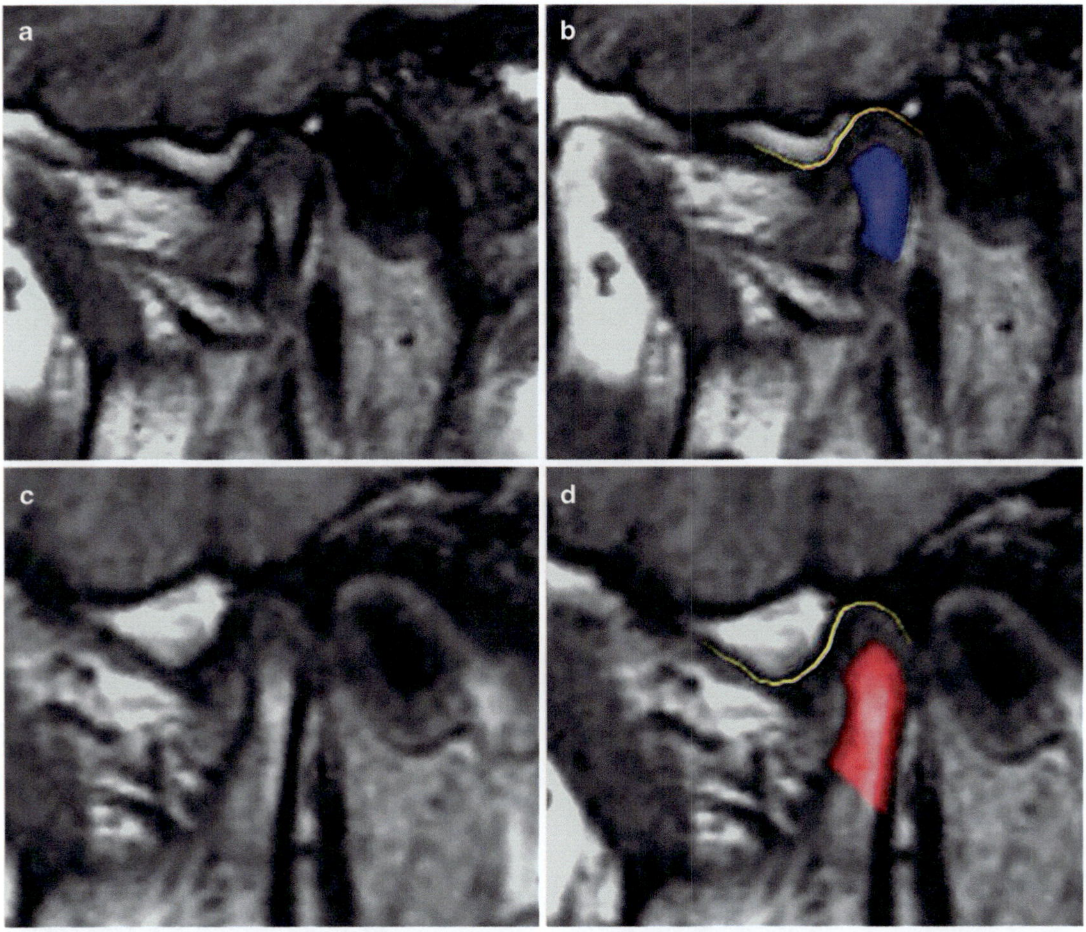

Fig. 21 MRI T1: Left and right TMJ sagittal slice, closed mouth before treatment

logical lordosis apparent in the patient's cervical spine image; however, an improvement can be seen (Fig. 32). The mouth opening of the patient improved from 32.9 to 38.9 mm and also reached an optimum speed regarding mouth opening and closing (Figs. 33 and 34).

The SEMG after the two phases of treatment demonstrates the symmetry between the anterior temporal muscles and between the masseter muscles. There is very low digastric muscle activity (Fig. 35a). The habitual trajectory is not coincident with the neuromuscular trajectory seen before the treatment Fig. 35b. The habitual trajectory is tridimensionally coincident with the neuromuscular trajectory after treatment. Tridimensional orthodontics needs to maintain the tridimensional position of the mandible in balance with its osseous and muscular planes as close as possible to the result obtained in the first phase. The conductive hearing loss resulting from Eustachian tube dysfunction initiated by temporomandibular disorders is often not considered (Fig. 36). The early detection of this deficiency is vital.

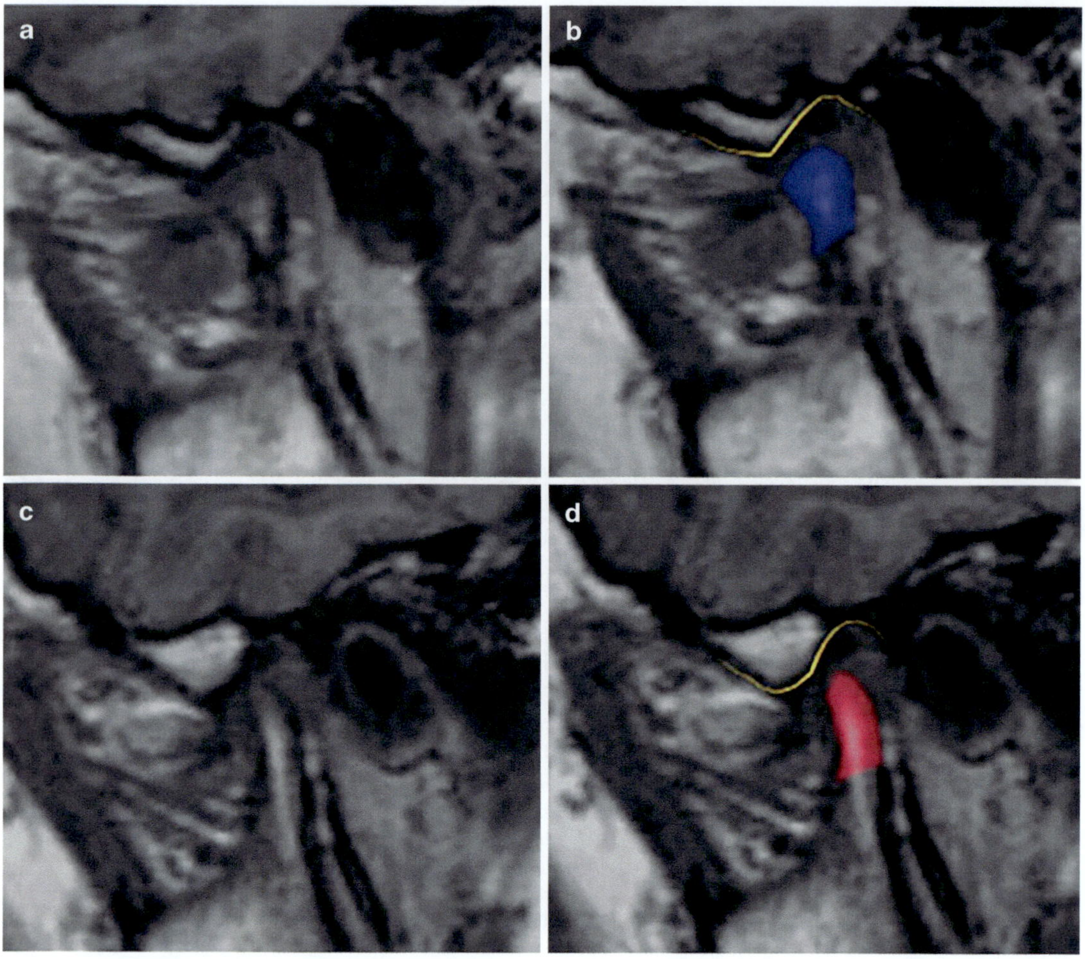

Fig. 22 MRI T1: Sagittal slice, left and right TMJ open mouth before treatment

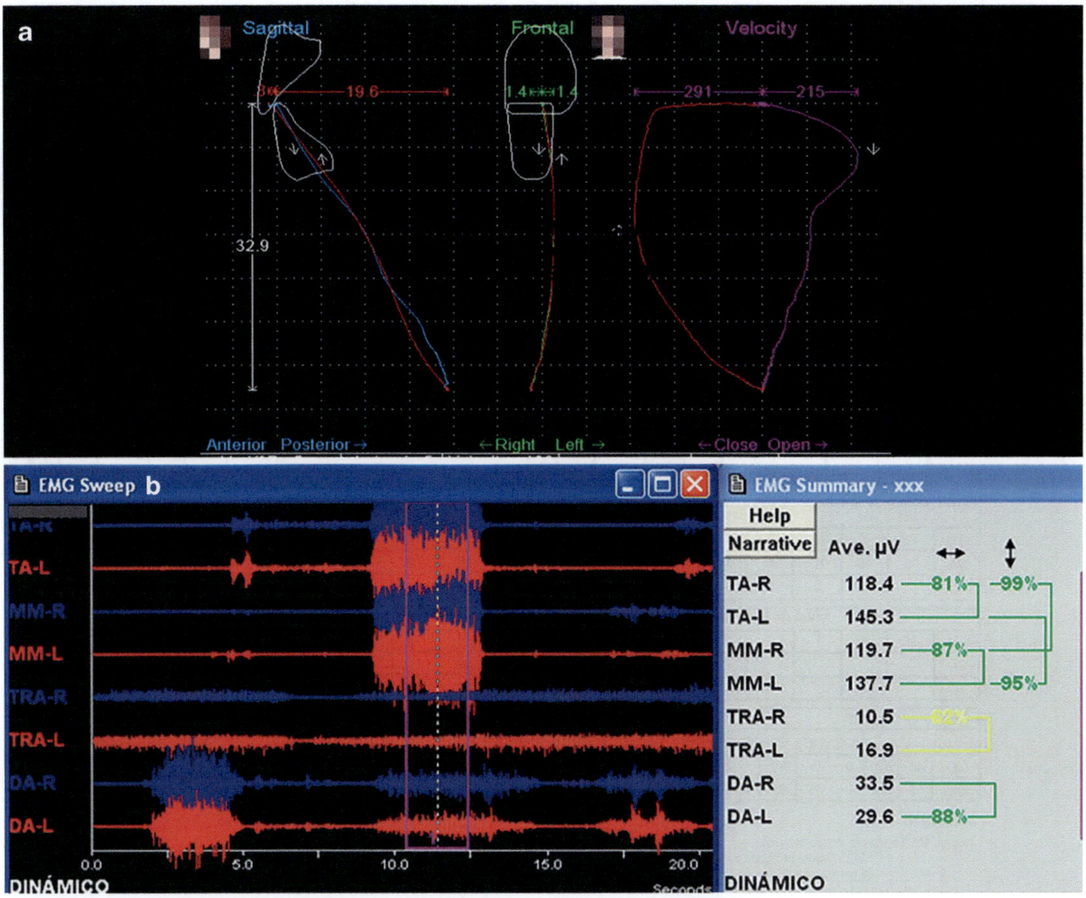

Fig. 23 (**a**) Initial kinesiographic and (**b**) initial electromyographic record. In the kinesiographic record (**a**), there is a reduced speed when the patient opens and closes his mouth, and limited mouth opening to only 32.9 mm. There is no coincidence between the opening and closing trajectories in the sagittal view of the record

AUDIOMETRIA TONAL LIMINAR

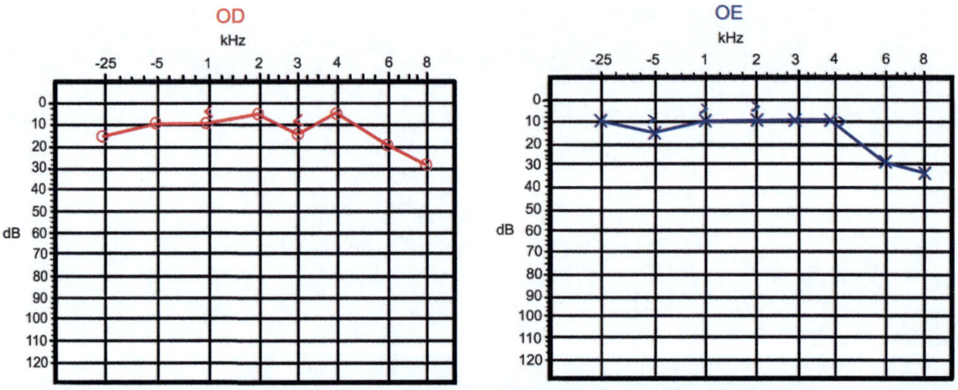

OD

Limiar									
kHz	-25	-5	1	2	3	4	6	8	
VA	15	10	10	5	15	5	20	30	dB
VO		10	5	5	10	5			dB

Nível de Mascaramento									
kHz	-25	-5	1	2	3	4	6	8	
VA									dB
VO									dB

IRF						
			MONOS		DISSIL	
OD	45	dB	0	%	96	%
OE	45	dB	0	%	96	%

RINNE		
kHz	-25	-5
OD		
OE		

OE

Limiar									
kHz	-25	-5	1	2	3	4	6	8	
VA	10	15	10	10	10	10	30	35	dB
VO		10	5	5	10	10			dB

Nível de Mascaramento									
kHz	-25	-5	1	2	3	4	6	8	
VA									dB
VO									dB

WEBER						
kHz	-25	-5	1	2	4	

LFR		
OD	0	dB
OE	0	dB

Conclusão:

AUDIOMETRIA: Na presente data:
O.D.: discreta hipoacusia a 8 KHz.
O.E.: Leve hipoacusia a 6 e 8 KHz.

RE : = Mild hearing loss 8 kHz

LE: Moderate hearing loss 6 e 8 kHz

Fig. 24 Threshold tonal audiometry

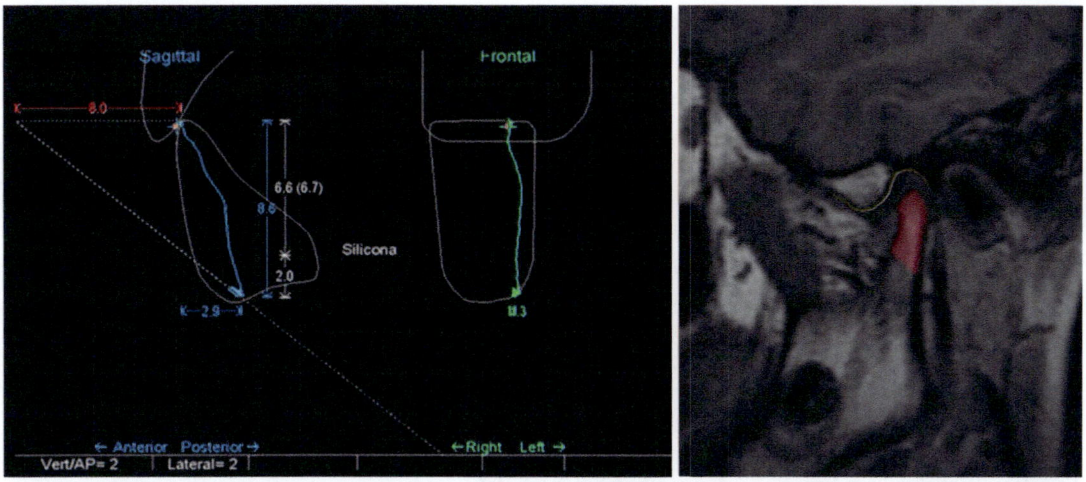

Fig. 25 Graphic for mandible tridimensional position after electronic deprogramming together with the MRI image of the left TMJ, which was more compromised

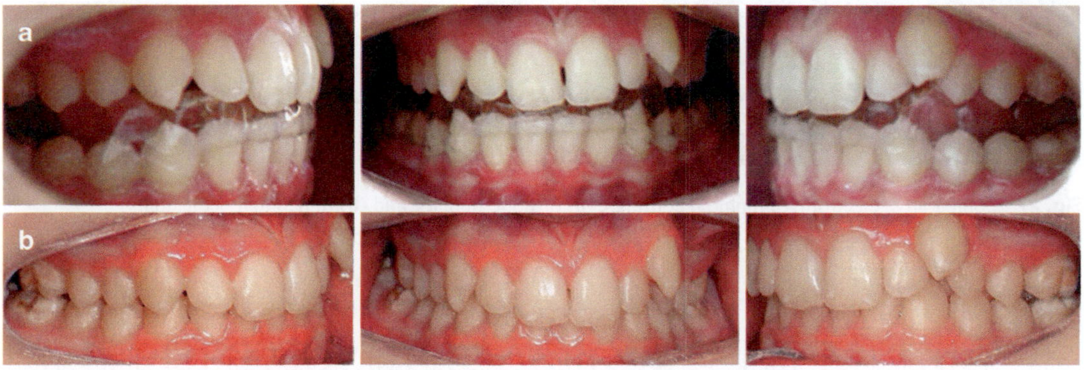

Fig. 26 Patient's comparative occlusions (**a**) with the orthotic and (**b**) habitual occlusion

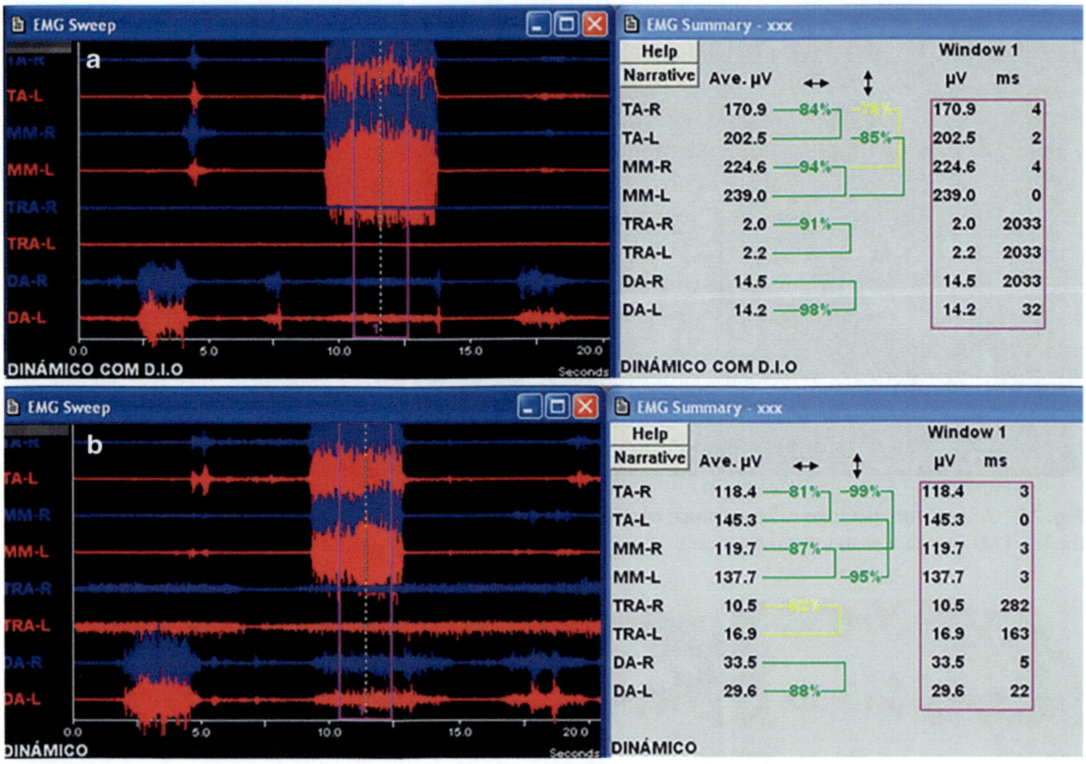

Fig. 27 Comparative electromyographic recordings, (**a**) orthotic in place and (**b**) in habitual occlusion

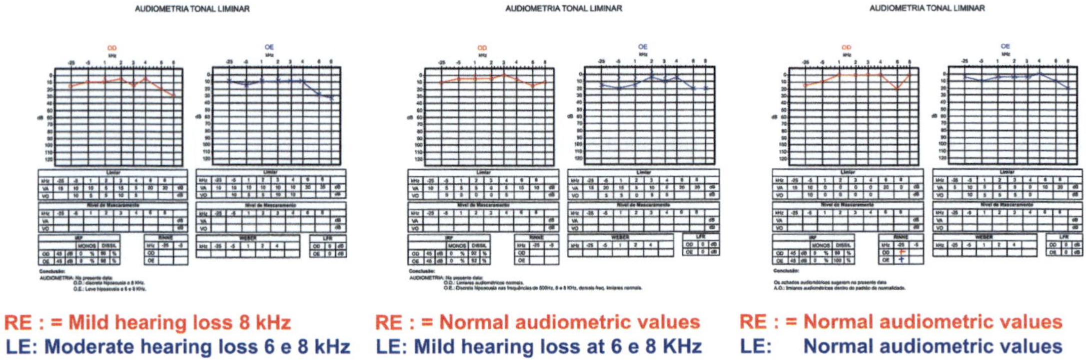

Fig. 28 Comparison of patient's first, second, and third audiometry during treatment

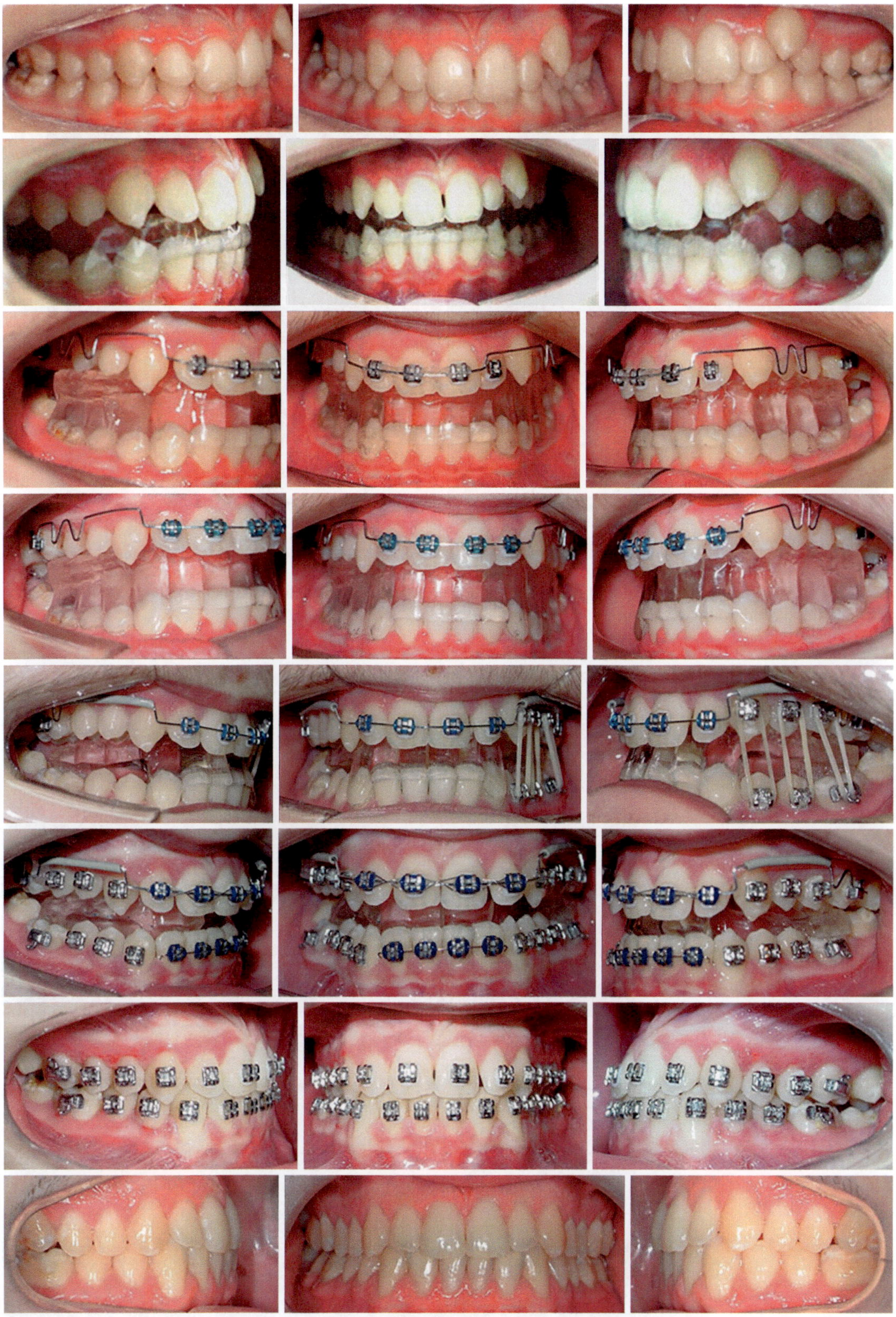

Fig. 29 From top to bottom, a sequence of three-dimensional orthodontics in the second phase of the treatment of TMJ disorders

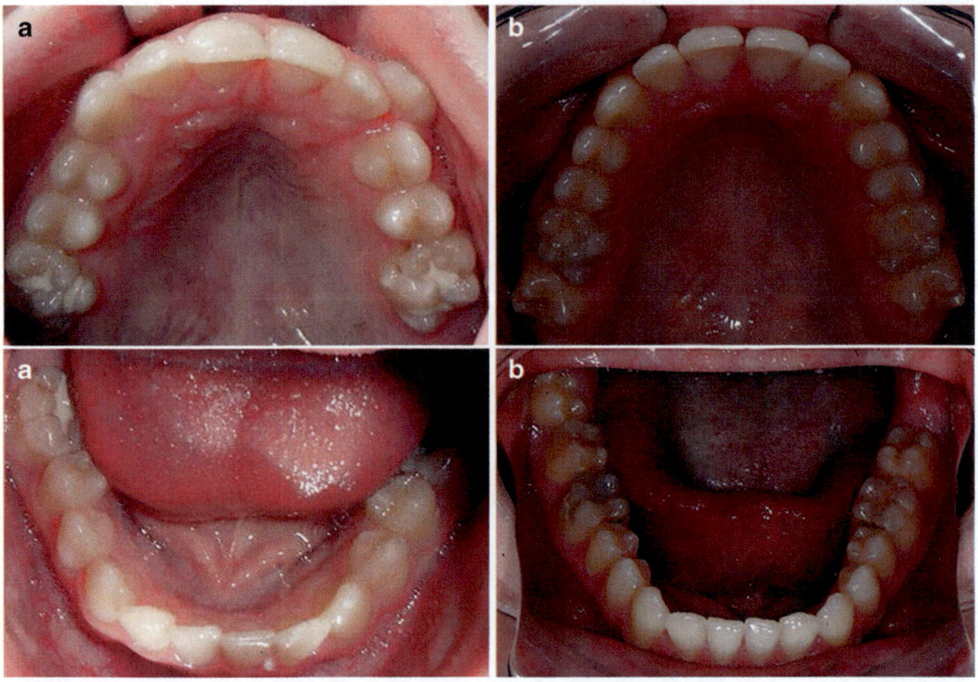

Fig. 30 Patient's comparative images of the upper and lower occlusal views before (**a**) and (**b**) after completion of the first- and the second-phase treatment

Fig. 31 Comparative panoramic radiographs: (**a**) before treatment and (**b**) after completion of the three-dimensional orthodontics

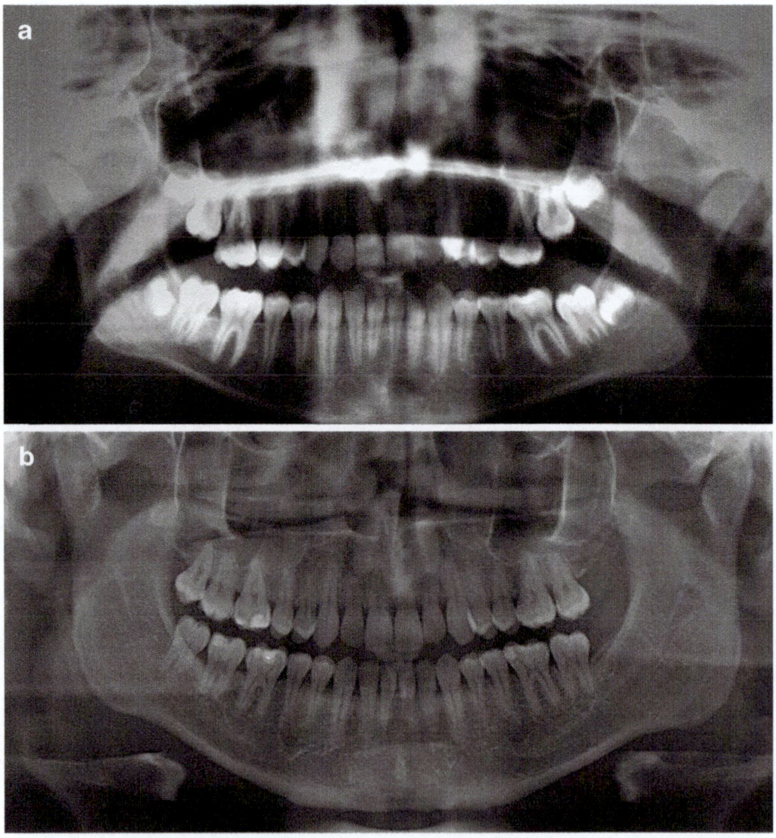

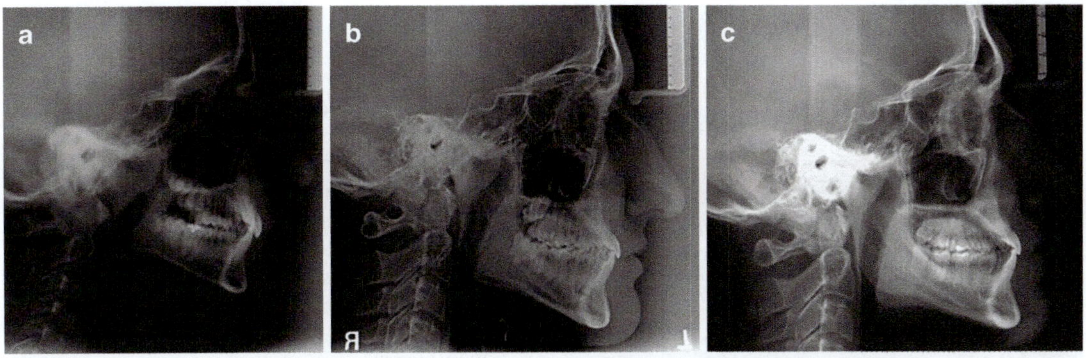

Fig. 32 Comparative lateral radiographs of the patient: (**a**) at the beginning of the treatment in habitual occlusion, (**b**) after the completion of the three-dimensional orthodontic, and (**c**) 6 years after treatment conclusion

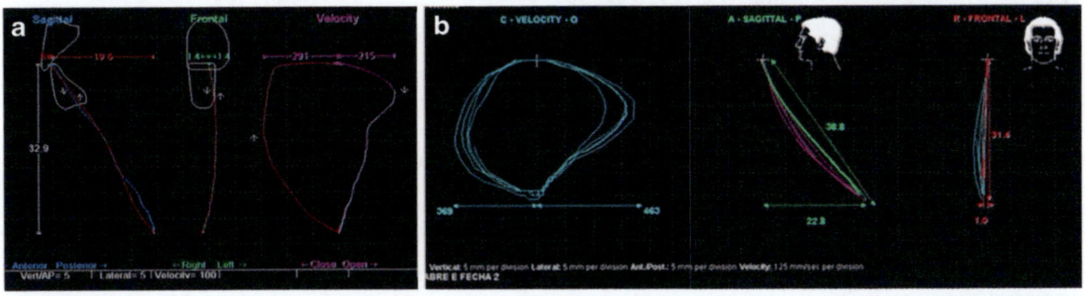

Fig. 33 Patient's kinesiographic records' comparison: before and after the two phases of orthodontic treatment

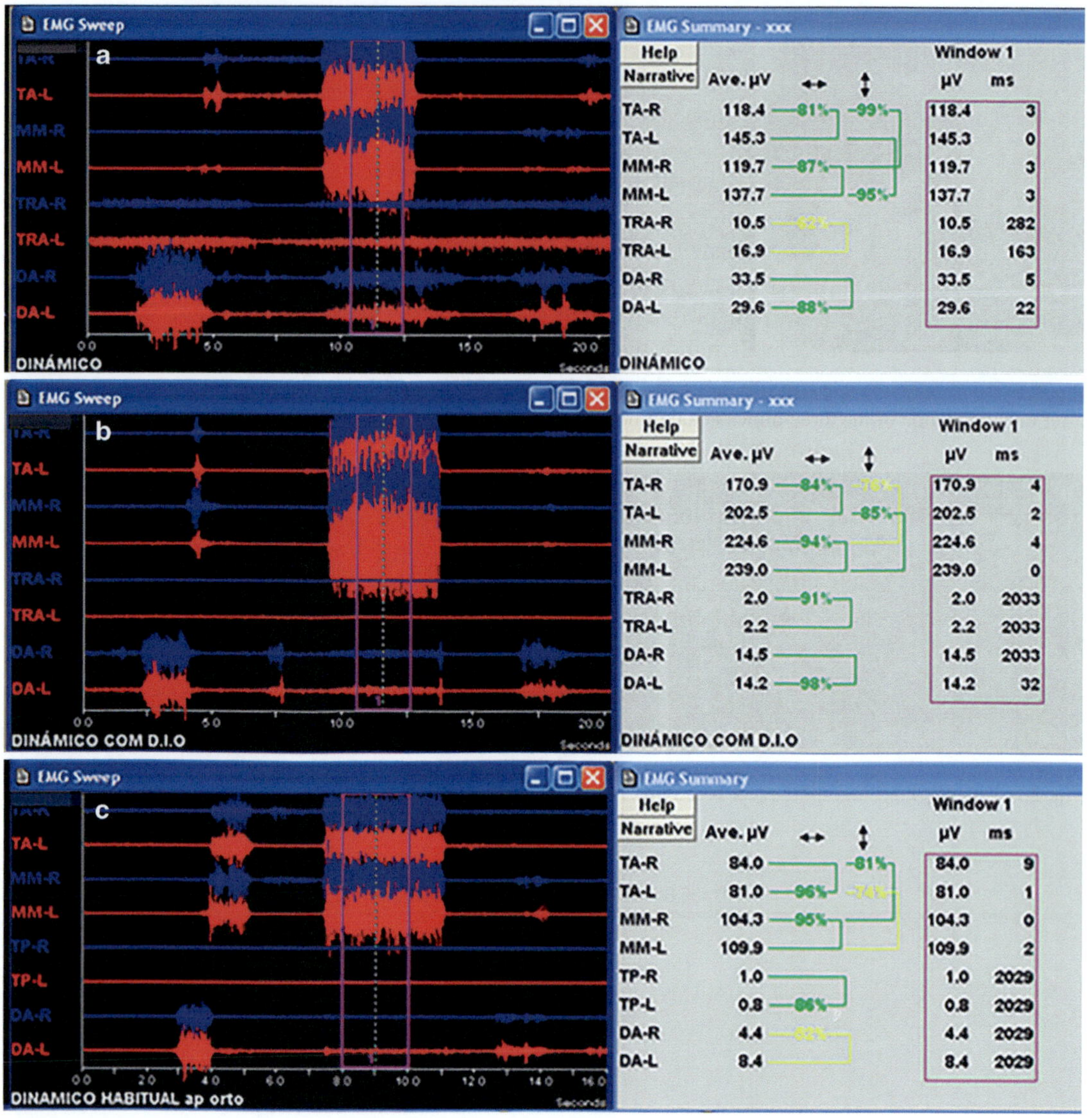

Fig. 34 Patient's electromyography comparison: (**a**) before, (**b**) during the first phase with the orthotic, and (**c**) after the completion of the orthodontic treatment

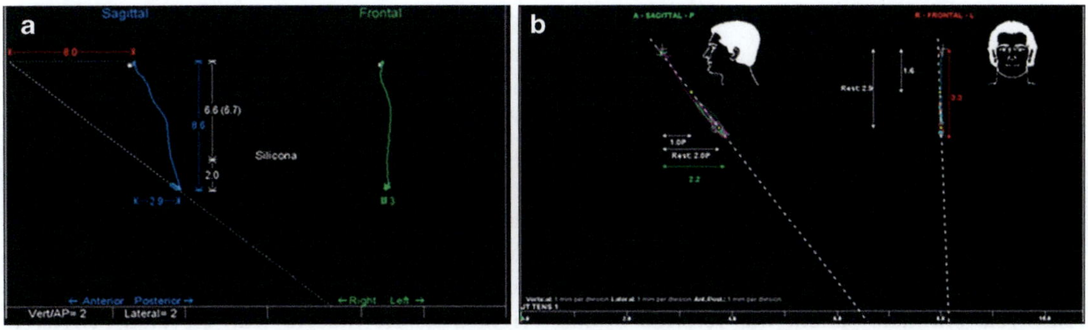

Fig. 35 Patient's kinesiographic records' comparison after electronically mandibular deprogramming (**a**) before treatment and (**b**) after treatment

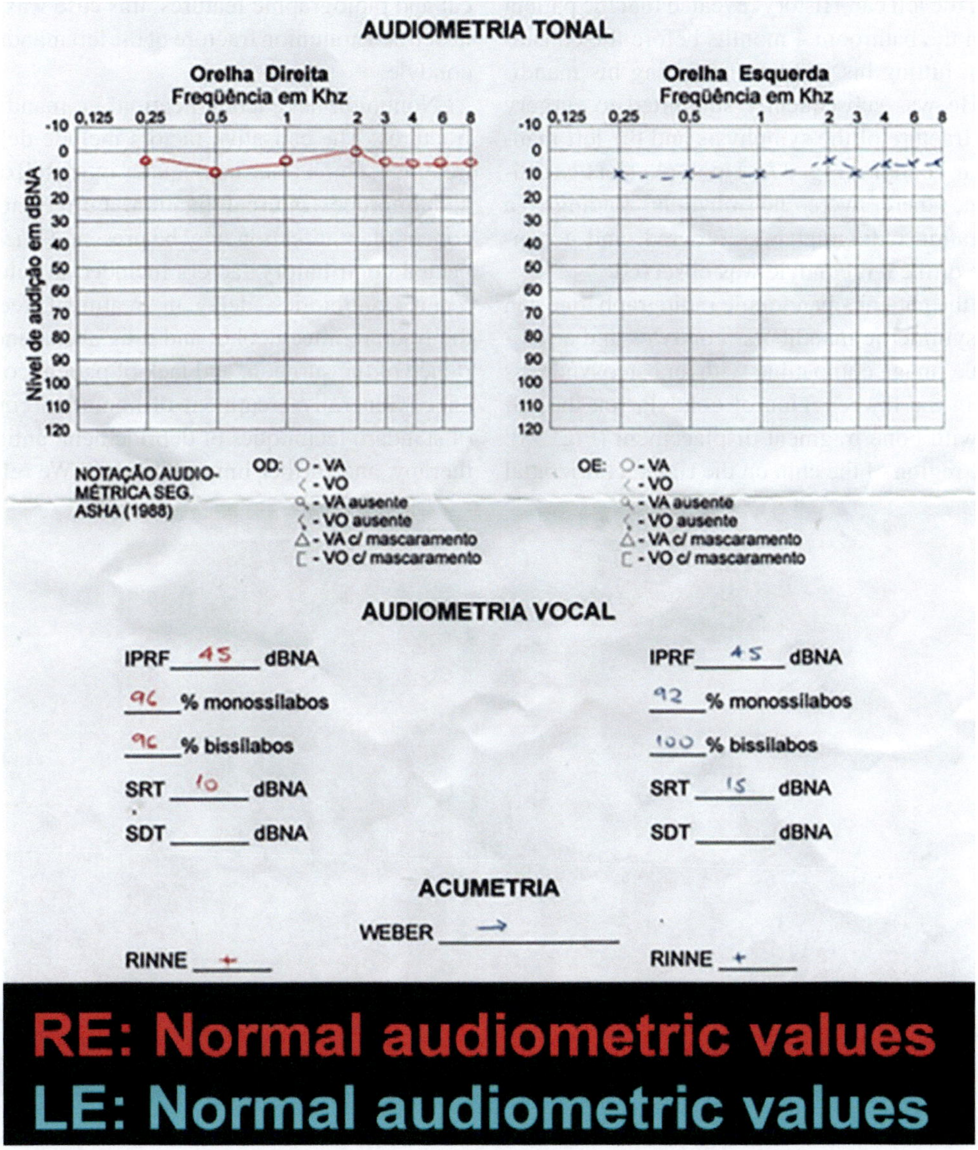

Fig. 36 Threshold tonal audiometry 6 years after the completion of the two phases of TMJ treatment

4 Case 3

4.1 Mandible Condyle Fracture Consolidation by Neuromuscular and Physiological Alignment of the Segments, 4 Months After Unsuccessful Surgery

A 57-year-old male patient was referred by his dentist. His principal complaints were lack of strength when chewing, difficulty in opening the mouth, cervical pain, pain in the TMJs, and ringing in the left ear. History revealed that the patient fell in the bathroom 4 months before the consultation, hitting his jaw and fracturing his mandible. He was subsequently submitted to surgery for a fracture of the symphysis and the left mandibular condyle (Fig. 37). Upon physical examination, there were no obvious findings, a panoramic radiograph was ordered, and a nonunion of the left condyle was observed.

In the patient's panoramic radiograph, one can see asymmetric mandibular condyles and a radiopaque image compatible with an osteosynthesis wire in the lower region of condylar on the left side with bone fragment displacement (Fig. 38). In the region of the chin on the right, a horizontal radiopaque image compatible with an osteosynthesis device for repair of the fracture of the anterior symphysis can be seen. Dental abnormalities included missing dentition and a posterior open bite on the left side (Fig. 39).

A CT was ordered (Figs. 40 and 41). The surface electromyographic record before electronic deprogramming showed the right and left masseter muscles, the right trapezius muscle, and the right digastric muscle with elevated activity at rest. The activity of most of these muscles lowered after electronic deprogramming (Fig. 42). Based on the case history and its clinical and radiographic features, this case was diagnosed as a nonunion fracture of the left mandibular condyle.

Nonunion is a complication in mandibular fractures. The causative factors include delay in treatment, infection, inadequate immobilization, and improper internal fixation. Furthermore, a concomitant infection may be present. Other suspected contributory factors included a failure to receive antibiotics, delay in treatment, teeth in the fracture line, alcohol and drug abuse, inexperience of the surgeon, and lack of patient compliance. Generally, treatment of nonunion consists of standard techniques of debridement, antibiotic therapy, and further immobilization. We referred

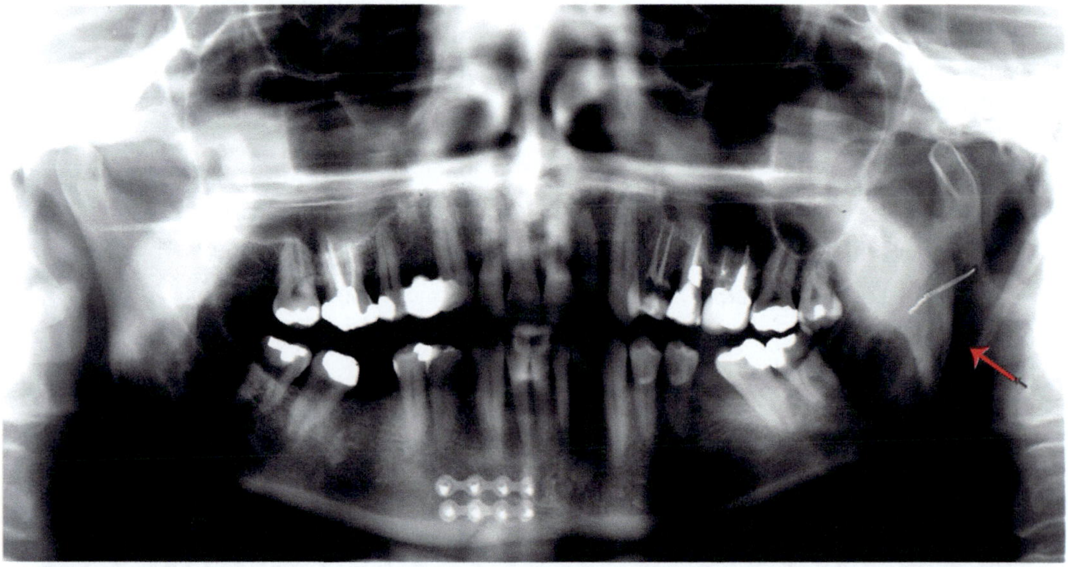

Fig. 37 Patient's panoramic radiograph on the day of consultation showing a nonunion of the left condyle (arrow)

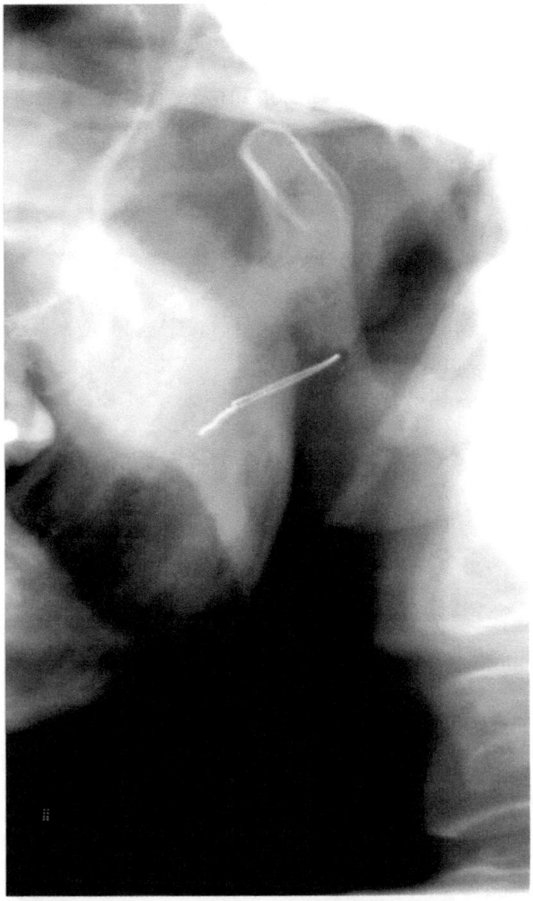

Fig. 38 Magnification of the left mandibular condyle on the panoramic radiograph demonstrating attempted wire synthesis

the patient back to the surgeon where a new surgical procedure was proposed. The patient refused to undergo another surgical procedure.

Considering the patient's refusal of revision surgery, a conservative approach was then proposed. The patient was informed about possible limitations due to his age. Ultralow-frequency and low-amplitude transcutaneous electrical neural stimulation (TENS) of the mandibular division of the trigeminal nerve (V) was used to relax the masticatory muscles to record the rest position of the mandible. The mandibular rest position was recorded after electronic deprogramming, together with the information from the MRI to orient bite registration, and a three-dimensional orthotic was fabricated (Fig. 43). The patient had a pathological free space of 6.4 mm and 4.3 mm of mandibular retro-position. This tridimensional mandible rest position was recorded in the form of a bite occlusal registration, which was later used to construct an orthotic (Fig. 44). This removable mandibular appliance must be worn during the day and night. This intraoral appliance tested by electromyography and kinesiographically supports the neuromuscular physiological position. The patient was asked to wear the intraoral appliance full-time and to remove it only for cleaning. The dynamic evaluations improved, and the patient felt no more pain or chewing difficulty. During the treatment, new orthotics in neuromuscular physiological position were constructed (Fig. 45).

A second panoramic radiograph was taken after 3 months. The new panoramic radiograph (Fig. 46b) showed an improvement in the condyle position. Finally, 4 months after the second panoramic radiograph, a third image (Fig. 46c) was ordered where union of the fracture was demonstrated. These images show (a) the day of the first consultation with the habitual occlusion; (b) 3 months later with the first orthotic; and (c) 7 months after the first consultation with a new orthotic; an improvement of condyle position and the bone union can clearly be seen. It is important to note the changes not only in the images but also in the occlusion with the orthotics as the muscles adjust to a more physiological position. A new CT was ordered (Fig. 47) and clearly showed the union of the fracture without subjecting the patient to a second surgery and without using any maxillomandibular fixation (MMF).

Fractures of the mandibular condyle are one of the most commonly occurring mandibular fractures. Management of these fractures has always been a controversial issue. One of the complications of mandibular condyle fracture is nonunion. Fractures, where the muscles tend to draw fragments together, are more favorable than those fractures where the muscles tend to draw fragments apart. The distraction of fracture fragments is observed in many mandibular condyle fractures. The most observed type is the displacement of the condyle head to the anteromedial

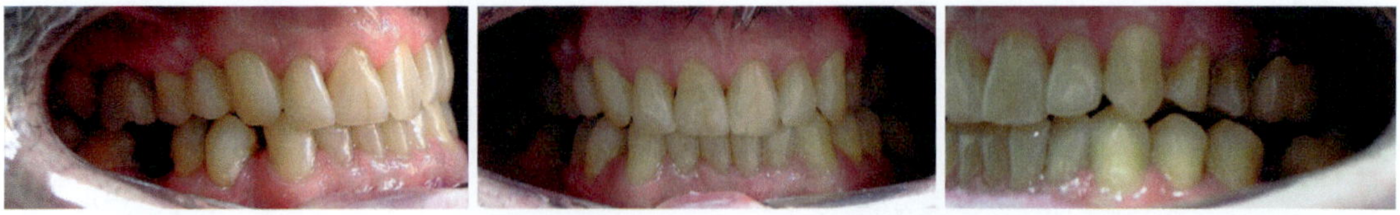

Fig. 39 Patient's habitual occlusion on the day of consultation

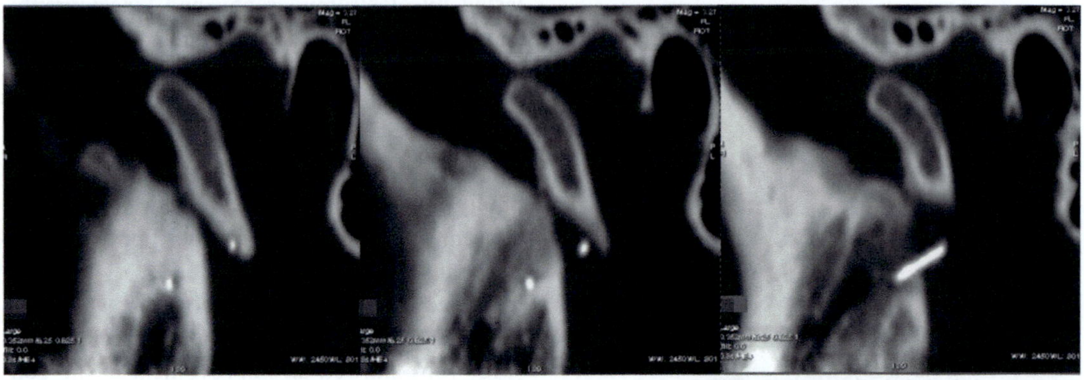

Fig. 40 CT sagittal slices confirming the **nonunion of the mandibular condyle fracture 4 months after surgery**

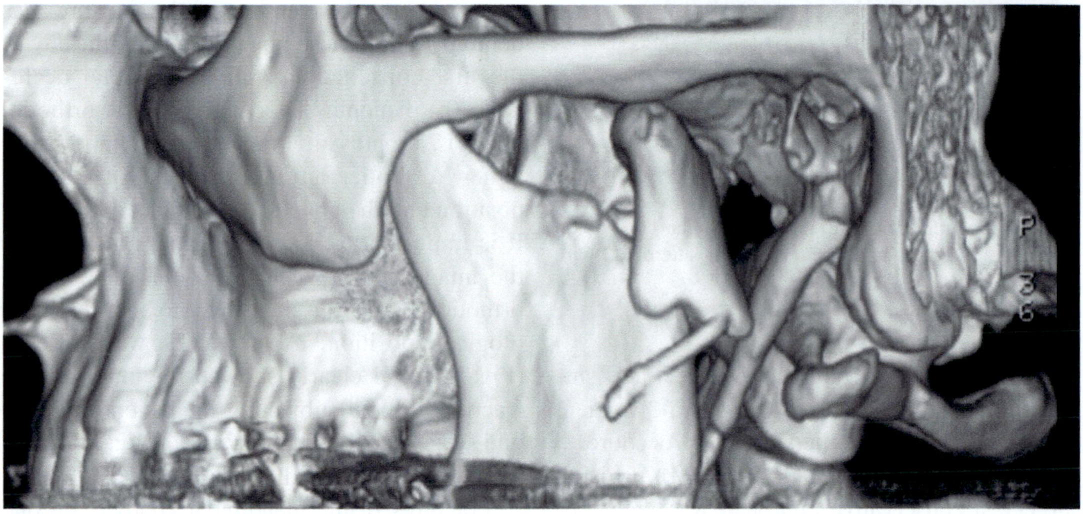

Fig. 41 3D reconstruction showing **nonunion of the mandibular condyle fracture 4 months after surgery**

side because of lateral pterygoid muscle action. The ability to place the mandible in a spatial relationship by measuring the masticatory muscles at their resting length can be an important auxiliary tool to assist in the rehabilitation of condylar fractures.

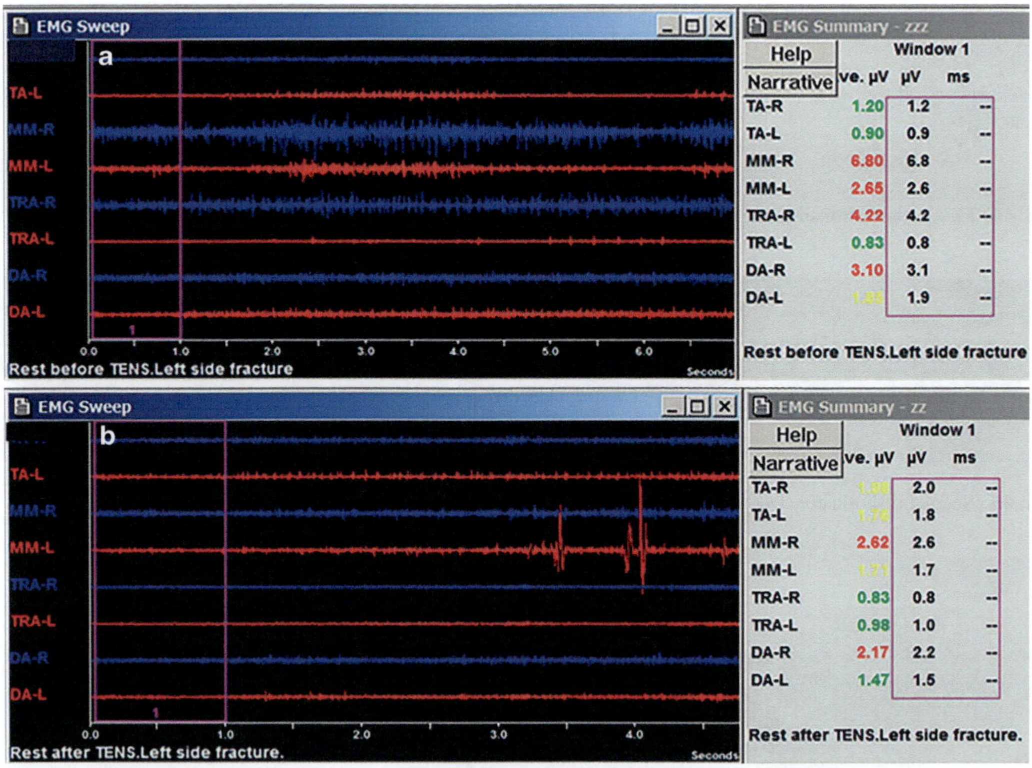

Fig. 42 Comparative rest electromyography (**a**) before and (**b**) after electronic deprogramming

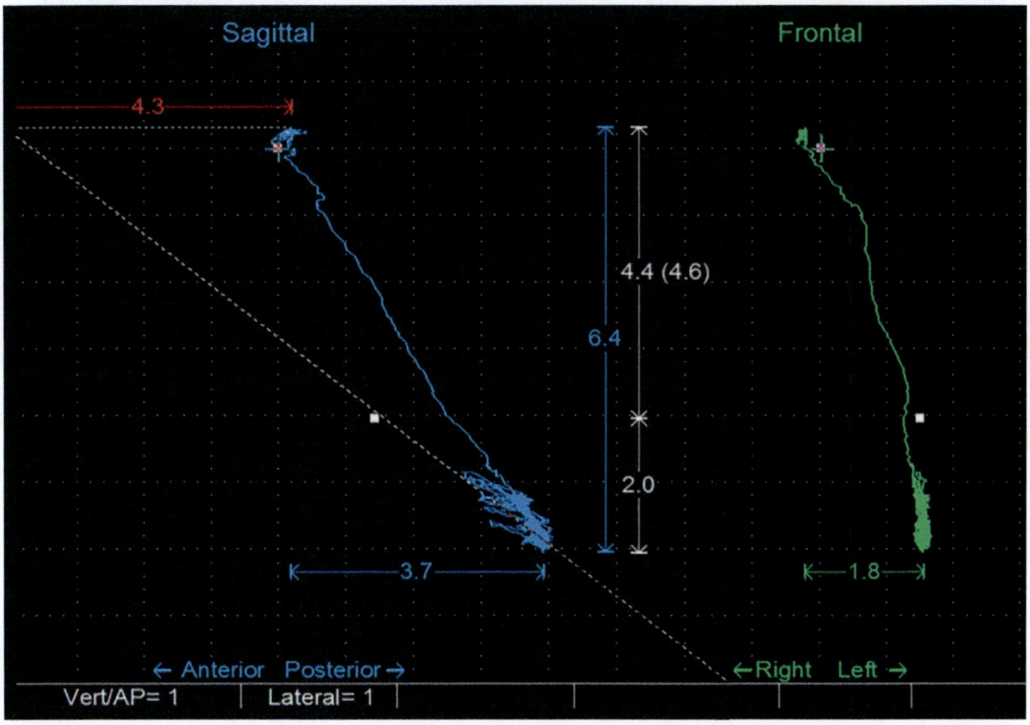

Fig. 43 Graphic record of the mandible tridimensional position after electronic deprogramming

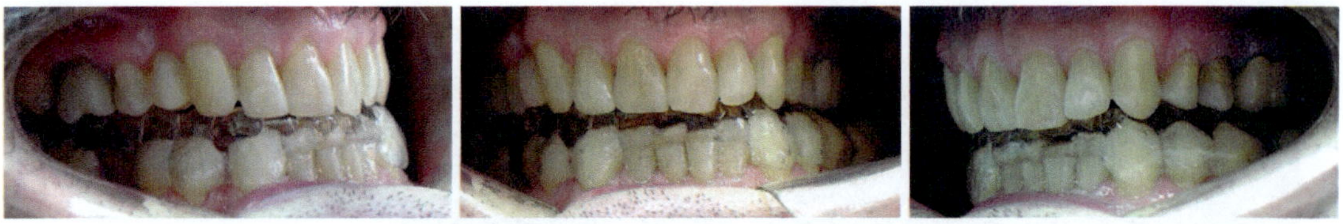

Fig. 44 First orthotic constructed in a neuromuscular and physiological position

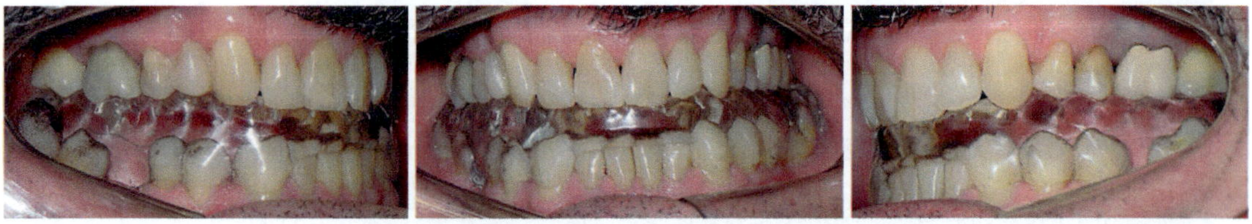

Fig. 45 Second orthotic constructed in a neuromuscular and physiological position

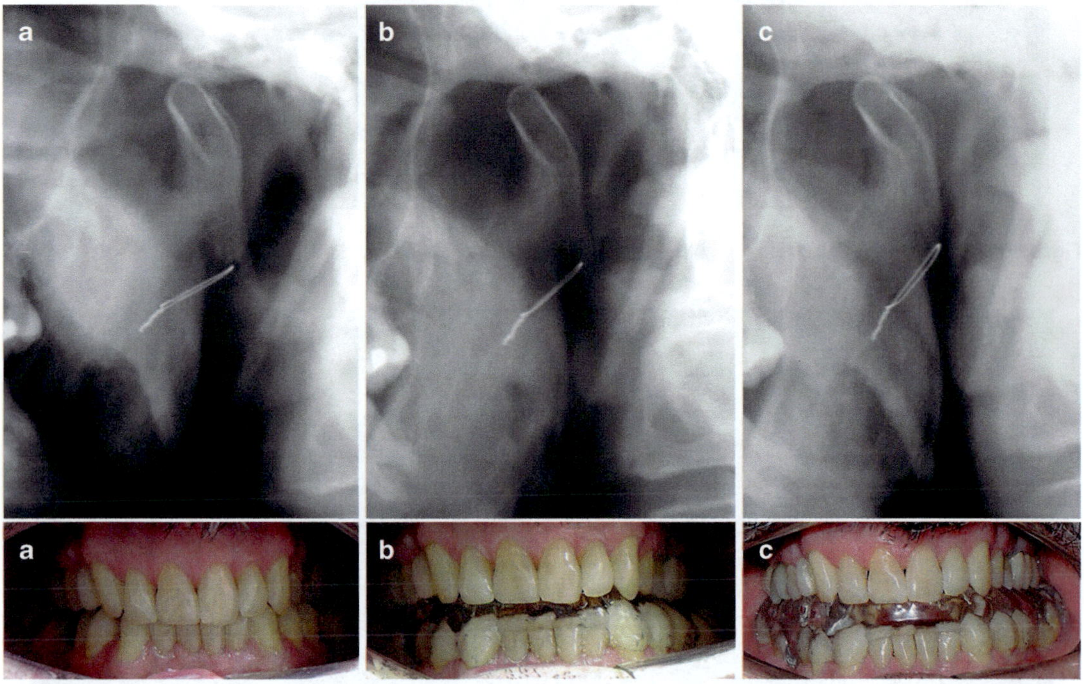

Fig. 46 Comparative images of the first (**a**), second (**b**), and third (**c**) left condyle on the section of the panoramic radiographs

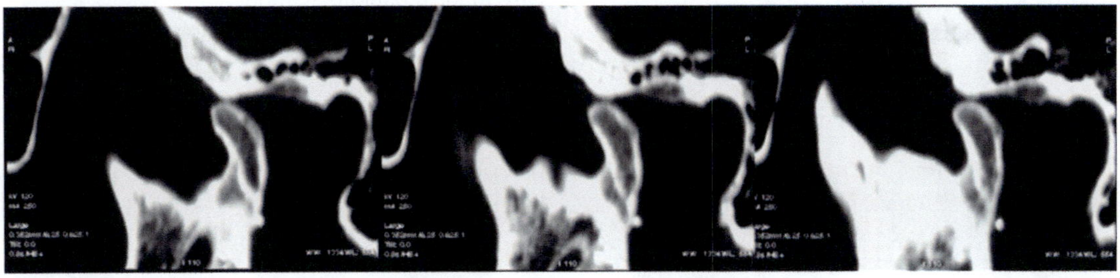

Fig. 47 CT sagittal slices confirming the union of the mandibular condyle fracture following treatment

5 Case 4

5.1 Patient with Autoimmune Disease and a Compressive Noninflammatory TMJ Pathology

A 40-year-old female patient, with a diagnosis of seronegative spondyloarthropathy, later diagnosed as ankylosing spondylitis, came to the clinic referred to by her rheumatologist. The patient was complaining of intense pain of the TMJ, dysesthesias of the head, and mouth opening limitation. Seronegative spondyloarthropathies refer to a group of diseases that share common characteristics including the occurrence of inflammation in the spine, peripheral joints, and, in various peri-articular tissues, entheses (where tendons and ligaments insert onto bones). The outstanding feature of seronegative spondyloarthropathies is the absence of rheumatoid factor and autoantibodies in the laboratory tests. Seronegative spondyloarthropathies have a strong association with human leukocyte antigen HLA-B27. The patient reported that she had been diagnosed at age 39 with arthritis when all her major joints, such as the knee and elbow, on the left side suddenly became inflamed. Swelling, redness, and intense pain prevented her from performing simple movements such as standing and extending her arm.

When she started to feel pain in the TMJ, she consulted an orthodontist and facial orthopedist who informed her that she had "bruxism" and that she needed to use a device to place her tongue in the correct position. She wore the appliance for a month, and then her TMJ locked. She could not open her mouth and felt an extreme pain in her entire head. At this point, she no longer knew what hurt more, the joints of the body or her head and mouth. She stressed that there was no medication that could ease the pain she felt in the TMJ and in the cervical spine. Her rheumatologist was apprehensive that she could have arthritis in the TMJ and immediately referred her.

She reported clicking on the right TMJ, difficulty opening the mouth, difficulty and pain with chewing, and bruxism. She also felt strong headaches, neck pain, pain in the right eyebrow, pain behind the eyes, pain in the right shoulder, and pain in both temporomandibular joints, stronger in the right joint (Figs. 48 and 49). In the first consultation, the patient reported that she had initiated treatment for bruxism and that upon her orthotic being changed, she began to feel a very intense pain and her mouth locked.

The radiographic image of the joint (Figs. 50 and 51) shows the superior and posterior positioning of the articular process on the left side (highlighted in red) in the joint cavity when the jaw is in maximal intercuspation. In the maximum opening position, there is a flattening of the posterior and anterior surface of the left mandibular condyle process (highlighted in red) and a flattening of the superior and anterior surface of the right mandibular condyle process (highlighted in blue). The right side also presents an alteration of the growth axis of the mandibular condyle.

Opening and closing computerized kinesiographic records show that the patient can open only 32 mm, which is a significant limitation. The skull model image shows the difference in the translation of the mandibular condyles

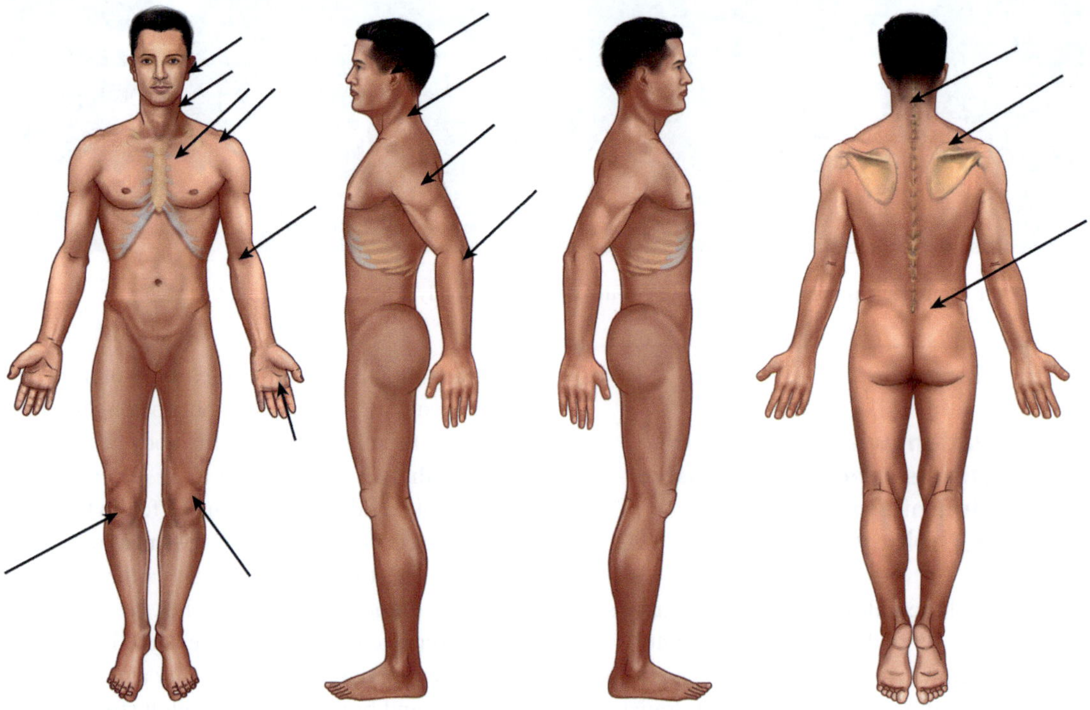

Fig. 48 A record of the patient's most significant points of pain as drawn by the patient

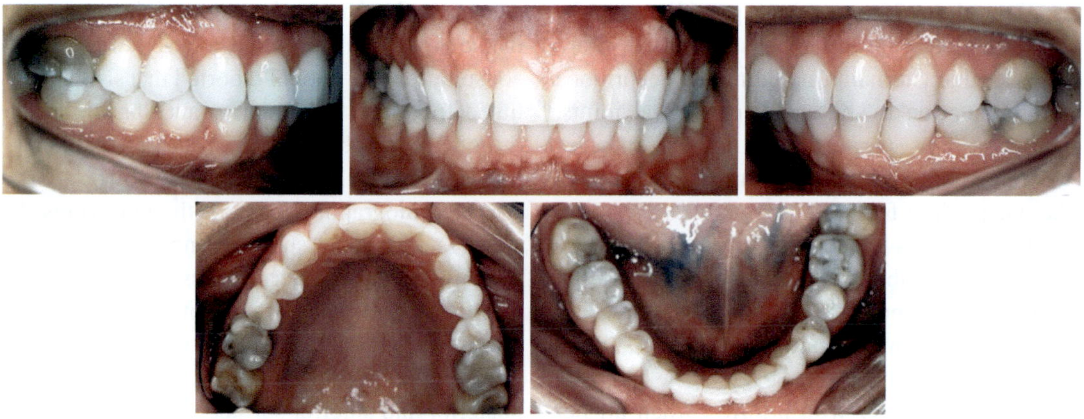

Fig. 49 Patient's habitual occlusion, frontal, right, and left lateral views (above). The superior and inferior occlusal view shows the anterior wear of the teeth (below)

when the patient is in maximum mouth opening (Figs. 52 and 53). In this surface electromyography record (Fig. 54), the patient could not clench when she was asked to bite hard and to maintain the teeth at maximum intercuspation. At the beginning of the record when asked to open the mouth, it is important to note the different activity between the right and left digastric muscles. Records of surface electromyography and computerized kinesiography alone do not provide a diagnosis; however, they are tools to assist in the diagnosis, together with images, clinical history, and examination. Furthermore, these data help to objectively compare and control mandibular position during the treatment.

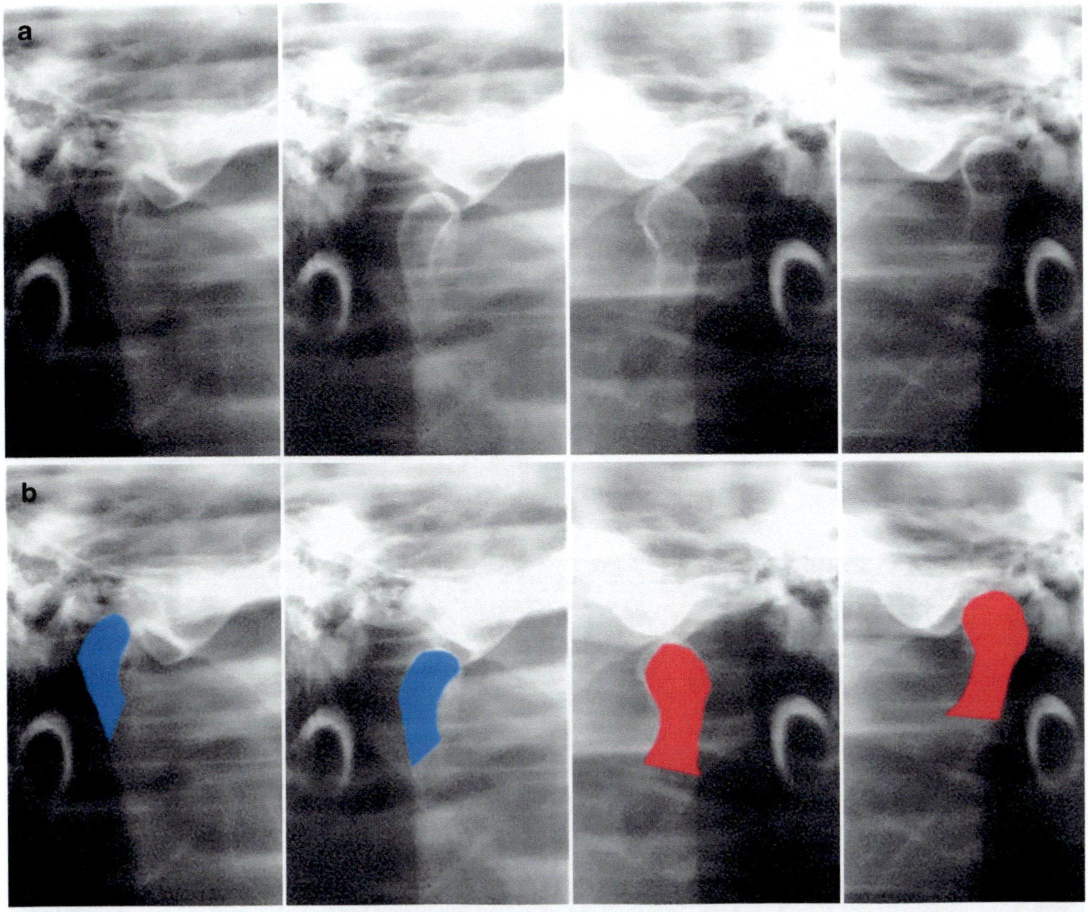

Fig. 50 (**a**) Patient's initial laminography and (**b**) the same images color highlighted

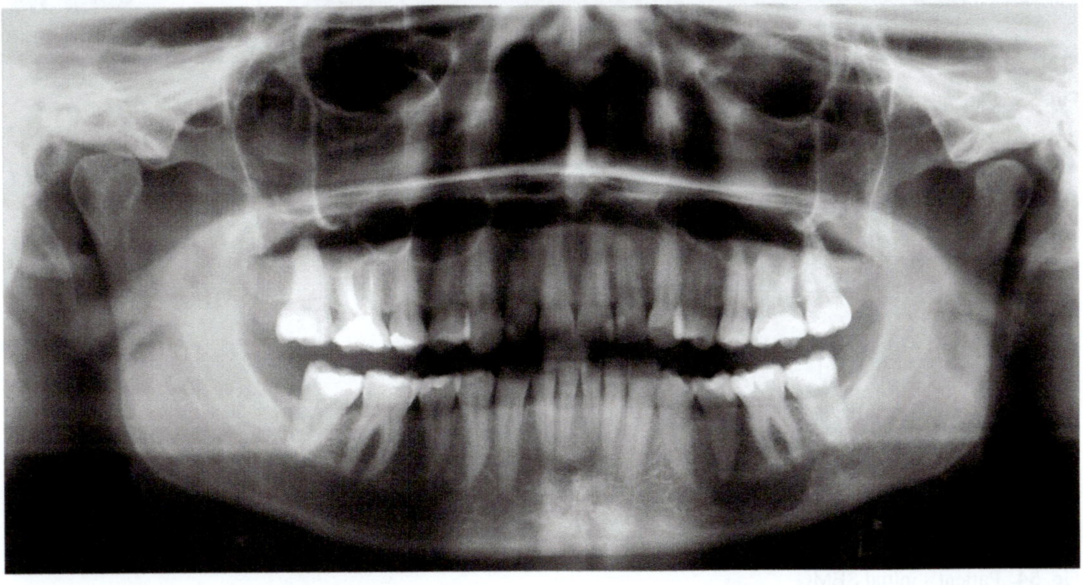

Fig. 51 Patient's panoramic radiograph

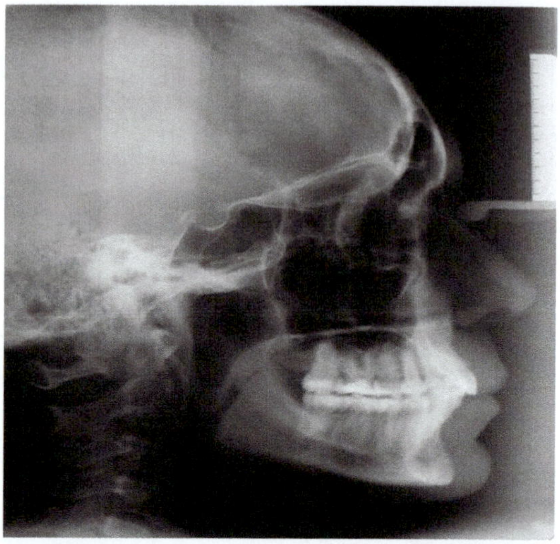

Fig. 52 Patient's lateral radiograph

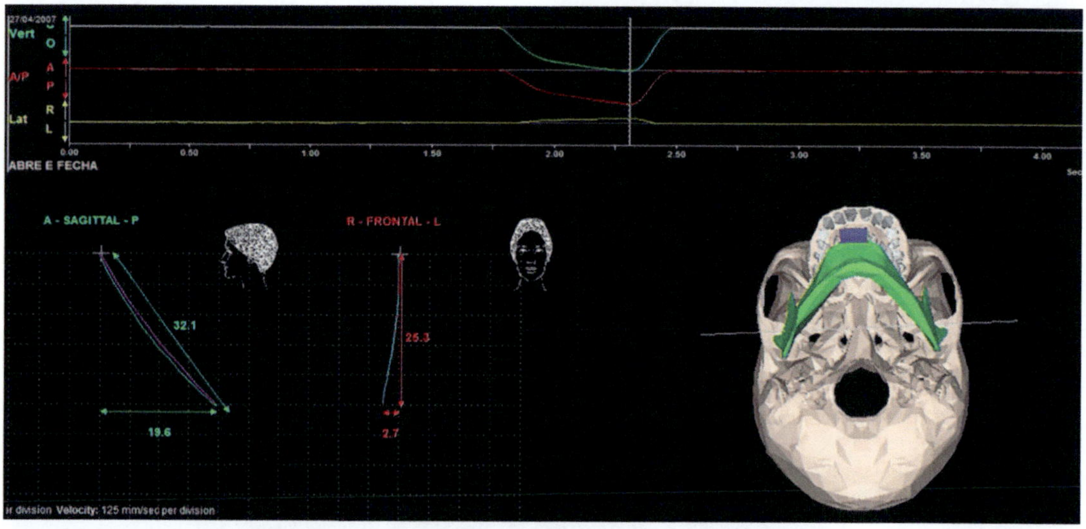

Fig. 53 Patient's range of motion (ROM) and 3D skull model

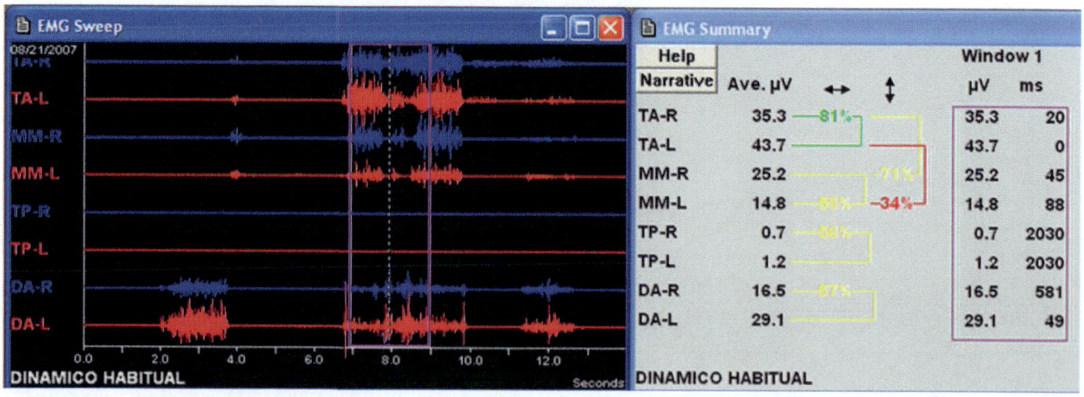

Fig. 54 Patient's initial SEMG

A TMJ MRI was requested, but when the patient filled out the clinical record for the MRI, she reported that she had had a tattoo done a month prior, which prevented the performance of the MRI until 3 months after the tattoo was done. Tattoos have pigments that may contain metal, which in an MR scanner could heat up and cause burns. With the information of the laminography and the bioinstrumentation, we constructed a temporary splint until the MRI was performed. One could easily assume that a patient who suffered from a systemic nonspecific inflammatory arthritis could also have TMJ involvement.

With regard to the systemic disease, it is the rheumatologist who decides on therapy. Dentists are to promote a non-compressive position of the TMJ where the masticatory muscles may perform without loading the joint and where the patient can fulfill all the functions of the stomatognathic system. The patient underwent the MRI examination. Figure 55 (a, b) Two slices of the right TMJ closed mouth: the articular disc is anteriorly displaced; there is a change in the growth axis of the mandibular condyle (greenstick fracture). (c, d) Two slices of the right TMJ open mouth: limitation in mouth opening. (e, f) Two slices of the left TMJ closed mouth: the articular disc is anteriorly displaced; there was a change in the growth axis of the mandibular condyle (greenstick fracture). (g, h) Two slices of the left TMJ open mouth: limitation in mouth opening.

Images in T1 are perfect for anatomy, T2, and STIR images are fundamental for detecting joint effusions, and there was no evidence of inflammatory signs. It is important to remember that in the first consultation, the patient reported that she had initiated treatment for the bruxism problem and that at one point with the device change, she began to feel very strong pain in the joint and the mouth locked. The patient remembers that the reason for the device change was to align the median line of the upper incisors to the median line of the lower incisors. This should serve as a cautionary warning to not carry out joint treatments without knowing the internal condition of the TMJ.

The masticatory muscles of the patient were electronically deprogrammed, and the rest position was recorded with a computerized kinesiograph (Fig. 56). This record was challenging to achieve because of trismus and pain. Therefore, a low orthotic was made, leaving an interocclusal free space of 1 mm, which would normally be too narrow (Fig. 57). After 2 weeks and with the patient already able to open her mouth, a new record was made and a new orthotic was constructed. The difference between the two records (a) and (b) is remarkable (Figs. 58 and 59). Improvement of the patient's mandibular opening was (b) from 32.1 to (a) 38.2 mm, and also, she had an increased velocity (Fig. 60).

Figure 61a, b two slices of the right TMJ with a closed mouth: articular disc in habitual position, with the orthotic in place. (c, d) Two slices of the right TMJ open mouth: Resolution of the opening limitation, with the orthotic in place. (e, f) Two slices of the left TMJ closed mouth: articular disc in habitual position, with the orthotic in place. (g, h) Two slices of the left TMJ open mouth: resolution of the opening limitation, with the orthotic in place. The patient no longer suffered pain nor opening limitations, and it was decided to continue with the orthotic and not to perform phase 2 treatment as she did not mind wearing the orthotic permanently; however, she did ask to restore the worn teeth that aesthetically bothered her. As a patient with an active but controlled autoimmune disease, she knew that the TMJ was not shielded from her disease. She continued rheumatology therapy, and, for the moment, the TMJ remains in a good position and free of inflammatory processes. The orthotic continues to be controlled and is calibrated when necessary.

There are many patients with an autoimmune disease without the inflammatory disease affecting the TMJ but with severe symptoms caused by compressive positions of the condyle, which in turn are caused by different etiologies. These are the patients that can benefit from TMD treatment.

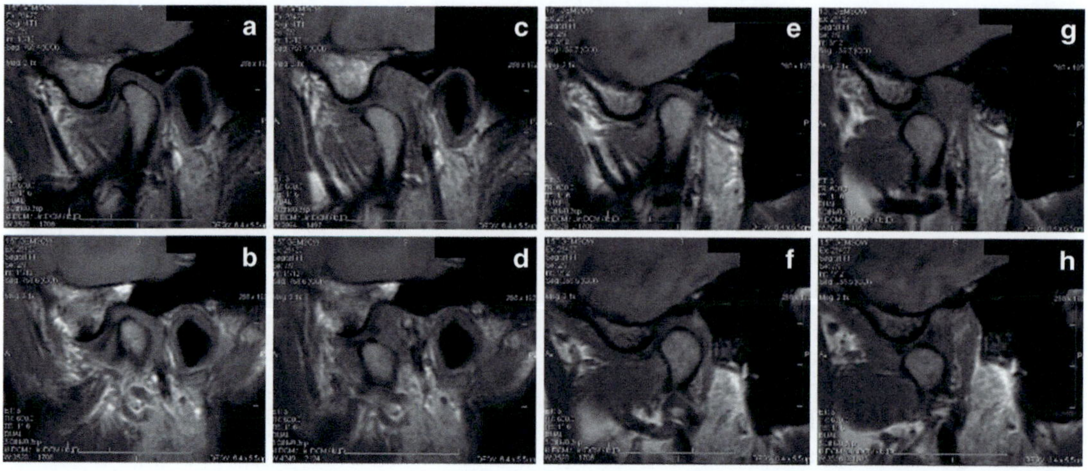

Fig. 55 MRI of the more significant sagittal slices of the right and left TMJ in closed- and open-mouth positions

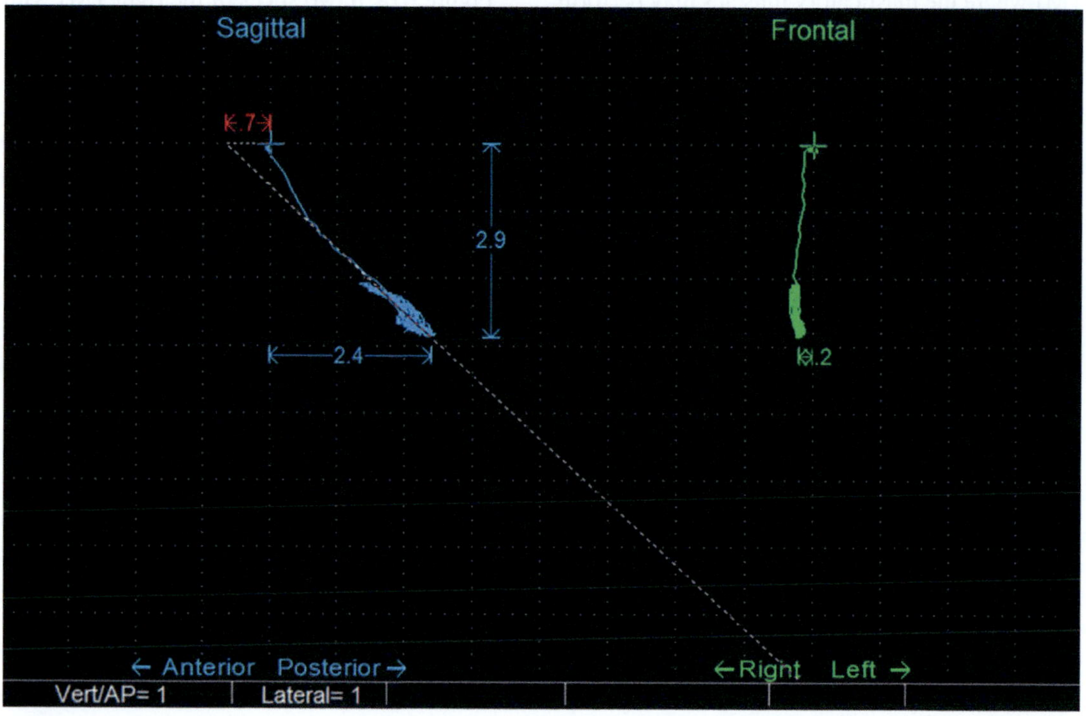

Fig. 56 Graphic for the record of the mandible tridimensional position after electronic deprogramming

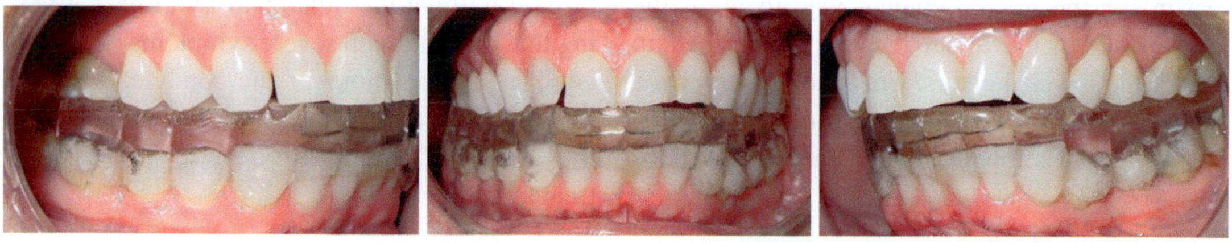

Fig. 57 Patient's occlusion with the new orthotic installed

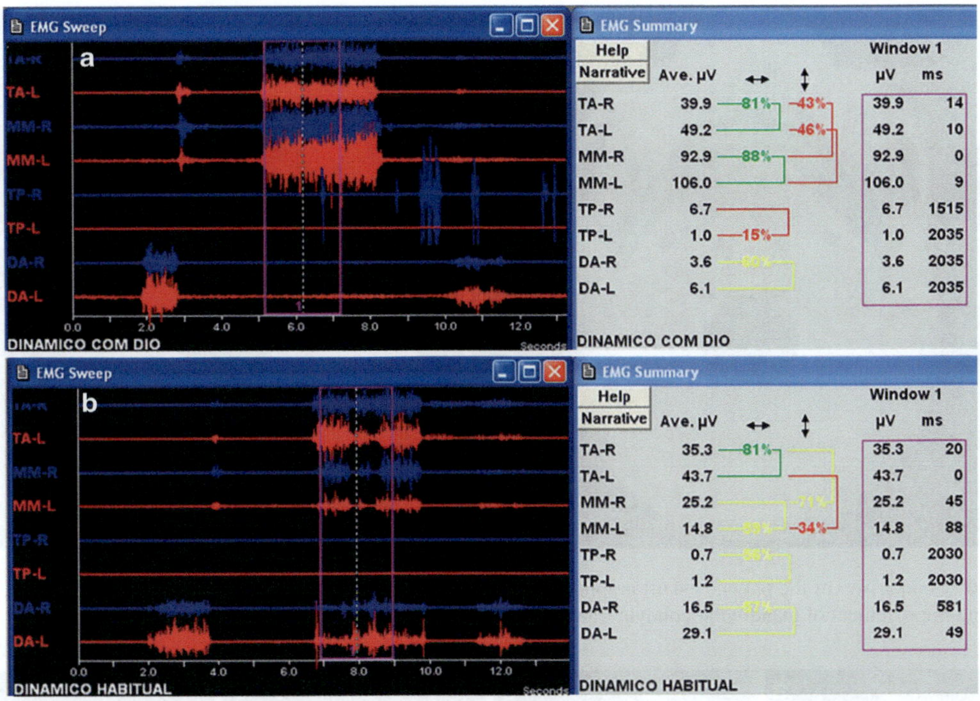

Fig. 58 Comparison of the patient's SEMG records (**a**) using the orthotic and (**b**) in habitual occlusion

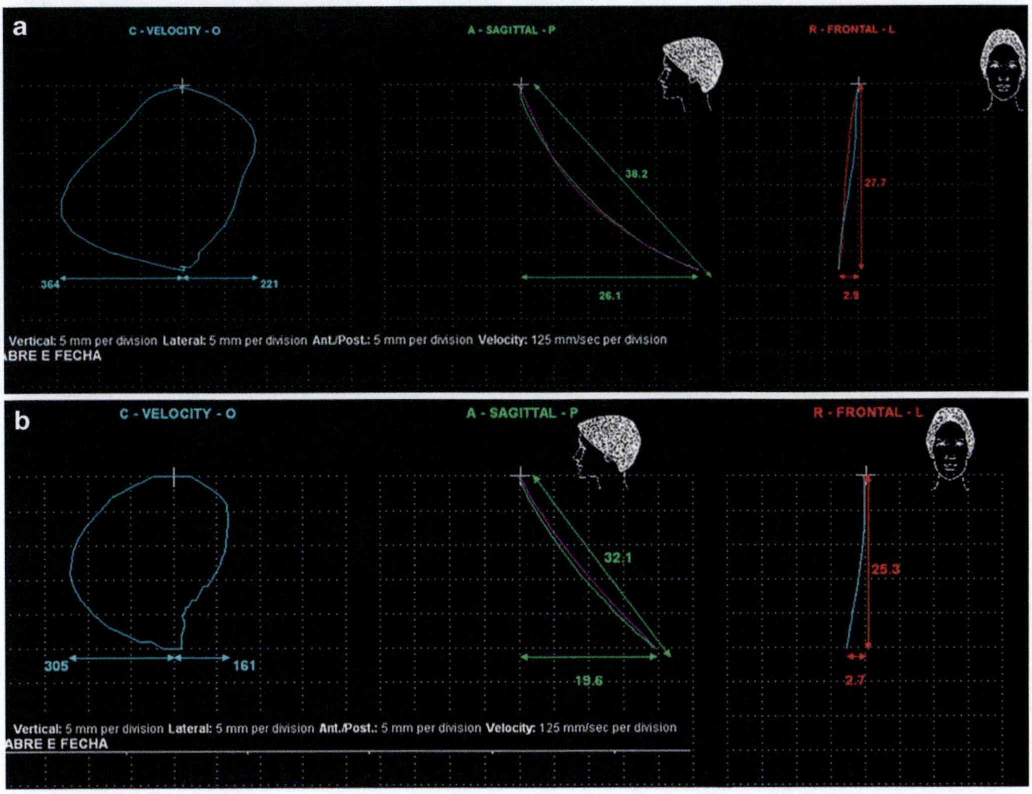

Fig. 59 Patient's comparative kinesiographic records (**a**) using the orthotic and (**b**) in the habitual occlusion

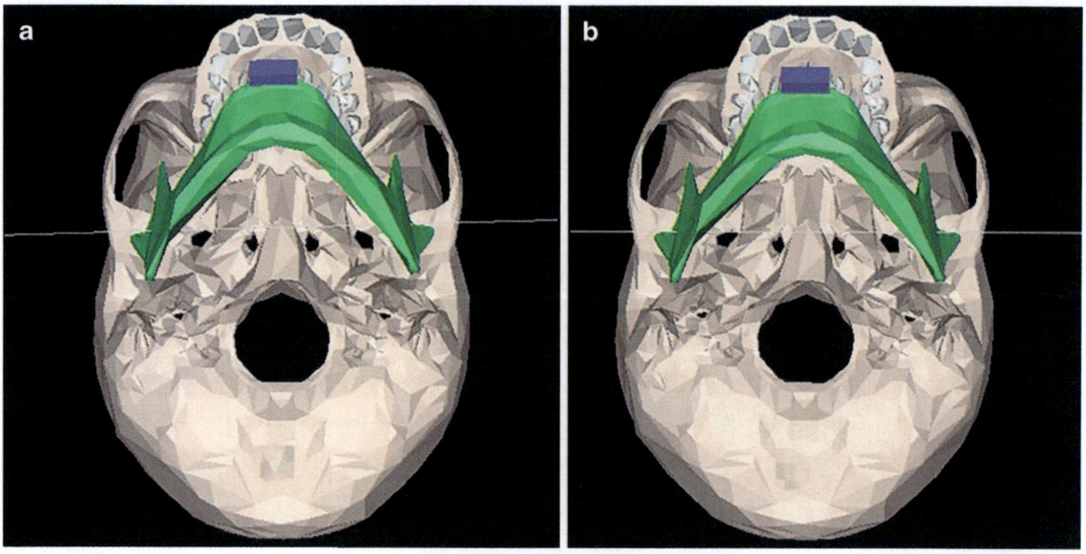

Fig. 60 Comparison of the patient's skull graphic model animation in 3D, (**a**) before treatment and (**b**) with orthotic showing improvement of mandibular condyle translation. Patient in maximum mouth opening

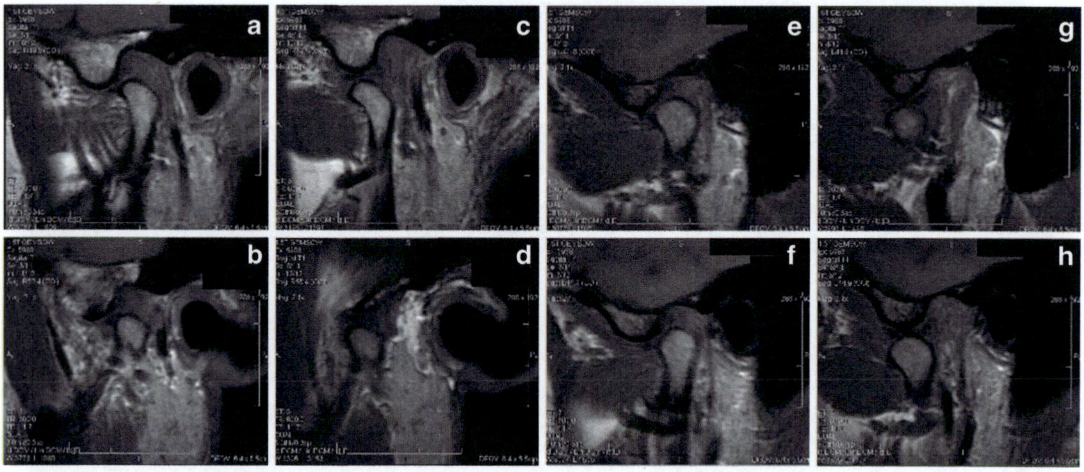

Fig. 61 MRI of same sagittal cuts as shown before in Fig. 55 of the right and left TMJ closed and open mouth with the orthotic in place

6 Summary

Four different clinical cases were presented with images and details of the clinical histories as well as records of bioinstrumentation. In one of the cases, the three-dimensional orthodontics of the second phase was reported. Without a doubt, patients like these are searching for help all around the world. It was a goal for this publication to highlight the "red flags" that can be found in simple images and investigate the clinical documentation for nuances that are often overlooked.

Acknowledgments I would like to thank Dr. Brendan C. Stack, Jr., and Dr. Anthony B. Sims for the opportunity to participate in this project in honor of Dr. Brendan C. Stack, Sr. hoping that, wherever he is, he will smile, review, and like this book.

Suggested Readings

1. Adib F. The efficacy of EMG, jaw tracking, and joint sound recording technologies in the evaluation of TMD. Oral Surg Oral Med Oral Pathol Oral Radiol Endod. 2011;111(4):409. https://doi.org/10.1016/j.tripleo.2010.11.005. Epub 2011 Jan 15.
2. Moses AJ. Controversy in temporomandibular disorders: clinicians' guide to critical thinking. Futa Book Publishers; 1997.
3. Arabshahi B, Baskin KM, Cron RQ. Reactive arthritis of the temporomandibular joints and cervical spine in a child. Pediatr Rheumatol Online J. 2007;5:4. https://doi.org/10.1186/1546-0096-5-4. PMID: 17550629; PMCID: PMC1869027.
4. Bag AK, Gaddikeri S, Singhal A, Hardin S, Tran BD, Medina JA, Curé JK. Imaging of the temporomandibular joint: an update. World J Radiol. 2014;6(8):567–82. https://doi.org/10.4329/wjr.v6.i8.567. PMID: 25170394; PMCID: PMC4147437.
5. Basmajian JV, De Luca Carlo J. Muscles alive: their functions revealed by electromyography. Williams & Wilkins; 1985.
6. Bayar N, Kara SA, Keles I, Koç MC, Altinok D, Orkun S. Temporomandibular joint involvement in rheumatoid arthritis: a radiological and clinical study. Cranio. 2002;20(2):105–10. https://doi.org/10.1080/08869634.2002.11746198.
7. Brenkert DR. Orthodontic treatment for the TMJ patient following splint therapy to stabilize a displaced disk(s): a systemized approach. Part I, TMJ orthodontic diagnosis [Erratum in: Cranio. 2010 Oct;28(4):264.]. Cranio. 2010a;28(3):193–9. https://doi.org/10.1179/crn.2010.027.
8. Brenkert DR. Orthodontic treatment for the TMJ patient following splint therapy to stabilize a displaced disk(s): a systemized approach. Part II. Cranio. 2010b;28(4):260–5.
9. Cedströmer AL, Andlin-Sobocki A, Abbu N, Hedenberg-Magnusson B, Dahlström L, Berntson L. Condylar alterations and facial growth in children with juvenile idiopathic arthritis. J Orofac Orthop. 2020;81(3):163–71. https://doi.org/10.1007/s00056-020-00216-8. Epub 2020 Feb 20. PMID: 32077980; PMCID: PMC7186245.
10. Cooper BC, Kleinberg I. Establishment of a temporomandibular physiological state with neuromuscular orthosis treatment affects reduction of TMD symptoms in 313 patients. Cranio. 2008a;26(2):104–17. https://doi.org/10.1179/crn.2008.015.
11. Cooper BC. The role of bioelectronic instruments in the management of TMD. N Y State Dent J. 1995;61(9):48–53.
12. Cooper BC, International College of Cranio-Mandibular Orthopedics (ICCMO). Temporomandibular disorders: a position paper of the International College of Cranio-Mandibular Orthopedics (ICCMO). Cranio. 2011;29(3):237–44. https://doi.org/10.1179/crn.2011.034.
13. Simmons HC, American Academy of Craniofacial Pain. Craniofacial pain: a handbook for assessment, diagnosis and management. 3rd ed. Chroma, Incorporated; 2009a.
14. Rozencweig D, Gerdolle D, Delgoffe C, Stricker M. Imagerie de l'ATM: aide au diagnostic des troubles cranio-mandibulaires. Editora Cahiers de prothèses éditions; 1995.
15. David MH, editor. Neuromuscular dentistry in the next millennium. Anthology, vol. 5. The International College of Cranio-Mandibular Orthopedics.
16. Langlade M. Diagnostic orthodontique. Maloine; 1981.
17. Ortu E, Pietropaoli D, Adib F, Masci C, Giannoni M, Monaco A. Electromyographic evaluation in children orthodontically treated for skeletal class II malocclusion: comparison of two treatment techniques. CRANIO®. 2017;37:129. https://doi.org/10.1080/08869634.2017.1393916.
18. Antonio MV, Gil JG. Enfermedades reumaticas extrarticulares. Masson; 1998.
19. Kasman GS, Cram JR, Wolf SL. Clinical applications in surface electromyography: chronic musculoskeletal pain. Gaithersburg: Aspen; 1998.
20. Grummons D. Orthodontics for the TMJ/TMD patient. Scottsdale: Wright & Co. Publ.; 1994.
21. Hickman DM, Stauber W. Mapping mandibular rest in humans utilizing electromyographic patterns from masticatory muscles. Cranio. 2007;25(4):264–72. https://doi.org/10.1179/crn.2007.040.
22. Isberg A, Widmalm SE, Ivarsson R. Clinical, radiographic, and electromyographic study of patients with internal derangement of the temporomandibular joint. Am J Orthod. 1985;88(6):453–60. https://doi.org/10.1016/s0002-9416(85)80044-0.
23. Jankelson B. Three-dimensional orthodontic diagnosis and treatment. A neuromuscular approach. J Clin Orthod. 1984;18(9):627–36.
24. Jankelson RR. Sensitivity/specificity: straw men, red herrings, and dental politics. Cranio. 2013;31(3):156–8. https://doi.org/10.1179/crn.2013.023.
25. Witzig JW, Spahl TJ. ISBN 978-0884165583.
26. Effat KG, Berty A. A comparative clinical study of temporomandibular disorder patients in the otolaryngology clinic versus a rheumatology clinic. CRANIO®. 2018; https://doi.org/10.1080/08869634.2017.1422846.
27. Kamyszek G, Ketcham R, Garcia R Jr, Radke J. Electromyographic evidence of reduced muscle activity when ULF-TENS is applied to the Vth and VIIth cranial nerves. Cranio. 2001;19(3):162–8.
28. Lous I, Sheik-Ol-Eslam A, Moller E. Postural activity in subjects with functional disorders of the chewing apparatus. Scand J Dent Res. 1970;78(5):404–10. https://doi.org/10.1111/j.1600-0722.1970.tb02089.x.

29. Masi M, Lederman HM, Yamashita HK, de Arruda Aidar LA. Temporomandibular joint evaluation with magnetic resonance imaging in children with functional unilateral posterior crossbite, treated with rapid maxillary expansion. Am J Orthod Dentofac Orthop. 2009;136(2):207–17. https://doi.org/10.1016/j.ajodo.2007.10.048.
30. Maulén-Yáñez M, Meeder-Bella W, Videla-Jiménez PJ, González-Arriagada WA. Assessment of association between muscular diagnosis in temporomandibular disorders with mandibular kinematics. CRANIO®. 2018; https://doi.org/10.1080/08869634.2018.1465513.
31. Monaco A, Cattaneo R, Marci MC, Marzo G, Gatto R, Giannoni M. Neuromuscular diagnosis in orthodontics: effects of TENS on maxillo-mandibular relationship. Eur J Paediatr Dent. 2007a;8(3):143–8.
32. Robert RJ. Neuromuscular dental diagnosis and treatment hardcover. Ishiyaku Euroamerica; 1990.
33. Hickman DM, editor. Neuromuscular dentistry the next millennium anthology, vol. 5. The International College of Cranio-Mandibular Orthopedics; 1999.
34. Skármeta NP, Araneda L, Araya C. Destructive psoriatic arthritis of the temporomandibular joint: a clinical case, an overview of the pathophysiology and its differential diagnoses. CRANIO®. 2018.
35. Paparella M. Otorrinolaringologia. Ciencias basicas y disciplinas afines. editorial medica panamericana; 1998.
36. Sih T. Otorrinolaringologia pediatrica. Springer; 2000.
37. da Costa SS, Cruz OL, de Oliveira JA. Otorrinolaringologia princípios e prática. 2006
38. Pinho JC, Caldas FM, Mora MJ, Santana-Penín U. Electromyographic activity in patients with temporomandibular disorders. J Oral Rehabil. 2000;27(11):985–90. https://doi.org/10.1046/j.1365-2842.2000.00571.x.
39. Rocha MJ, Almeida. Reabsorção Condilar Progressiva após cirurgia ortognática-revisão sistemática com meta-análise. Diss: Universidade de Coimbra; 2017.
40. Saldanha AD, Hilgenberg PB, Pinto LM, Conti PC. Are temporomandibular disorders and tinnitus associated? Cranio. 2012;30(3):166–71. https://doi.org/10.1179/crn.2012.026.
41. Schmid W, Deregibus A, Mongini F. Conservative treatment of craniomandibular asymmetries during growth. A long term study. Prog Orthod. 2007;8(1):62–73.
42. Mummolo S, Nota A, Tecco S, Caruso S, Marchetti E, Marzo G, Cutilli T. Ultra-low-frequency transcutaneous electric nerve stimulation (ULF-TENS) in subjects with craniofacial pain: a retrospective study. CRANIO®. 2018a; https://doi.org/10.1080/08869634.2018.1526849.
43. Spahl TJ, Witzig JW. The clinical management of basic maxillofacial orthopedic appliances, vol. 1: mechanics first. Littleton: PSG Publishing Co.; 1987.
44. Jacobson A. The clinical management of basic maxillofacial orthopedic appliances, vol. III temporomandibular joint. 1992.
45. Langlade MM. Thérapeutique orthodontique. 1978.
46. Travell JG, Simons DG. Myofascial pain and dysfunction: the trigger point manual. Lippincott Williams & Wilkins; 1990.
47. Tuna EB, Dündar A, Cankaya AB, Gençay K. Conservative approach to unilateral condylar fracture in a growing patient: a 2.5-year follow up. Open Dent J. 2012;6:1–4. https://doi.org/10.2174/1874210601206010001. Epub 2012 Jan 12. PMID: 22276078; PMCID: PMC3263469.
48. Vieira e Silva CA, da Silva MA, Melchior MD, de Felício CM, Sforza C, Tartaglia GM. Treatment for TMD with occlusal splint and electromyographic control: application of the FARC protocol in a Brazilian population. Cranio. 2012;30(3):218–26. https://doi.org/10.1179/crn.2012.033.
49. Voudouris JC, Kuftinec MM. Improved clinical use of Twin-block and Herbst as a result of radiating viscoelastic tissue forces on the condyle and fossa in treatment and long-term retention: growth relativity. Am J Orthod Dentofac Orthop. 2000;117(3):247–66. https://doi.org/10.1016/s0889-5406(00)70231-9.
50. Yavich LG. Alterações na orientação do côndilo mandibular devido a traumatismos na primeira infância. JBA. 2001a;1(4):270–9.
51. Yavich LG. Eletromiografia de superfície no diagnóstico e controle do tratamento das disfunções temporomandibulares. JBA. 2001b;1(3):193–8.
52. Yavich LG. Paciente com disfunção temporomandibular apresentando assimetria condilar e micro nódulos no terço anterior das pregas vocais. JBA. 2002a;2(5):12–9.
53. Yavich LG. Princípios neuromusculares na Odontologia, trajetória de fechamento habitual coincidente com a trajetória de fechamento neuromuscular. JBA. 2002b;2(6):101–11.
54. Yitschaky O, Yitschaky M, Zadik Y. Case report on trial: do you, doctor, swear to tell the truth, the whole truth and nothing but the truth? J Med Case Rep. 2011;5:179. https://doi.org/10.1186/1752-1947-5-179. PMID: 21569508; PMCID: PMC3113995.

Transformation of Trigeminal Nerve Stimuli into Movement Disorders: A Series of Cases

Anthony B. Sims

Abbreviations

ABCFP	American Board of Craniofacial Pain
DHS	Doctor of Humanitarian Services
IMD	Integrative Medical Doctor
WONM	World Organization of Natural Medicine

1 Introduction

The TMJ has its innervation from the mandibular division (V3) of the CN5 and the auriculotemporal (AT) branch of that nerve. The AT runs behind the mandibular condylar portion of the mandible. It is believed that when this nerve is damaged, irritated, or compressed, the movement disorders begin to manifest themselves. As seen in Fig. 1, the nerve innervates the TMJ and its capsule and other areas within the joint. When trauma occurs, the signal goes through the spinal cord, and then to the brain through multiple tracts. But, in fact, there are other pathways CN5 travels to different parts of the brain, brainstem, and spinal cord connections. CN5 is the only cranial nerve that has direct connections to the CNS by entering the reticular formation (RF). CN5 has connections to the cerebellum and the basal ganglia as well.

Reduced inhibition can be observed in the central nervous system (CNS), especially within the sensorimotor cortex, basal ganglia, brainstem, spinal cord, and cerebellum, in neurophysiological studies of individuals with dystonia. Additionally, anatomical, neurophysiological, and medical research implies that the trigeminal sensory nuclear complex (TSNC) plays a role in some cases of dystonia that impacts the muscles of the face and neck. Multiple afferents supplying various structures in the head and neck that are involved in sensory and non-nociceptive communication support neurons in the TSNC, which in turn extend to the somatosensory cortex.

Seeing the benefits of clinical intervention in movement disorder patients is crucial for both clinician and patient. This chapter is illustrated with case report videos (Video 1). These videos can be found at URL.

Supplementary Information The online version contains supplementary material available at https://doi.org/10.1007/978-3-031-57563-1_14.

A. B. Sims (✉)
Columbia, MD, USA

B. C. Stack Jr. et al. (eds.), *Craniofacial Pain*, https://doi.org/10.1007/978-3-031-57563-1_14

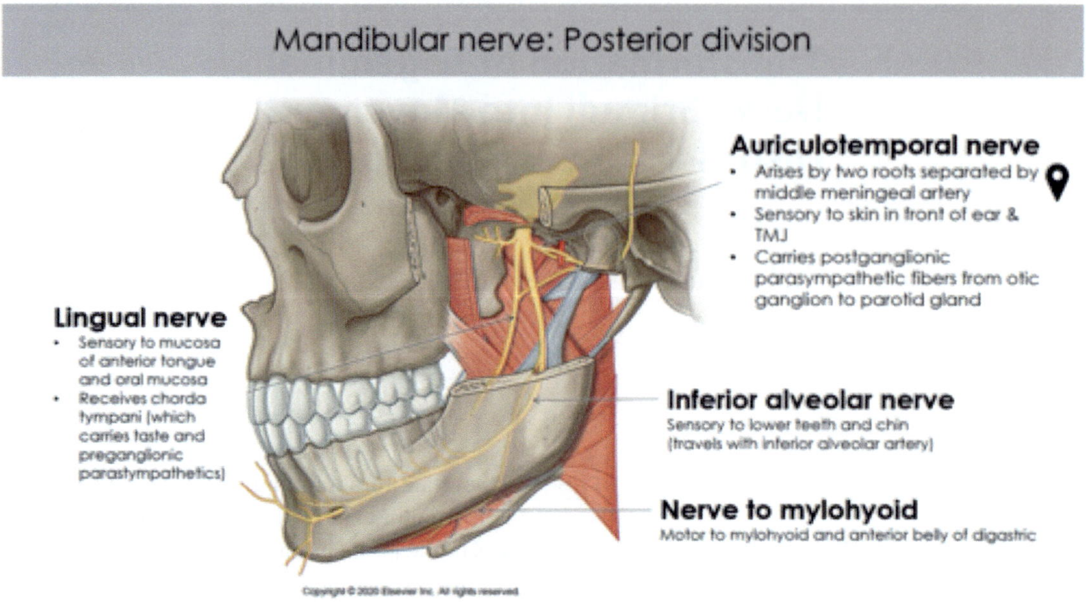

Fig. 1 Auriculotemporal nerve. (**Courtesy of Quizlet:** https://quizlet.com/513723165/innervation-of-the-temporal-and-infratemporal-fossa-flash-cards/)

2 Dystonias

A neurological disorder termed primary focal dystonia generates involuntary repetitive or infrequent muscle contractions that twist and create an abnormal posture in a body component. Blepharospasm and oromandibular, laryngeal, lingual, cranial, and cervical dystonia, among others, are common variations on focal dystonia which influence the muscles of the head and neck. There is currently no known single causative characteristic, and onset typically occurs between the ages of 40 and 60. Approximately 20 out of every 100,000 people globally suffer from primary focal dystonia, the third most prevalent movement disorder.

2.1 Blepharospasm

Any aberrant tightening of the orbicularis oculi muscle is called blepharospasm. It is important to differentiate this condition from myokymia, or fasciculation, the more prevalent and milder involuntary fluttering of an eyelid. The symptoms of blepharospasm typically last a few days before disappearing completely on their own without treatment. In certain cases, the muscle twitching is chronic and persistent, posing problems for an extended period of one's life. The symptoms in these situations are frequently serious enough that they lead to functional blindness. The person's eyes feel as though they are clamping shut and are difficult to open. Despite having vision, a few individuals experience temporary blindness because they cannot raise their eyelids. The reflex blepharospasm, on the other hand, is brought on by any kind of discomfort in or near the eye. It occurs in a couple of different forms: reflex and critical blepharospasm.

Benign essential blepharospasm (BEB), a neurological movement disorder, causes involuntary, persistent spasms of the muscles situated around the eyes. Though fatigue, tension, or an irritant may have contributed, the word vital suggests an unidentified cause.

Despite the lack of a cure, botulinum toxin injections may offer momentary relief. A surgical procedure called a myomectomy may be beneficial. BEB is a relatively uncommon condition that affects 1 in 20,000 people in the United States.

Some people who experience blepharospasm have a history of dry eyes, light sensitivity, and even tiredness. Others assert that their symptoms began without any visual problems.

Some drugs, particularly those used to treat Parkinson's disease and hormone therapies like estrogen replacement for menopausal women, can cause blepharospasm. Blepharospasm may also occur as a severe withdrawal symptom from benzodiazepines. Long-term benzodiazepine use is also a known risk factor for blepharospasm.

The following are cases in which it is believed to be originating from the TMJ/CN5.

2.1.1 Case 1

A 70-year-old right-handed male was diagnosed with blepharospasm. He had difficulty driving. He cannot keep eyes open. There was closure or spasm for over a minute. There was no tear formation. His past medical history includes car whiplash in 2004, noticed eyes slowly closing in 2005, bilateral eye pain, eye lens removed, and scaffolding accident in 2010. He was seen by the best ophthalmologists in his city without relief. His allergist stated that he could not find any problems. He was seen at a famous east coast teaching hospital for special light-blocking scleral glasses without no relief. He was on naltrexone eye drops when he presented.

Initial examination revealed eye closure for 30 s to 1.5 min normally, photophobia, bilateral TMJ pain, and bilateral neck stiffness. Imaging (MRI) showed left lateral meniscal displacement, left condylar early degeneration, and right meniscal ankylosis (Fig. 2).

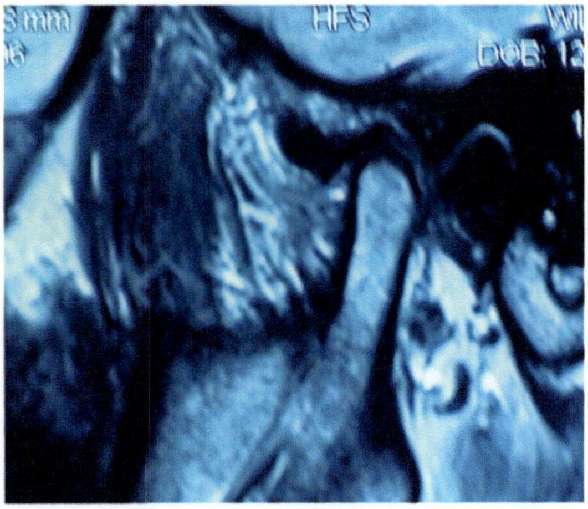

Fig. 2 Sagittal MR of left TMJ in case 1

The patient had a mandibular orthotic made to the exact dimensions both anteriorly and posteriorly with an additional vertical dimension that would decompress the nerve effecting eyelid closure (cranial nerve 7). Upon decompression, the muscles (orbicularis oculi) and the oculomotor nerve branches to the superior levator palpebrae muscle normalized, the aberrant signal discontinued, and the blepharospasm stopped.

Results: Immediate resolution of blepharospasm, head tremor, and bilateral eye pain. Resolution occurred after 1 month (Figs. 3, 4 and 5). The patient was able to drive. The patient shared his recovery experience in a letter:

> Dr. X:
> Last week I went fishing with my brother in eastern Washington and we fished 4 lakes and covered 700 miles in 6 Days. The fishing was great … but the big news is I DROVE THE CAR OVER 700 MILES (with my brother riding shotgun). So the obvious conclusion is that the blepharospasm is much less of a problem and that the Dr. Sim's mouth appliance is helping. I have been taking the naltrexone eye drops for a month now, so it is still too early to judge what effect they may have.
> Sandy and I take off on a car trip next Monday and will drive 650 miles to see our children and grand kids in Idaho. For the first time in a number of years Sandy won't have to shoulder the whole driving task and we can trade off like we used to. This really helps on long trips. Thanks for all your help.
> Your grateful patient, D (Videos 2 and 3).

2.1.2 Case 2

The patient's chief complaint was jaw and facial pain, headaches, tinnitus, blurred vision, eye pain, jaw clicking, and teeth clenching. Past medical history was a mouth guard and orthodontics. His family history included sleep apnea, diabetes, and high blood pressure.

On exam, he had severe pain in right temporalis, lateral TMJ capsule, right masseter muscle, sternocleidomastoid muscles (SCM) bilaterally, and trapezius muscles bilaterally. Maximum mouth opening: 40 mm (normal = 50–55 mm). Lateral mouth shift bilaterally: 8 mm (normal = 12 mm).

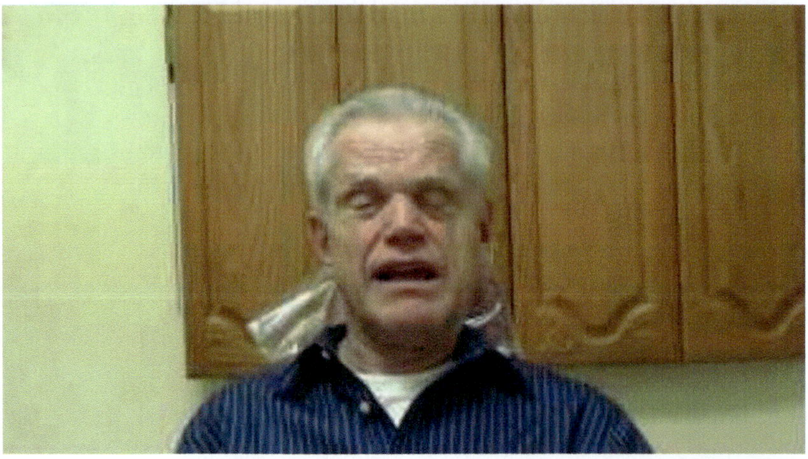

Fig. 3 Case 1 upon presentation without occlusal appliance

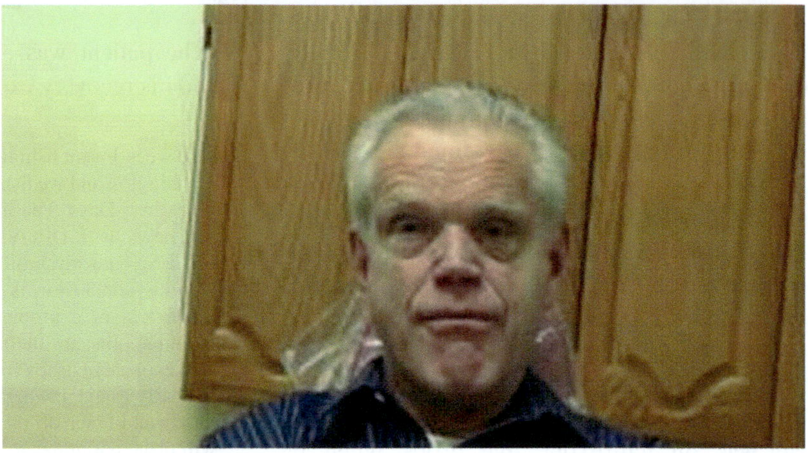

Fig. 4 Case 1 upon presentation with occlusal appliance

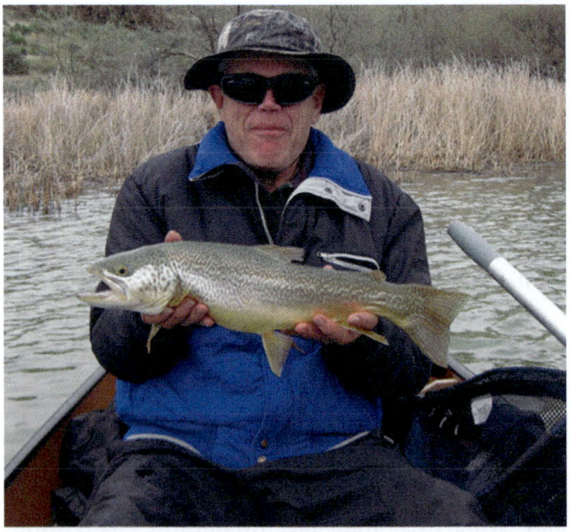

Fig. 5 Case 1 return to a normal lifestyle

An oral orthotic was made for this patient to decompress and reposition the lower neck muscles to their original length. Upon decompression and placing the lower neck muscles into the proper position, this patient's torticollis symptoms diminished greatly (Video 4).

2.2 Torticollis

A dystonic illness known as torticollis, often known as a "wry neck," is defined by an abnormal, asymmetrical position of the head or neck that can be caused by a wide range of etiologies. The most common scenario involves pain and difficulty rotating the head without obvious cause. Torticollis is static or dynamic, head or cervical tilt, and rotation or extension. The type of torticollis can be determined by how the head and neck are positioned (Table 1). Frequently, a combination of these motions can be seen (Table 2). In addition to being a symptom of other diseases, torticollis can be a disorder in and of itself.

Congenital muscular torticollis is the most common kind of torticollis, which manifests at birth. Congenital muscle torticollis is the third most common congenital musculoskeletal abnormality in babies. The cause of congenital muscular torticollis is unknown. Birth trauma or prenatal malposition is thought to have harmed the sternocleidomastoid muscle in the neck. A hard mass that usually appears between the ages of 1 and 4 weeks represents congenital torticollis. It is often detected with ultrasonography together with a physical evaluation of the infant's passive cervical range of motion. The reported incidence of congenital torticollis is 0.3–2.0%. Plagiocephaly is a rare consequence of congenital torticollis, and it may not resolve on its own. Secondary problems of congenital muscular torticollis include visual impairments, facial asymmetry, delayed development, cervical scoliosis, and vertebral wedge degeneration, all of which will negatively impact the child's appearance and mental health.

Table 1 Types of torticollis

• Laterocollis: tilting of the head toward the shoulder
• Rotational torticollis: the head rotates toward the shoulder along the horizontal line
• Anterocollis: the head and neck bend forward along with the chin moving in toward the torso
• Retrocollis: bringing the rear of the head toward the back [5] while hyperextending the head and neck backward

Table 2 Additional signs of torticollis

• Tremor in the head
• Unequal shoulder heights
• Periodic development of a neck mass
• Thickened or tight sternocleidomastoid muscle
• Tenderness on the cervical spine
• Reduced neck movement

Benign paroxysmal torticollis, a rare disorder, can affect infants. The interval between repeated episodes can be up to a week. The problem improves with age. The underlying factor is thought to be genetics.

Non-congenital (acquired) muscle torticollis can be brought on by a number of disorders, including adenitis, tonsillitis, rheumatoid arthritis, enlarged cervical glands, retropharyngeal abscess, or cerebellar tumors. Other causes include muscle spasms, injuries, scarring, or cervical spine illnesses. It could be chronic or cyclic (spasmodic/tonic). The latter type might be brought on by Pott's disease (spinal tuberculosis).

Torticollis, sometimes known as "stiff neck," is a common condition that affects one or more sore neck muscles and is a self-limiting, naturally occurring disorder. Usually, it takes 1–4 weeks for it to go away on its own. Typically, the sternocleidomastoid or trapezius muscles are involved. Occasionally, draughts, colds, or odd postures may be to blame, but frequently, there is no apparent cause. These incidents are regularly seen by physicians.

Untreated dental occlusal dysfunction brought on by teeth clenching and grinding (bruxism) during sleep is the most common cause of this self-limiting type. Once the occlusion has been treated, it will completely dissolve away. To produce the intended effects, occlusal appliances and dental equilibration are used during treatment. Other differential diagnoses to consider include the following:

1. Tumors in the posterior fossa: These can obstruct the nerve supply to the neck and cause torticollis and need to be surgically removed.
2. Infections in the posterior pharynx: These can aggravate the nerves supplying the neck muscles and might result in torticollis. Antibiotics can be used to treat infections that are not too dangerous, but in cases where they are, surgical debridement may be required.
3. Ear infections.
4. Surgical removal of adenoids: 3 and 4 can both result in Grisel's syndrome, a sublux-

ation of the upper cervical joints, most notably the atlantoaxial joint, caused by inflammatory laxity of the ligaments brought on by an infection.
5. Pharmaceuticals: These include antipsychotics and phenothiazines, a type of neuroleptic antiemetics, which might cause torticollis.

Spasmodic torticollis is characterized by repeated, fleeting contractions of the neck muscles, particularly the sternocleidomastoid. Depending on the underlying reason, the terms "intermittent torticollis," "cervical dystonia," and "idiopathic cervical dystonia" are synonyms.

2.2.1 Case 3

M.E. was a 47-year-old female with complaints of dystonia of hands and feet. She had 12 prescriptions. She experienced difficulty walking and used a wheelchair. She reported photophobia, nausea, vomiting, fatigue, migraines, multiple allergies, dizziness, chest pain, and neck pain. She was diagnosed with a functional/psychogenic movement disorder. She had negative genetic testing. She had exploratory surgery on the abdomen and esophagus. She was relegated to a dystonia support group. On examination, it was easy for her to walk backward. She had foot inversion, a diplegic gait, and TMJ pain. Her previous oral splint was worn down. Previous MRIs of TMJ showed bilateral anterior dislocation of TMJ discs, w/o recapture and degenerative changes in both mandibular condyles.

This patient had an orthotic fabricated to the correct vertical dimension so that there was no further compression of the temporomandibular joint nerves that had influenced the cervical nerves and the spinal cord interrelationship that was the basis of her symptoms. This demonstrated that the symptoms were not psychosomatic or a functional disorder (Video 5).

2.2.2 Case 4

The patient complained of pain daily and weakness. She would lose consciousness when trying to fight her symptoms. She reported difficulty breathing. She denied seizures. Her history included breast cancer, 5 mm, with metastases to the left neck. She had two previous neck fusions prior to her cancer diagnosis. There were no family neuro issues. Her prescriptions included Advil, Ativan, and Cymbalta.

On physical exam, the patient had a left-hand inversion lock with clenching and upper arm contraction. The neck flexed to the left. There was rib cage tensing, which migrated to neck and shoulder. Her gait was slow with decreased arm swinging. She had a tremor. Imaging included a panorex (Fig. 6), a normal MRI of brain and spine, and a normal, whole-body positron emission tomography (PET).

This patient, seen by multiple physicians, hospitals, and clinics, was told that this was a functional disorder and she needed to live it. Upon making a lower and upper orthotics for the patient, her mandible and maxilla were aligned and the temporomandibular joint stabilized. Her

Fig. 6

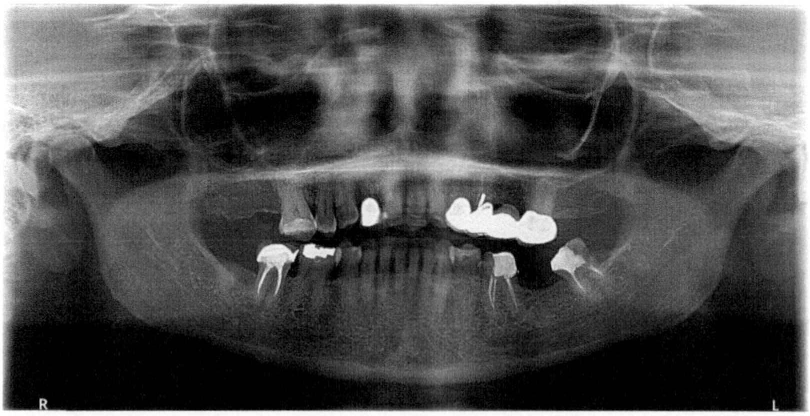

symptoms discontinued and that was later recognized by the treating hospital and physicians (Videos 6 and 7).

2.3 Gait Disorders

The action made when walking or running is referred to as your gait. Walking is a complex sequence of motions that calls for the cooperation of your heart and lungs, as well as your brain, bones, and muscles. The capacity to walk may be impacted if any of those systems experience a problem. Gait dysfunction is the term for this. Disorders of gait may be signs of another disease. Older people tend to experience them more frequently. A gait disorder can reduce your quality of life and increase your risk of stumbling and getting hurt.

2.3.1 Typical Gait Disorders

Movement can be observed by physicians who can determine what kind of gait problem a patient may be displaying. They can learn more about the root cause of movement disorders by watching how their body moves. They can use this to identify the problem and determine treatment plans. There are variations among each gait disorder type, so no two individuals will experience the same symptoms. When examining gait disorders, doctors will be attempting to identify broad characteristics of how a patient moves.

Hemiplegic Gait

Hemiplegic gait refers to a condition where just one side of the body is afflicted. One limb will remain immovable at the side of the body while walking. The patient drags the limb on the same side. Hemiplegia is a common outcome of a stroke.

Diplegic Gait

This gait condition affects both sections of your body. The knees and pelvis may also be bent, as well as the ankles. Every step one takes while moving around will generate a swing. A person may walk with a diplegic gait if they have cerebral palsy, a stroke, or brain damage.

Myopathic Gait

Also referred to as a waddling gait, it is a side-to-side motion used while walking. It frequently happens as a result of pelvic area weakness. It is possible that myopathic posture is caused by hip problems that have existed since infancy. It can be a symptom of muscular dystrophy, spinal atrophy, or another illness that affects the muscles.

Ataxic Gait

This is distinguished by a staggered gait when walking. One could find it difficult to walk straight and instead stagger from side to side. A person may also lose their balance while standing, which will make them wobble even when they are not moving. When one quits drinking, their ataxic gait will improve from alcohol intoxication. Some medications may also cause an ataxic gait.

Parkinsonian Gait

You might walk with a Parkinsonian posture, hunching forward and bending the neck and back. Instead of taking lengthy strides, it might take a few short ones (shuffle). Parkinson's illness frequently manifests as Parkinsonian gait.

Neuropathic Gait

Neuropathic posture, sometimes known as a foot drop, is unnatural. Due to the fact that one foot flops down as the other lifts up, it is vital to pull the knee up high enough to prevent the toes from dragging on the ground when you walk. Neuropathic walking is a symptom of multiple sclerosis (MS), amyotrophic lateral sclerosis (ALS), and a peripheral neuropathy.

2.3.2 Other Gait Disorders

Walking could be difficult for someone for other reasons. Chronic pain brought on by conditions like arthritis or previous injuries may affect one's ability to move. Pain or weakness may be coming from the ankles. Imbalance issues could be a movement-related inner ear disorder. The way a person moves can be impacted by obesity and other medical conditions that have an impact on breathing, heart health, and mobility.

2.3.3 Case 5

A 36-year-old female was involved in a motor vehicle accident and sustained a traumatic brain injury (TBI). She had difficulty walking and slurred speech. Her shoulders were frozen bilaterally. She was diagnosed: generalized dystonia of arms and hands. She had years of physical therapy.

This patient had a mandibular repositioning device fabricated to remove the pressure on the auriculotemporal nerve. Once that was completed, her movements of arms, legs, shoulders, and even better cognition were improved. She eventually went and received her license to drive again (Video 8).

2.3.4 Case 6

The patient was a 74-year-old female who had difficulty walking and used a wheelchair. She had sustained multiple falls and cannot walk up stairs. She had polypharmacy (30 prescriptions) and complained of photophobia, phonophobia, fatigue, headaches, dizziness, chest and neck pain, multiple allergies, and difficulty breathing. She had negative genetic testing and had previous dentures that did not wear at this time and heart surgery.

Patient was edentulous in the maxilla and had to be assisted by hospital orderlies each time she was to go to physical therapy. On examination, she had foot inversion, a diplegic gait, missing all maxillary teeth, TMJ pain, collapsed vertical occlusion, and a positive Romberg test. She had been diagnosed as having a functional/psychogenic movement disorder and relegated to home and support groups. Imaging revealed bilateral anterior dislocation of TMJ discs, without recapture and degenerative changes in both mandibular condyles.

Upon making a maxillary complete denture and restoring the proper vertical dimension between the maxilla and mandible, her symptoms discontinued. Her gait was restored, her Romberg signs resolved, and she was able to raise her hands and arms above her head.

2.4 Paroxysmal Kinesigenic Dyskinesia (PKD)

PKD is a hyperkinetic movement condition marked by episodes of uncontrollable shaking that are brought on by abrupt voluntary movements. Attack frequency may rise during adolescence and fall between the ages of 20 and 30. Involuntary movements, which can include chorea, dystonia, or ballism, typically only impact one side of the body or one specific limb. With PKD accounting for 86.8% of all paroxysmal dyskinesia types and affecting more men than women, this rare disorder only affects about 1 in 150,000 individuals.

Primary and secondary PKDs are the two varieties. There are two types of primary PKD: familial and random. Although sporadic instances of PKD are also seen, familial PKD—which means the person has a family history of the condition—is more prevalent. Multiple sclerosis (MS), stroke, pseudohypoparathyroidism, hypocalcemia, hypoglycemia, hyperglycemia, damage to the central nervous system, or trauma to the peripheral nervous system are just a few of the other medical conditions that can result in secondary PKD.

There are several genes that have been found where mutations can cause paroxysmal kinesigenic dyskinesias, which are frequently inherited in an autosomal dominant manner. The genes usually produce ion channels, ion transporters, or proteins known to be involved in synaptic transmission. A complete explanation of PKD's pathogenesis is lacking. So far, the following methods have been proposed: imbalance of gamma-aminobutyric acid (GABA), abnormal dopamine degradation in the basal ganglia, substantia nigra dysfunction, and an epileptic subtype. The small sample size is the primary issue with many studies looking at the pathophysiology of the disorder, and the results of the studies cannot be applied to the complete patient population.

2.4.1 Case 7

A 31-year-old male was diagnosed with paroxysmal kinesigenic dyskinesia following an accident when riding a roller coaster and his head hit a beam. The patient had a diminished gait and walked with the aid of a cane. He had difficulty concentrating, his hands turned medially, he had dystonic posturing and tremors, foot inversion, facial grimacing, and difficulty walking. His contorted positions would be maintained for several hours to several days. He had been prescribed Artane and Baclofen with no effect. He was told that it was "all in his head" or is a "functional disorder."

His major concern was that he was not able to play with his 3-year-old daughter. A test was utilized to determine if he had Munchausen syndrome. After adding a vertical component to his lower mandibular teeth, the vertigo and balance stabilized, and the patient was able to exhibit normal balance without vertigo.

2.4.2 Case 8

A 36-year-old female was diagnosed with paroxysmal kinesigenic dyskinesia. She had anterocollis with head tremor, lip twitch/tic, and hand and leg inversion and soreness. She complained of dyspnea and sinus infections requiring allergy injections. She was unable to run or drive a vehicle. She was told that her symptoms were "all in her head" and a "functional disorder." Examination demonstrated neck tenderness, finger numbness bilaterally, and temporalis tenderness. MRI imaging demonstrated a left TMJ disc anteriorly and medially displaced and a right TMJ disc anteriorly displaced.

An oral orthotic was fabricated to decompress the temporomandibular joint and prevent compression of the auriculotemporal and deep temporal nerves. The patient wore the appliance 4 weeks consistently and then returned. Upon reevaluation, the patient was able to run 2 miles and work in her yard without symptoms. The patient was to have orthodontic treatment to complete treatment but never returned (Video 9).

2.5 Parkinsonism

The term "Parkinsonism" is used to refer to a variety of brain conditions that cause sluggishness, rigidity, and tremors. These illnesses can be brought on by a wide range of causes, including infections, drug interactions, and genetic changes.

2.5.1 What Sets Parkinson's Disease Apart from Parkinsonism?

A number of conditions, including Parkinson's disease, that have similar signs and symptoms are collectively referred to as Parkinsonism. However, accounting for nearly 80% of all cases, Parkinson's disease is by far the most common form of Parkinsonism. Parkinson's disease is the second most common age-related degenerative brain disease (behind Alzheimer's disease). It is also the most common motor (movement-related) brain condition. Patients over 60 in the world make up at least 1% of those who are affected. Parkinsonism essentially is a condition linked to aging; nevertheless, it can appear much earlier in life. The average age at which teenage Parkinsonism begins is 17.

Parkinsonism encompasses additional disorders such as multiple system atrophy and corticobasal degeneration. There are treatable or even curable reasons for Parkinsonism. Some of the causes of Parkinson's disease may resolve on their own. Depending on the cause, Parkinsonism can have various consequences. Many Parkinsonian disorders impact the brain's motor centers. Movement is more slow and tremulous due to muscular tremors. The following are the main signs of Parkinsonism: moving slowdown (bradykinesia), tremors, rigidity, or rigor. Parkinsonism is always accompanied by these conditions: unsteady posture or a staggered gait; posture that is bent, hunched, or stooped; and freezing (being unable to move when trying to walk).

Along with its motor (movement-related) symptoms, Parkinson's condition has several non-motor symptoms. Many of these influence how the body functions internally. Examples include constipation, decreased smell sensitivity, and sleep problems.

Parkinsonism is caused by vascular disease: This condition typically causes early coordination and movement problems. Dysarthria, a speech disorder, can make it challenging to swallow and speak (dysphagia). Babinski's sign, which causes their toes to stretch and fan out rather than curl when the bottom of their foot is touched, is more frequent.

Drug-induced patients with Parkinson's disease usually experience symptoms equally on both sides of their body. Typically, one side of a person with Parkinson's disease will experience more severe symptoms. Toxin-induced Parkinsonism is characterized by a more pronounced "cogwheel rigidity," or jerky pattern to their movements. Their muscles cause slower motion and make going backward difficult.

Different things can cause Parkinsonism depending on the condition's particular subtype.

Parkinson's disease. The brain typically uses neurotransmitters to control how brain cells (neurons) communicate with one another. Parkinson's disease patients lack dopamine, one of the most important neurotransmitters. The basal ganglia, a crucial part of the brain, begin to degrade when dopamine is not present. They lose the powers they once had as they proceed.

Secondary Parkinsonism is a disease that develops because of another illness. Secondary Parkinsonism examples include:

Vascular Parkinsonism: This type of Parkinsonism develops when certain parts of the brain do not receive enough blood supply. The brain suffers damage to the affected areas as a result, which produces Parkinsonian symptoms.

Post-traumatic Parkinsonism arises from repeated head trauma, which injures the brain. Boxing, football, and other high-contact sports are particularly prone to it.

Drug-induced Parkinsonism occurs when a substance (whether prescribed or used recreationally) alters how your body generates or uses dopamine. Parkinsonism may be brought on by toxic agents that particularly target and eliminate particular types of brain cells. When such specific brain cells are dopamine-sensitive neurons in the basal ganglia, Parkinsonism symptoms may appear. Infection-related cerebral inflammation known as encephalitis can cause postencephalitic Parkinsonism. It might happen after a condition that causes encephalitis, such as Parkinson's disease.

2.5.2 Case 9

A 53-year-old male who traveled from Jordan for treatment was a cab driver. He was diagnosed with Parkinsonism and dystonia. He had a history of a previous MVA. His symptoms were a gait disorder, shoulder contracture with limited arm swing, unable to move head off right shoulder, dysphasia, dyspnea, dysarthria, bilateral temporal headaches, and tinnitus of the right ear. MRI demonstrated bilateral TMJ dislocation. The right image showed anterior-medial dislocation with moderate condylar degeneration, and the left showed anterior dislocation.

The son of the patient was an oral and maxillofacial surgeon at a local university. The video shows that he also had compression of the auriculotemporal nerve with involvement of the cervical nerves 1 and 2, which activated the torticollis symptoms that were presented. The gait difficulty was likely due to noxious innervation into the upper spinal cord. Once the orthotic was received, the aberrant signals were discontinued and there was relief of his malady (Video 10).

2.6 Complex Regional Pain Syndrome (CRPS)

Complex regional pain syndrome (CRPS) is a condition that causes discomfort, skin color changes, and other symptoms in a specific area of the body, usually your extremities. One's extremities include things like their arm, leg, hand, and foot. The symptoms of CRPS can have a substantial influence on a person's emotional well-being, sleep, everyday activities, and function of the affected limb.

The central or peripheral nervous systems may malfunction to cause CRPS, according to doctors. The central nervous system is made up of the spinal nerves and the brain. Through their peripheral nerve systems, the brain and spinal cord transmit information to the organs, limbs, legs, fingers, and toes. The central nervous system overreacts to pain impulses due to faulty functioning and is unable to turn them off.

CRPS has two subtypes:

Type I: This kind does not result in nerve injury. It takes place following a disease or injury that did not immediately harm a nerve. Reflex sympathetic dystrophy was the previous name for type I.

Type II: This kind develops following documented nerve damage. It used to be referred to as causalgia.

Additionally, CRPS may be either acute (short-term) or persistent (lasting longer than 6 months). Usually, it is curable. CRPS affects adults more commonly than it does young children. The largest onset happens around age 40. CRPS affects people assigned as female at birth more frequently than it affects people assigned as male. Between 66 and 80% of instances are seen in people of European descent.

CRPS is a rare condition. In the USA, it affects roughly 200,000 people annually. Symptoms of CRPS might emerge for no apparent reason, but they typically do so 4–6 weeks after an injury, fracture, or surgery. CRPS's most common and noticeable symptom is pain. The pain, which may be constant or intermittent, is characterized by burning, stinging, or ripping feelings. Frequently, it is located deep within the injured extremity. In the affected region, sensory changes are also typical and may include heightened sensitivity to unpleasant stimuli (a pinch may feel more painful than usual) and experiencing discomfort from events that are typically painless (such as just touching the skin).

Additional signs of CRPS include the following: skin swelling which may be intermittent or persistent; reduced mobility and/or increased stiffness in the affected extremity which are possible symptoms of decreased function; challenge in applying weight to the limb or joint that is symptomatic; variations in skin temperature where one extremity's skin may feel warmer or colder than the other; skin tone changes such as blotchy, pale, purple, or red; skin structure modifications including thinning, glossy skin, or excessive perspiration; and change in nail and hair growth, either growing quickly or not at all.

More than 90% of the time, CRPS is caused by a limb-specific nerve lesion or trauma that damages the smallest sensory and autonomic nerve fibers. This is why the symptoms of CRPS usually improve over time. These minute fibers provide sensations of pain, itchiness, and temperature. Additionally, they control the conditions of the adjacent cells and tiny blood arteries. The most common injury associated with the onset of CRPS is a bone fracture, typically a wrist fracture. Pressure from a cast or a bone that has broken or dislocated might cause nerve damage.

The following common wounds can also result with CRPS: surgery can result in scarring from sutures and incisions, all of which have the potential to harm nerves; sprains; and strains. When connective tissues are damaged, the joint may move too much, stretching the nearby nerves in the process; cuts, bruises, and burns are all mechanisms that may have the potential to affected deeper nerves; CRPS can also appear without any apparent wounds or as a result of extended immobility.

2.6.1 Case 10

A 38-year-old female was diagnosed with CRPS. The patient was a nurse at a major hospital in the northeast. Her chief complaint was that she could not walk and/or sit without pain in her arms and legs. Her symptoms included tenderness to light touch, gait imbalance (see below), and an inability to work. Previous TMJ problems existed since high school, 20 years of constant headaches, and restless leg syndrome. She had been previously treated with seven ketamine infusions. She took 14 medications daily, of which 3x/day were for pain. MRI revealed a right TMJ disc which was displaced anteriorly and a retrognathic mandible.

The CRPS symptoms caused her to discontinue working, and she was confined to her home. She explored multiple medications, and none worked. Upon evaluation, it was found that she had severe bruxism and that she had chronic TMJ pain. Placing an orthotic at the calculated vertical dimension relieved her CRPS symptoms.

This patient's symptoms were distinct from the normal constellation of TMD symptoms. The patient was extremely sensitive to temperature changes, particularly cooling. This manifested itself as inward turned feet, which severely affected her gait. These findings arise from stimulation of the rostral ventral medial reticular formation. The trigeminal nerve is the only one of all cranial nerves that has direct synapsing with reticular formation. The patient also reported cardiac symptoms (chest pain and palpitations), which were improved by TMD treatment (Fig. 7). The trigeminal vagus cardiac reflex, akin to the vasovagal response, demonstrates the connection between CNs V and X. TMD as a noxious stimulus to the trigeminal nerve can adversely affect vagal innervated organs (Video 11).

2.6.2 Case 11

A 28-year-old female was diagnosed with CRPS. She suffered from right foot and left arm inversion. She had experienced a severe loss of strength. Environmental barometric changes caused severe reactions. Her CRPS symptoms caused inversion of the feet. She had chest pain due to irritation of the intercostobrachial nerve, which can occur in those who have CRPS that affects the upper limbs which she demonstrated. Testing showed a loss of vertical height within the oral cavity and was confirmed by an MRI showing a dislocated TMJ disc.

She had a history of multiple physicians and hospitalizations. Lidocaine knee patches and ketamine injections were prescribed. She was scheduled for a ketamine coma 5 days after her consultation. MRI revealed a left TMJ disc which was anteriorly displaced and a collapsed occlusal

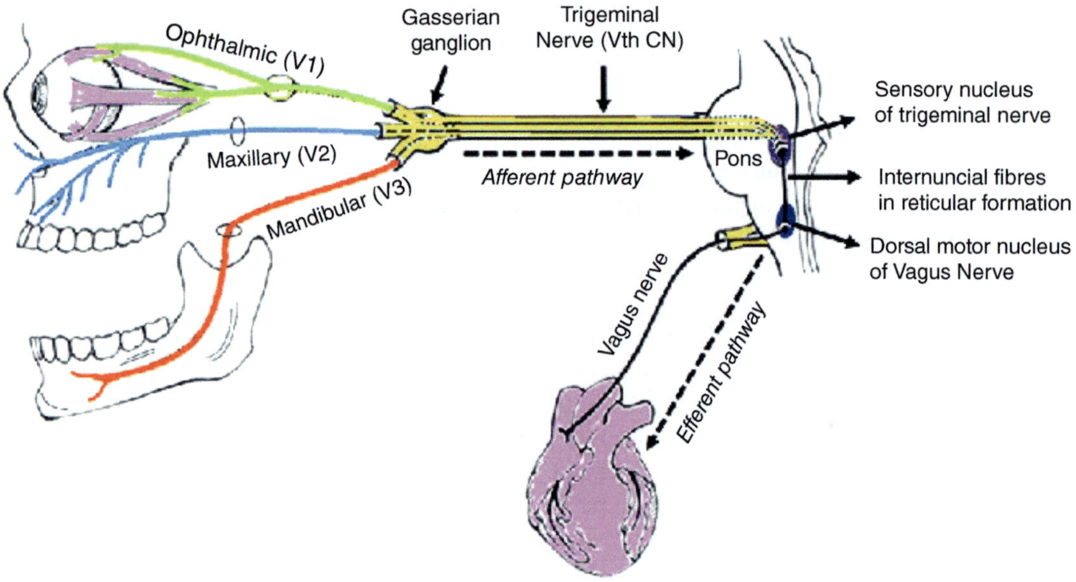

Fig. 7 Trigeminocardiac reflex. Trigeminocardiac reflex (TCR) is a well-established neurogenic reflex, although its exact mechanism and clinical significance remain unclear. This reflex may be incited by stimulation of the trigeminal nerve anywhere along its course starting from the peripheral distribution to the central nucleus. It usually manifests as bradycardia and asystole. (Singh GP, Chowdhury T, Bindu B, Schaller B. Sudden Infant Death Syndrome - Role of Trigeminocardiac Reflex: A Review. Front Neurol. 2016 Dec 5;7:221. doi: 10.3389/fneur.2016.00221. PMID: 27994573; PMCID: PMC5136573)

vertical dimension. Upon placing an orthotic to the right vertical dimension, her symptoms diminished greatly, so that she did not have to have any further ketamine injections.

2.7 Tourette Syndrome

Tics, unexpected, unwanted, uncontrollable, quick, and repetitive movements or vocalizations, can be caused by the neurological disorder known as Tourette syndrome (TS). TS is a disorder-related condition that affects the developing neurological system. The motor or vocal tics associated with TS might entail physical movement of the body or sounds made by a person, and they can change over time in terms of type, frequency, location, and severity. Some patients cannot make their bodies stop ticking once the tic commences. Between the ages of 5 and 10 years, the initial symptoms frequently manifest in the head and neck area. Their limbs, legs, and torso may eventually develop them. Typically, vocal tics emerge first and then physical tics.

Tourette syndrome affects more men than women. However, from late adolescence to early adulthood, tics typically reduce and can be controlled. Early adolescence is typically when TS patients have the worst tic symptoms. Some people with TS could have ongoing symptoms well into adulthood. Tics can occasionally worsen as people age. The disease is not degenerative; therefore, TS patients have a normal life expectancy, and it does not worsen over time.

One might encounter simple or complex motor tics if they have TS. Although many cases are mild, they can vary from extremely mild to severe. Simple tics are brief, repetitive motions that happen suddenly and only use a few muscles. They are more prevalent.

Simple motor tics include:

- Eye blinking and other eye movements
- Facial grimacing
- Shoulder shrugging
- Head or shoulder jerking

Simple vocal tics include:

- Repetitive throat clearing
- Sniffing
- Barking
- Grunting

Complex tics are distinct, coordinated patterns of movement involving several muscle groups in different parts of the body. Complex motor tics might include facial grimacing combined with a head twist and a shoulder shrug. Other complex motor tics may appear purposeful, including:

- Sniffing or touching an object
- Hopping
- Jumping
- Bending
- Twisting

Complex vocal tics may include:

- Repeating one's own words or phrases
- Repeating others' words or phrases (echolalia)
- Using vulgar, obscene, or swear words

One of the most severe and incapacitating tics can be a motor movement that results in self-harm, like hitting oneself in the face, or a vocal tic, such as echolalia or swearing. Some tics are preceded by an urge or sensation in the affected muscle area (a warning compulsion). One can think that a tic must be performed by a certain method or a certain number of times (coprolalia) to satiate the desire or diminish the sensation.

Some people can suppress or otherwise control their tics to decrease how much of an impact they have on everyday functioning, even though TS symptoms are unwanted and unplanned (i.e., involuntary). To the point that they believe the tic must be expressed, people with TS typically say that repressing their tics significantly raises their level of anxiety.

Like many people with TS, one can also experience co-occurring neurobehavioral disorders which are problems with how the brain affects emotion, behavior, and learning. These problems typically get worse before the tics occur. The most typical co-occurring diseases are as follows:

- **Attention deficit hyperactivity disorder (ADHD)**: TS patients may experience impulsivity, hyperactivity, and focus issues.
- **Obsessive-compulsive disorder or behaviors (OCD/OCB)**: People with TS may feel compelled to engage in certain behaviors frequently or in a particular manner because of unwanted thoughts, ideas, or sensations (obsessions and compulsions). Handwashing, checking things, and cleaning are some examples of repetitive behaviors that can be disruptive.
- **Anxiety**: When faced with a risky situation or event, people with TS may feel fear, dread, or apprehension.
- **Learning challenges**: Problems with math, reading, and writing that are experienced are unrelated to intellect.
- **Behavior**: Common issues include hostility, challenges with anger management, and trouble adjusting emotionally and socially.
- **Sleep disturbances**: Trouble falling or staying asleep as well as being too sleepy throughout the day.
- **Maintaining social connections**: They might have issues interacting with others and have limited social skills.
- **Sensory organization and response**: Some TS patients have trouble receiving and interpreting sensory data: touch, flavor, smells, sounds, or movement.

2.8 TS Diagnosis

A physician will inquire about whether a patient may have:

- Motor and verbal tics present, occurring regularly or irregularly, for at least a year.
- Tics start before the age of 18.
- Tics are not brought on by drugs, other chemicals, or illnesses.

Laboratory or imaging studies are not required for a TS diagnosis. Rarely, other diseases that might be mistaken for TS may be ruled out using neuroimaging tests like magnetic resonance imaging (MRI) or computerized tomography (CT), electroencephalogram (EEG) studies, or specific blood tests.

2.9 Treating TS

Currently, there is no accepted cure for TS, but treatments are available to help manage some symptoms.

2.9.1 Case 12

The patient started with his symptoms at 4.5 years, and in this video, he is now 15 years old. He was diagnosed with Tourette syndrome. His symptoms included blinking, leg twitching, throat clearing, and humming. He was considered to have ADD/ADHD. On presentation, he suffered from sniffles, knee bending, abdominal tics, and facial grimaces. His most recent MRI/CT scans demonstrated retrognathic mandible.

A mandibular oral orthotic was made to reposition his jaw downward and forward to remove pressure from the auriculotemporal nerve. Also, a maxillary expander was fabricated due to an insufficient growth. 90% of the tic symptoms dissipated immediately, and within 4 weeks, the tic symptoms were completely resolved. His follow-up was to have orthodontic treatment to maintain the jaw position that was established. He has been tic free since completion of orthodontic treatment (Video 12).

2.9.2 Case 13

This lady presents at 37 years with a history starting at age 30 of a Tourette syndrome diagnosis Her symptoms included blinking, head shaking, leg shaking, internal tics, and arm movements. She was on multiple medications upon presentation. On examination, she was noted to have vocal tics. Her MRI/CT scans demonstrated bilateral anteriorly displaced TMJ discs, a retrognathic mandible, and upper and lower teeth crowding.

She was made a mandibular oral orthotic and an upper expander, which reduced her tic symptoms by 85%, and was able to ride the subway without people believing that she had a mental illness. She is currently in orthodontic treatment to stabilize her jaw position. The appliances equalized the pressure within the TM joints that allowed a normal sensory signal to be expressed, and the disc was not compressed or irritated (Video 13).

2.9.3 Case 14

The patient presented at age 11, but in the video, he is of age 20. His diagnosis was Tourette syndrome. His symptoms included head twitching, eye rolling, blinking, and abdominal tics. He was on multiple medications that changed his personality. In the video, he presents with facial grimaces, vocal tics, shoulder shrugging, sniffles, coughing, and an ADHD phenotype. His MRI/CT scans revealed bilateral TMJ anterior disc and a displacement and a retrognathic mandible. All other treatment modalities proved ineffective. Medications made him drowsy such that he could not conduct his daily work schedule. He rejected an offer for deep brain surgery. He had a mandibular orthotic which reduced his symptoms without surgery or medication.

3 Summary

The trigeminal system can be impacted by the correct maxillomandibular interaction. Communications from the trigeminal network that reach the brainstem through the spinal trigeminal nucleus cross over brainstem fibers via the reticular formation, which is why it is important for individuals with movement disorders to improve. It has been demonstrated that the authors are able to treat the symptoms of pain and discomfort as well as those associated with neurological disorders, neurological dysfunctions, and dystonia by treating the temporomandibular disorder and influencing the maxillomandibular relationship with oral appliances. The auricular-temporal nerve, which innervates the posterior and lateral ligaments of the temporomandibular disc, is compressed or the aberrant signal is removed clinically to achieve this. In perspective of the preceding explanation, many neurological conditions have a strong connection to the architecture and physiology of the temporomandibular joint. This method of treatment provides a noninvasive way to address several movement disorders that may be related either directly or indirectly to TMD.

Suggested Readings

1. https://nei.nih.gov/health/blepha/blepharospasm.
2. Jordan DR, Patrinely JR, Anderson RL, Thiese SM. Essential blepharospasm and related dystonias. Surv Ophthalmol. 1989;34(2):123–32.
3. Tolosa E, Martí MJ. Blepharospasm-oromandibular dystonia syndrome (Meige's syndrome): clinical aspects. Adv Neurol. 1988;49:73–84.
4. Eckhardt B, McClean JM, Goodell H. Experimental studies on headache: the genesis of pain from the eye. Proc Assoc Res Nerv Ment Dis. 1943;23:209–27.
5. Lebensohn JE. Photophobia: mechanism and implications. Am J Ophthalmol. 1951;34:1294–300.
6. Schrag A, Bhatia KP, Quinn NP, Marsden CD. Atypical and typical cranial dystonia following dental procedures. Mov Disord. 1999;14(3):492–6.
7. Lo SE, Gelb M, Frucht SJ. Geste antagonistes in idiopathic lower cranial dystonia. Mov Disord. 2007;22(7):1012–7.
8. Brodal PR. The central nervous system: structure and function. 3rd ed. New York: Oxford University Press; 2004.
9. Tamai Y, Iwamoto M, Tsujimoto T. Pathway of the blink reflex in the brainstem of the cat: interneurons between the trigeminal nuclei and the facial nucleus. Brain Res. 1986;380(1):19–25.
10. Di Lazzaro V, Restuccia D, Nardone R, Tartaglione T, Quartarone A, Tonali P, Rothwell JC. Preliminary clinical observations on a new trigeminal reflex: the trigemino-cervical reflex. Neurology. 1996;46(2):479–85.
11. Dostrovsky JO, Hu JW, Sessle BJ, Sumino R. Stimulation sites in periaqueductal gray, nucleus raphe magnus and adjacent regions effective in suppressing oral-facial reflexes. Brain Res. 1982;252(2):287–97.
12. Bolton S, O'Shaughnessy CT, Goadsby PJ. Properties of neurons in the trigeminal nucleus caudalis responding to noxious dural and facial stimulation. Brain Res. 2005;1046(1–2):122–9.
13. Durham PL, Garrett FG. Emerging importance of neuron-satellite glia interactions within trigeminal ganglia in craniofacial pain. Open Pain J. 2010;3:3–1.
14. Thalakoti S, Patil V, Damodaram S, et al. Neuron-glia signaling in trigeminal ganglion: implications for migraine pathology. Headache. 2007;47:1008–23.

15. Pullicino PM, Jacobs L, McCall WD Jr, Garvey M, Ostrow PT, Miller LL. Spontaneous palpebromandibular synkinesia: a localizing clinical sign. Ann Neurol. 1994;35(2):222–8.
16. Jacobs L, Gossman MD. Three primitive reflexes in normal adults. Neurology. 1980;30(2):184–8.
17. Restless Legs Syndrome Fact Sheet | National Institute of Neurological Disorders and Stroke. Ninds.nih.gov. Accessed 7 July 2019.
18. Manconi M, Zavalko I, Bassetti CL, Colamartino E, Pons M, Ferri R. Respiratory-related leg movements and their relationship with periodic leg movements during sleep. Sleep. 2014;37(3):497–504.
19. Wassell R, Naru A, Steele J, Nohl F. Applied occlusion. London: Quintessence; 2008. p. 26–30.
20. Macedo CR, Macedo EC, Torloni MR, Silva AB, Prado GF. Pharmacotherapy for sleep bruxism. Cochrane Database Syst Rev. 2014;2014(10):CD005578.
21. Shetty S, Pitti V, Satish Babu CL, Surendra Kumar GP, Deepthi BC. Bruxism: a literature review. J Indian Prosthodont Soc. 2010;10(3):141–8.
22. Lavigne GJ, Huynh N, Kato T, et al. Genesis of sleep bruxism: motor and autonomic–cardiac interactions. Arch Oral Biol. 2007;52(4):381–4.
23. Lobbezoo F, Van Der Zaag J, Naeije M. Bruxism: its multiple causes and its effects on dental implants—an updated review. J Oral Rehabil. 2006;33(4):293–300.
24. Macedo CR, Machado MC, Silva AB, Prado GF. Pharmacotherapy for sleep bruxism". Cochrane Database Syst Rev. 2009.
25. Huynh N, Manzini C, Rompré PH, Lavigne GJ. Weighing the potential effectiveness of various treatments for sleep bruxism. J Can Dent Assoc. 2007;73(8):727–30.
26. Phillips CL, Grunstein RR, Darendeliler MA, Mihailidou AS, Srinivasan VK, Yee BJ, Marks GB, Cistulli PA. Health outcomes of continuous positive airway pressure versus oral appliance treatment for obstructive sleep apnea: a randomized controlled trial. Am J Respir Crit Care Med. 2013;187(8):879–87.
27. Bevilaqua Grossi D, Lipton RB, Bigal ME. Temporomandibular disorders and migraine chronification. Curr Pain Headache Rep. 2009;13(4):314–8.
28. Fernandes G, Franco AL, Gonçalves DA, Speciali JG, Bigal ME, Camparis CM. Temporomandibular disorders, sleep bruxism, and primary headaches are mutually associated. J Orofac Pain. 2013;27(1):14–20.
29. Cuccia AM, Caradonna C, Caradonna D. Manual therapy of the mandibular accessory ligaments for the management of temporomandibular joint disorders. J Am Osteopath Assoc. 2011;111(2):102–12.
30. George JS. Understanding the neuroanatomical organization of serotonergic cells in brain provides insight into the functions of this neurotransmitter. In: Agranoff BW, Fisher SK, Albers RW, Uhler MD, editors. Basic neurochemistry. 6th ed. Lippincott Williams and Wilkins; 1999.
31. Dickoff DJ. Primary restless limbs syndrome, migraine, and bruxism: a common clinical triad. Sleep Rev. 2015;
32. Aoki M, Mori S. Locomotion elicited by pinna stimulation in the acute precollicular post-mammillary decerebrate cat. Brain Res. 1981;214:424–8.
33. Beresovskii VK, Bayev KV. Locomotor regions of the brain stem: a new hypothesis of locomotion initiation. In: Armstrong DM, Bush BMH, editors. Locomotor neural mechanisms in arthropods and vertebrates. Manchester: Manchester University Press; 1991. p. 260–8.
34. Goulding M. Circuits controlling vertebrate locomotion: moving in a new direction. Nat Rev Neurosci. 2009;10:507–18.
35. Grillner S, Wallen P, Saitoh K, Kozlov A, Robertson B. Neural bases of goal-directed locomotion in vertebrates—an overview. Brain Res Rev. 2008;57:2–12.
36. Jordan LM, Liu J, Hedlund PB, Akay T, Pearson KG. Descending command systems for the initiation of locomotion in mammals. Brain Res Rev. 2008;57:183–91.
37. Li W-C, Roberts A, Soffe SR. Specific brainstem neurons switch each other into pacemaker mode to drive movement by activating NMDA receptors. J Neurosci. 2010;30:16609–20.
38. Li W-C, Soffe SR, Wolf E, Roberts A. Persistent responses to brief stimuli: feedback excitation among brainstem neurons. J Neurosci. 2006;26:4026–35.
39. Matesz C, Székely G. The motor column and sensory projections of the branchial cranial nerves in the frog. J Comp Neurol. 1978;178:157–75.
40. Noga BR, Kriellaars DJ, Jordan LM. The effect of selective brain-stem or spinal-cord lesions on treadmill locomotion evoked by stimulation of the mesencephalic or pontomedullary locomotor regions. J Neurosci. 1991;11:1691–700.
41. Orlovsky GN. Work of reticulo-spinal neurones during locomotion. Biophysics. 1970;15:761–71.
42. van Rooijen DE, Geraedts EJ, Marinus J, Jankovic J, van Hilten JJ. Peripheral trauma and movement disorders: a systematic review of reported cases. J Neurol Neurosurg Psychiatry. 2011;82(8):892–8. Epub 2011 Apr 14.
43. Kitsoulis P, Marini A, Iliou K. Symptoms of temporomandibular joint disorders. BMC Ear Nose Throat Disord. 2011;11:5.
44. Stocker SD, Steinbacher BC Jr, Balaban CD, Yates BJ. Connections of the caudal ventrolateral medullary reticular formation in the cat brainstem. Exp Brain Res. 1997;116(2):270–82.
45. Brodal A. Anatomical aspects of the reticular formation of the pons and medulla oblongata. Prog Neurobiol. 1956;2:240–55.
46. Frumker SC, Kyle MA. The dentist's contribution to rehabilitation of cervical posture and function: orthopedic and neurological considerations in the treatment of craniomandibular disorders. Basal Facts. 1987;9(3):105–9. Review.

47. Chan J, Brin MF, Fahn S. Idiopathic cervical dystonia: clinical characteristics. Mov Disord. 1991;6(2):119–26.
48. Jankovic J, Leder S, Warner D, Schwartz K. Cervical dystonia: clinical findings and associated movement disorders. Neurology. 1991;41(7):1088–91.
49. Canale ST. Congenital muscular torticollis. In: Canale ST, Daugherty K, Jones L, editors. Campbell's operative orthopaedics. 9th ed. St Louis: Mosby-Year Book; 1998. p. 1064–7.
50. Robin NH. Congenital muscular torticollis. Pediatr Rev. 1996;17(10):374–5.
51. Müller J, Wissel J, Masuhr F, Ebersbach G, Wenning GK, Poewe W. Clinical characteristics of the geste antagoniste in cervical dystonia. J Neurol. 2001;248(6):478–82.
52. Tecco S, Tetè S, D'Attilio M, Perillo L, Festa F. Surface electromyographic patterns of masticatory, neck, and trunk muscles in temporomandibular joint dysfunction patients undergoing anterior repositioning splint therapy. Eur J Orthod. 2008;30(6):592–7. Epub 2008 Nov 5.
53. Jiang T, Yang Z, Zhang Z, Feng H. Electromyography activities of the head, neck and upper trunk muscles with mandibular movement in normal adults. Zhonghua Kou Qiang Yi Xue Za Zhi. 2002;37(6):431–4.
54. Pinto ML, Olyntho-Tokunaga HH, Souccar C, Schoorlemmer GH, Lapa RC. The interstitial system of the trigeminal spinal tract projects to the red nucleus in mice. Somatosens Mot Res. 2007;24(4):221–5.
55. Mainero C, Zhang WT, Kumar A, Rosen BR, Sorensen AG. Mapping the spinal and supraspinal pathways of dynamic mechanical allodynia in the human trigeminal system using cardiac-gated fMRI. NeuroImage. 2007;35(3):1201–10. Epub 2007 Feb 4.
56. Siegel JM, Tomaszewski KS. Behavioral organization of reticular formation: studies in the unrestrained cat. I. Cells related to axial, limb, eye, and other movements. J Neurophysiol. 1983;50(3):696–716.
57. Davidson AG, Buford JA. Bilateral actions of the reticulospinal tract on arm and shoulder muscles in the monkey: stimulus triggered averaging. Exp Brain Res. 2006;173(1):25–39. Epub 2006 Feb 28.
58. Garone G, Capuano A, Travaglini L, Graziola F, Stregapede F, Zanni G, Vigevano F, Bertini E, Nicita F. Clinical and genetic overview of paroxysmal movement disorders and episodic ataxias. Int J Mol Sci. 2020;21(10):3603. https://doi.org/10.3390/ijms21103603. PMID: 32443735; PMCID: PMC7279391.
59. McGuire S, Chanchani S, Khurana DS. Paroxysmal dyskinesias. Semin Pediatr Neurol. 2018;25:75–81. https://doi.org/10.1016/j.spen.2017.12.007. Epub 2017 Dec 27.
60. Jannetta PJ, Whiting DM, Fletcher LH, Hobbs JK, Brillman J, Quigley M, Fukui M, Williams R. Parkinson's disease: an inquiry into the etiology and treatment. Neurol Int. 2011;3(2):e7. https://doi.org/10.4081/ni.2011.e7. Epub 2011 Aug 30. PMID: 22053261; PMCID: PMC3207233.
61. Li ST, Wang X, Pan Q, Hai J, Liu N, Shen F, Liu Z, Guan Y. Studies on the operative outcomes and mechanisms of microvascular decompression in treating typical and atypical trigeminal neuralgia. Clin J Pain. 2005;21(4):311–6. https://doi.org/10.1097/01.ajp.0000120790.69705.5b.
62. Tremblay C, Durand Martel P, Frasnelli J. Trigeminal system in Parkinson's disease: a potential avenue to detect Parkinson-specific olfactory dysfunction. Parkinsonism Relat Disord. 2017;44:85–90. https://doi.org/10.1016/j.parkreldis.2017.09.010. Epub 2017 Sep 11.
63. Heir GM, Nasri-Heir C, Thomas D, Puchimada BP, Khan J, Eliav E, Benoliel R. Complex regional pain syndrome following trigeminal nerve injury: report of 2 cases. Oral Surg Oral Med Oral Pathol Oral Radiol. 2012;114(6):733–9. https://doi.org/10.1016/j.oooo.2012.06.001. Epub 2012 Oct 24.
64. Sakamoto E, Shiiba S, Noma N, Okada-Ogawa A, Shinozaki T, Kobayashi A, Kamo H, Koike K, Imamura Y. A possible case of complex regional pain syndrome in the orofacial region. Pain Med. 2010;11(2):274–80. https://doi.org/10.1111/j.1526-4637.2009.00777.x.
65. Sims A, Stack B. Tourette's syndrome: a pilot study for the discontinuance of a movement disorder. Cranio. 2009;27(1):11–8. https://doi.org/10.1179/crn.2009.003.
66. Cheng JC, Tang SP, Chen TM, Wong MW, Wong EM. The clinical presentation and outcome of treatment of congenital muscular torticollis in infants—a study of 1086 cases. J Pediatr Surg. 2000;35(7):1091–6.
67. Ho BC, Lee EH, Singh K. Epidemiology, presentation and management of congenital muscular torticollis. Singap Med J. 1999;40(11):675–9.
68. Cheng JC, Au AW. Infantile torticollis: a review of 624 cases. J Pediatr Orthop. 1994;14(6):802–8.
69. Lundh H, Westesson PL. Clinical signs of temporomandibular joint internal derangement in adults. An epidemiologic study. Oral Surg Oral Med Oral Pathol. 1991;72(6):637–41.
70. Singer HS, Schucmolz U, Dcnclcla MB. Learning difficulties ill children with Tourette syndrome. J Child Neurol. 1995;10(Suppl 1):S58.
71. Hallett M. Tourette syndrome: update. Brain Dev. 2015;37(7):651–5. https://doi.org/10.1016/j.braindev.2014.11.005. Epub 2015 Jan 17. PMID: 25604739; PMCID: PMC4475482.
72. Müller-Vahl KR, Szejko N, Verdellen C, Roessner V, Hoekstra PJ, Hartmann A, Cath DC. European clinical guidelines for Tourette syndrome and other tic disorders: summary statement. Eur Child Adolesc Psychiatry. 2022;31(3):377–82. https://doi.org/10.1007/s00787-021-01832-4. Epub 2021 Jul 10. PMID: 34244849; PMCID: PMC8940881.
73. Lin WD, Tsai FJ, Chou IC. Current understanding of the genetics of Tourette syndrome. Biomed

J. 2022;45(2):271–9. https://doi.org/10.1016/j.bj.2022.01.008. Epub 2022 Jan 15. PMID: 35042017; PMCID: PMC9250083.

74. Abi-Jaoude E, Gorman DA. Tourette syndrome. CMAJ. 2013;185(3):236. https://doi.org/10.1503/cmaj.120628. Epub 2012 Oct 22. PMID: 23091179; PMCID: PMC3576443.

75. Murakami J, Tachibana Y, Akiyama S, Kato T, Taniguchi A, Nakajima Y, Shimoda M, Wake H, Kano Y, Takada M, Nambu A, Yoshida A. Oral splint ameliorates tic symptoms in patients with Tourette syndrome. Mov Disord. 2019;34(10):1577–8. https://doi.org/10.1002/mds.27819. Epub 2019 Aug 23. PMID: 31442353; PMCID: PMC6852427.

GPSR Compliance

The European Union's (EU) General Product Safety Regulation (GPSR) is a set of rules that requires consumer products to be safe and our obligations to ensure this.

If you have any concerns about our products, you can contact us on ProductSafety@springernature.com

In case Publisher is established outside the EU, the EU authorized representative is:

Springer Nature Customer Service Center GmbH
Europaplatz 3
69115 Heidelberg, Germany

Batch number: 10731385

Printed by Printforce, the Netherlands